Manual of Intracytoplasmic Sperm Injection in Human Assisted Reproduction

Manual of Intracytoplasmic Sperm Injection in Human Assisted Reproduction

With Other Advanced Micromanipulation Techniques to Edit the Genetic and Cytoplasmic Content of the Oocyte

Edited by

Gianpiero D. Palermo
Cornell Institute of Reproductive Medicine, New York

Zsolt Peter Nagy
Reproductive Biology Associates, Atlanta, GA

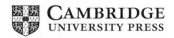
CAMBRIDGE
UNIVERSITY PRESS

CAMBRIDGE
UNIVERSITY PRESS

University Printing House, Cambridge CB2 8BS, United Kingdom

One Liberty Plaza, 20th Floor, New York, NY 10006, USA

477 Williamstown Road, Port Melbourne, VIC 3207, Australia

314–321, 3rd Floor, Plot 3, Splendor Forum, Jasola District Centre,
New Delhi – 110025, India

103 Penang Road, #05–06/07, Visioncrest Commercial, Singapore 238467

Cambridge University Press is part of the University of Cambridge.

It furthers the University's mission by disseminating knowledge in the pursuit of
education, learning, and research at the highest international levels of excellence.

www.cambridge.org
Information on this title: www.cambridge.org/9781108743839
DOI: 10.1017/9781108887595

First published 2022

Printed in the United Kingdom by TJ Books Limited, Padstow Cornwall

A catalogue record for this publication is available from the British Library.

Library of Congress Cataloging-in-Publication Data
Names: Palermo, Gianpiero D., editor. | Nagy, Zsolt Peter, editor.
Title: Manual of intracytoplasmic sperm injection in human assisted
reproduction : with other advanced micromanipulation techniques to edit
the genetic and cytoplasmic content of the oocyte / edited by Gianpiero
D. Palermo, Zsolt Peter Nagy.
Description: Cambridge, United Kingdom ; New York, NY : Cambridge
University Press, 2021. | Includes bibliographical references and index.
Identifiers: LCCN 2021009698 (print) | LCCN 2021009699 (ebook) | ISBN
9781108743839 (paperback) | ISBN 9781108887595 (ebook)
Subjects: MESH: Sperm Injections, Intracytoplasmic – methods | Gene
Editing – methods | Cytological Techniques | Laboratory Manual
Classification: LCC QH581.2 (print) | LCC QH581.2 (ebook) | NLM WQ 25 |
DDC 571.6–dc23
LC record available at https://lccn.loc.gov/2021009698
LC ebook record available at https://lccn.loc.gov/2021009699

ISBN 978-1-108-74383-9 Paperback

Contents

v

Contributors

Simona Alfano MSc
Clinica Ruesch, GENERA Center for Reproductive
Medicine, Naples, Italy

Erminia Alviggi MSc
Clinica Ruesch, GENERA Center for Reproductive
Medicine, Naples, Italy

Carly Barber BSc MSc
Reproductive Biology Associates, Atlanta, GA, USA

Annekatrien Boel PhD
Department for Reproductive Medicine, Ghent
University Hospital, Ghent, Belgium

Guy Cassuto MD
ART Unit, Laboratoire Drouot, Paris, France

Stephanie Cheung BSc
The Ronald O. Perelman & Claudia Cohen Center for
Reproductive Medicine, Weill Cornell Medicine,
New York, NY, USA

Danilo Cimadomo MSc PhD
Clinica Valle Giulia, GENERA Center for Reproductive
Medicine, Rome; Clinica Ruesch, GENERA Center for
Reproductive Medicine, Naples, Italy

Jacques Cohen PhD HCLD
ART Institute of Washington, Althea Science,
Hudson, NY, USA

Paul Couke PhD
Department for Reproductive Medicine, Ghent
University Hospital, Ghent, Belgium

Marta Czernik PhD
Laboratory of Embryology, Faculty of Veterinary
Medicine, University of Teramo, Teramo, Italy

Changsheng Dai PhD
Department of Mechanical & Industrial
Engineering, University of Toronto, Toronto,
Ontario, Canada

Thomas Ebner PhD
Kepler University, MedCampus IV, Linz, Austria

Gemma Fabozzi MSc
Clinica Valle Giulia, GENERA Center for
Reproductive Medicine, Rome, Italy

Steven D. Fleming MSc PhD
Department of Anatomy & Histology, School of
Medical Sciences, University of Sydney, Sydney,
NSW, Australia

Helena Fulka PhD
Institute of Experimental Medicine, Prague, Czech
Republic

Josef Fulka Jr PhD
Institute of Animal Science, Prague, Czech Republic

Mounia Haddad MD
The Ronald O. Perelman & Claudia Cohen Center for
Reproductive Medicine, Weill Cornell Medicine,
New York, NY, USA

Lauren E. Hamilton PhD
Department of Biomedical & Molecular
Sciences, Queen's University, Kingston, Ontario,
Canada

Katsuhiko Hayashi PhD
Department of Stem Cell Biology & Medicine,
Graduate School of Medical Sciences, Kyushu
University, Fukuoka, Japan

Björn Heindryckx PhD
Department for Reproductive Medicine, Ghent
University Hospital, Ghent, Belgium

Laura Hewitson PhD
The Johnson Center for Child Health & Development,
Austin, TX, USA

Kenichiro Hiraoka PhD
Kameda Medical Center, Kamogawa-shi,
Japan

Romain Imbert MD
Centre Hospitalier Inter Régional Cavell, Braine-l'Alleud-Brussels, Belgium

Kiyotaka Kawai MD PhD
Kameda Medical Center, Kamogawa-shi, Japan

Derek Keating BA
The Ronald O. Perelman & Claudia Cohen Center for Reproductive Medicine, Weill Cornell Medicine, New York, NY, USA

Sherina Lawrence BS
The Ronald O. Perelman & Claudia Cohen Center for Reproductive Medicine, Weill Cornell Medicine, New York, NY, USA

Pasqualino Loi DVM PhD
Laboratory of Embryology, Faculty of Veterinary Medicine, University of Teramo, Teramo, Italy

Roberta Maggiulli MSc
Clinica Valle Giulia, GENERA Center for Reproductive Medicine, Rome, Italy

Tetsunori Mukaida MD
Hiroshima HART Clinic, Hiroshima, Japan

Maximillian Murtinger MD
Nextclinics, IVF Centers Prof. Zech, Bregenz, Austria

Zsolt Peter Nagy MD PhD
Reproductive Biology Associates, Atlanta, GA, USA

Vivian Kimble BSc MSc
Reproductive Biology Associates, Atlanta, GA, USA

Richard Oko PhD
Department of Biomedical & Molecular Sciences, Queen's University, Kingston, Ontario, Canada

Luca Palazzese PhD
Laboratory of Embryology, Faculty of Veterinary Medicine, University of Teramo, Teramo, Italy

Gianpiero D. Palermo MD PhD
The Ronald O. Perelman & Claudia Cohen Center for Reproductive Medicine, Weill Cornell Medicine, New York, NY, USA

Alessandra Parrella MSc
The Ronald O. Perelman & Claudia Cohen Center for Reproductive Medicine, Weill Cornell Medicine, New York, NY, USA

Csaba Pribenszky PhD
University of Veterinary Science, Budapest, Hungary

Alexandrea Ramsey BSc
Reproductive Biology Associates, Atlanta, GA, USA

Laura Rienzi BSc MSc
Clinica Valle Giulia, GENERA Center for Reproductive Medicine, Rome; Clinica Ruesch, GENERA Center for Reproductive Medicine, Naples, Italy

Zev Rosenwaks MD
The Ronald O. Perelman & Claudia Cohen Center for Reproductive Medicine, Weill Cornell Medicine, New York, NY, USA

Shahad Sabti MBBS
King's College, London, UK

Pier Augusto Scapolo DVM
Laboratory of Embryology, Faculty of Veterinary Medicine, University of Teramo, Teramo, Italy

Guanqiao Shan MSc
Department of Mechanical & Industrial Engineering, University of Toronto, Toronto, Ontario, Canada

Yu Sun PhD
Department of Mechanical & Industrial Engineering, University of Toronto, Toronto, Ontario, Canada

Alastair G. Sutcliffe MD PhD MRCP FRCPCH
Institute of Child Health, University College London, London, UK

Peter Sutovsky PhD
Division of Animal Sciences, College of Food, Agriculture & Natural Resources; Department of Obstetrics, Gynecology & Women's Health, School of Medicine, University of Missouri, Columbia, MO, USA

Mao-Xing Tang PhD
Department for Reproductive Medicine, Ghent University Hospital, Ghent, Belgium

Filippo Maria Ubaldi MD PhD
Clinica Valle Giulia, GENERA Center for
Reproductive Medicine, Rome; Clinica Ruesch,
GENERA Center for Reproductive Medicine, Naples,
Italy

Pierre Vanderzwalmen Bio.Eng. MSc
Centre Hospitalier Inter Régional Cavell, Braine-
l'Alleud-Brussels, Belgium; Nextclinics, IVF Centers
Prof. Zech, Bregenz, Austria

June Wang BA
The Ronald O. Perelman & Claudia Cohen Center for
Reproductive Medicine, Weill Cornell Medicine,
New York, NY, USA

Hideaki Watanabe PhD
Sugiyama Clinic, Tokyo, Japan

Barbara Wirleitner PhD
Nextclinics, IVF Centers Prof. Zech, Bregenz, Austria

Philip Xie BSc
The Ronald O. Perelman & Claudia Cohen Center for
Reproductive Medicine, Weill Cornell Medicine,
New York, NY, USA

Zhuoran Zhang PhD
Department of Mechanical & Industrial
Engineering, University of Toronto, Toronto,
Ontario, Canada

Foreword

"If I have seen further than others, it is by standing upon the shoulders of giants." – Isaac Newton

This exhaustive manual entitled *Manual of Intracytoplasmic Sperm Injection in Human Assisted Reproduction: With Other Advanced Micromanipulation Techniques to Edit the Genetic and Cytoplasmic Content of the Oocyte*, edited by Gianpiero Palermo and Zsolt Peter Nagy, is the apotheosis of two pioneers of our field, who themselves were tutored and inspired by the giants of ART. Dr. Palermo, when recounting the development of his revolutionary work on intracytoplasmic sperm injection, often mentions that he was inspired by IVF pioneers Drs. Robert Edwards, Susan Lanzendorf, and André Van Steirteghem, among others. Both Dr. Palermo and Dr. Nagy were members of the Belgian team at the Free University in Brussels, where Dr. Palermo described the first successful implementation of ICSI in the human. The editors, themselves academic stars, have put together a superb manual, which addresses seminal aspects of ART-associated micromanipulation techniques. This volume is a thoughtful, in-depth collection of contributions by world authorities representing the current status of intracytoplasmic sperm injection and contemporary oocyte and embryo micromanipulation techniques. The editors, students of pioneers in our field, with whom I have worked and interacted for almost three decades, have in their own right become contemporary giants who are now teachers and mentors of the next generation of ART practitioners.

Although this volume is touted as a manual of micromanipulation techniques, it is in fact a compendium of manuscripts that describe the physiology of early fertilization and post-fertilization cellular and molecular events. It elegantly reviews how and when intracytoplasmic sperm injection was developed in humans, as well as contemporary modifications or enhancements of ICSI. Several contributions address the impact of ICSI on the treatment of male infertility, as well as its impact on the health and well-being of ICSI children. This manual endeavors to describe the early developments of micromanipulation instruments and microscopes in both animals and humans, along with a description of contemporary state-of-the-art instrumentation, while giving credit to the scientists involved in their development. The historical aspect of the development of micromanipulation instruments is most interesting and provides the reader with an appreciation for the complexity of these procedures. This is especially evident in the descriptions of recent innovative nuclear transfer procedures, including germline nuclear transfer technology to overcome mitochondrial diseases and female infertility, mitochondrial replacement therapy, and the prospects of developing manufactured oocytes from stem cells.

All in all, this should be a must-read for all clinicians and scientists involved in the assisted reproductive technologies.

Zev Rosenwaks

Chapter

1

In Vitro Fertilization and Micromanipulation
The History That Changed the Treatment of Male Factor Infertility

Jacques Cohen

Male Factor Infertility: Historical Aspects Before 1980

Not everything in medical science has a clear beginning. The first realization of infertility and putative remedies remain shrouded in contextual history, but likely goes back to the dawn of our species, well before there was a written record. Childlessness was, and is still, considered a burden in some communities. Early feminism and medical enlightenment in the nineteenth century, such as the discovery of the ovum in 1827 by Von Baer [1] and the observation of the mammalian fertilization process in sea urchins by Oskar Hertwig in 1876 and rabbit by Leopold Schenk in 1878 [2], laid the foundations for our understanding of the role of spermatozoa and oocytes in reproduction, although the concept of the infertile man was not deeply explored or reported until the late 1920s [3,4]. Sperm function studies commenced only after the Second World War, with semen analysis becoming a systematic and published diagnostic method using mathematical endpoints in a similar approach to that of blood chemistry laboratories [5–7]; mammalian spermatozoa being successfully cryopreserved by Polge and co-workers in 1949 [8] and later in the human by Bunge and Sherman in 1953 [9]; and the maturation processes which spermatozoa had to undergo after meiosis being described in some detail [10,11]. Since the early 1970s there has been an increase in the development of new assays studying seminal chemistry, male pronuclear formation, membrane fusion, genetics and complex morphology, but despite much progress, many aspects of spermatozoa and the fertilization process remain unexplored [12,13]. Microscopic semen analysis provided medical fertility specialists interested in andrology with tools for diagnosis and possible treatment, and even in the relative absence of a scientific basis and medical literature in the 1930s, some open-minded practitioners taught Obstetrics and Gynecology residents about the reality of male infertility. When Patrick Steptoe was a pre-war registrar at St. George's Hospital in London, his clinical supervisor in the National Health Service, consultant Mr. Gwillim, explained that as many as one-third of clinical infertility cases could be traced back to male factor [14], but demographic publications were hardly available. It would be another 40 years before a suitable and universal treatment was found in in vitro fertilization (IVF) and particularly once the egg was microsurgically prepared to promote fertilization using fledgling new micromanipulation procedures [15–20]. This culminated in the development of a definitive solution (although not a remedy) for male factor infertility, first successfully applied at the Free University of Brussels in Belgium: the direct injection of a single immobilized spermatozoon into the ooplasm, a procedure the authors described as intra-cytoplasmic sperm injection (ICSI) [21]. This chapter reviews the brief but intense period of the exploration of male factor treatment using IVF and derived micromanipulation technologies before the Brussels team's publication of ICSI in 1992.

Natural procreation is a dance that involves two partners, although historically, women were blamed for unwanted childlessness unless the male partner was impotent. The latter was often confused with infertility [22]. The existence of male infertility was abjured by public individuals such as George Washington, who decried his spouse's alleged infertility even though she had children from a prior marriage. Male factor infertility in contemporary reproductive medicine is considered to be either the trigger or a secondary factor of involuntary childlessness. Contemporary studies over the past 20 years show that infertility is directly or indirectly affected by male factor in as many as 30–50% of cases [23].

Before the advent of in vitro fertilization (IVF) in the late 1970s, male factor infertility was rarely taught in medical class. The field of andrology appeared to be of no interest among most male specialists dominating gynecological research, and so it is perhaps not surprising that the causes and treatment for male infertility were not well studied until the routine application of IVF. In IVF and other derivatives since, the female partner is often the focus of the procedures, not because of the probable underlying etiology, but because it is much more complicated to obtain female gametes – at least in the vast majority of couples. Following the birth of Louise Brown, when embryologists were able to show that fertilization could be established in couples with male factor infertility, there was a surge of interest in sperm function and the physiological role of men in reproduction [24–26]. Though some male factor cases were successful, the method of IVF as an alternative treatment was not clearly shown to be more successful than artificial insemination or even natural procreation [27]. No randomized clinical trials were conducted comparing the various routes of alleged treatment, and prospective trials of male factor infertility treatment by IVF or modifications using micromanipulation were not performed. This was typical for the entire period of investigation of male factor treatment using assisted reproduction methods between 1980 and 1995. It is remarkable that the standard of the randomized controlled trial in the IVF laboratory was only explored from 1990 onward [28,29], and the first systematic reviews in infertility research also date from the early 1990s. A well-documented systematic review of infertility treatment and research, conducted by the University of Leeds in 1993, showed that randomized methodology was introduced relatively late in infertility practice compared to other branches of medicine [30]. An exponential rise in identified controlled trials with pregnancy as an outcome occurred only after 1990, alongside a simultaneous increase in the routine practice of assisted reproductive technology in multiple countries. Treatment of idiopathic oligo-astheno-teratozoospermia was investigated broadly without assisted reproduction, as was artificial insemination by partner or donor spermatozoa for male factor infertility. Only 60 trials were identified for male factor treatment without assisted reproduction till 1993, with fewer than 3000 patients tested [30]. Oocyte and embryo preparation or culture were tested in another 17 trials, mostly involving comparisons of embryo culture media. Sperm preparation trials were only reported in four investigations and none involved a comparison of IVF with either artificial insemination or micromanipulation of the oocyte. In the period between 1980 and 1992, preceding ICSI, there was a series of studies of IVF insemination in cases of male factor infertility and the first attempts at microsurgical fertilization [17,18], but without systematic comparison involving control groups and randomization. These studies included patients who either had failed fertilization during previous attempts of IVF or where the male partner had a diagnosis of abnormal semen analysis and so were considered inappropriate for further clinical treatment without some form of assisted reproduction. Results of the experimental procedures were compared with prior unsuccessful attempts, or the procedure was simply performed based on poor semen analysis, a very low yield of spermatozoa after semen preparation and male factor history. This approach may be considered archaic from an evidence-based point of view, but the use of a control group would have meant that participants had either no treatment or a treatment that was known not to work well in those years, such as artificial insemination in cases of extreme male factor infertility. As a consequence, the use of prospective series investigations of new experimental approaches seemed to be the only ethical alternative at the time. The relatively low outcomes following conventional IVF in most patient groups undoubtedly played a role as well.

In Vitro Fertilization: A Treatment for Male Factor Infertility?

When the genius population geneticist Haldane gave a private lecture for a group of Cambridge (UK) academics on the future of society and technology in 1923, he contemplated oddly on the history of the future of technology by projecting it retrospectively from hundreds of years into the future, and on the possibility of the processes of IVF, embryo culture and artificial gestation [31]. He branded the process as an apparent obvious solution for population planning and called it "ectogenesis," a name that surprisingly was not popularized. Not too many details were given, but his friend, the journalist and author Aldous Huxley filled in a few gaps a decade later with the publication of the novel *Brave New World* in 1932. Neither predicted that ectogenesis would have its origin by treating less fertile individuals, nor did the authors distinguish between preimplantation and postimplantation development.

The possibility of IVF as a treatment for infertility was first suggested in 1937, in a short editorial in *The New England Journal of Medicine* by Dr. John Rock, a highly regarded ObGyn at Harvard University who would later become a key scientist in the development of the anti-conception pill. He and his laboratory partner Miriam Menkin were presumably the first to isolate and attempt to fertilize human oocytes in vitro [32]. At the time of the 1937 editorial, however, the idea of IVF was perceived to be so outrageous that even the author avoided claiming it, and the editorial was published anonymously. The concept of assisted procreation had matured from being proposed as a futuristic method of general reproduction for anyone (Haldane and Huxley), into a clinical treatment for "barren" women with tubal disease. There was no mention of treating male factor infertility by in vitro fertilization in Rock's letter. The possibility of treating infertile men this way may have been contemplated by IVF pioneers in the UK, Australia and the USA in the 1970s, but there is no clear mention of it in Steptoe's and Edwards' book *A Matter of Life*, which tells the story of their 11-year collaboration prior to establishing the world's first purpose-built IVF clinic at Bourn Hall near Cambridge in the latter half of 1980 [33]. Nor was it suggested in Edwards' famous view of the future of assisted reproduction in 1965 [34] or in the short letter to the *Lancet* announcing the birth of Louise Brown [14], which described the case of Leslie Brown and her husband and characteristic tubal infertility. The entire series of cases performed before the birth of baby Louise was only evaluated in depth in a group of articles published in 2013 in *Reproductive Biomedicine Online* (RBMO) by Elder and Johnson, after the death of the pioneers, Purdy, Edwards and Steptoe. However, four of the pregnancies established in Oldham, of which only two led to births in 1978 and 1979, were described in a full-length paper by Edwards, Steptoe and Purdy in 1980 [35]. In characteristically understated prose they postulated that *"There seems no reason why similar methods of [IVF and embryo culture] treatment should not be applied in cases of infertility arising in some men with oligospermia, because so few spermatozoa are needed for fertilization in vitro."* Some experts at the time reacted disapprovingly to this, although it does not seem that they confronted the authors publicly in writing. There was a fear among experts that morphologically and functionally abnormal spermatozoa could lead to congenital malformations, but this was soon put to rest when the first studies of treating infertile men by IVF were published. This fear was founded in terms of anomalies of somatic cell morphology, as abnormally shaped somatic cells and cells with differing physiology have classically been associated with disease. Poikilocytosis and anisocytosis are examples of abnormally shaped blood cells associated with forms of vitamin deficiency, iron-deficient anemia and other malfunctions.

The first references to, and description of, treating male factor infertility by in vitro fertilization are included in the proceedings of the first human conception in vitro meeting (this was before the general terminology of IVF was accepted internationally). This meeting was held at Bourn Hall Clinic in 1981 and the proceedings, edited by Bob Edwards and Jean Purdy, were published in the spring of 1982 [24]. In this, the emerging possibility of using IVF to treat oligospermia and immunological infertility was described by Fishel and Edwards. The first two babies from oligospermic men were reported in a series of 182 infertile couples, and the likely limitations of treating severe oligospermia with IVF were also discussed by Mettler's team from Germany. In a series of eight oligospermic cases reported by Fishel and Edwards, five had one oocyte fertilized, but details of semen analysis were not presented, although sperm quality in the insemination droplets was provided, and one case was presented as having severe oligospermia, without further details. It is presumed that this patient had less than 5 million spermatozoa per mL in his semen. The general fertilization rate with "acceptable" spermatozoa was 85%. In 31 patients, observations of the spermatozoa in the insemination droplets identified features that were considered to reduce fertilization. It is unknown how many of those cases were classified as male factor infertility: formal diagnosis was not always evident in those days, routine semen analyses not universal, and most early IVF clinics did not have male reproductive specialists on staff. All of these patients had natural cycles or some clomiphene was given during the early follicular phase. Of the 33 mature oocytes, 14 (42%) were fertilized, and sperm agglutination was reported to be compatible with fertilization. During the discussion between the participants, Simon Fishel commented that fertilization was still possible at concentrations of 1 million spermatozoa, albeit at a much lower rate (it is possible that he referred to the prepared specimen and not the initial semen sample). Fertilization was apparently normal in cases of unexplained infertility. In the contemporaneous series of 25 couples with abnormal semen analysis reported in the same book by Mettler, no embryo cleavage was observed after IVF, perhaps indicating that there were differences between laboratories and their ability to obtain motile spermatozoa for in vitro insemination from men with adverse semen analyses. The two teams apparently did not delve into the differences of their approaches. Regardless of these modest results during the early days of IVF, the establishment of pregnancy and live birth reported by Fishel and Edwards suggested that male factor could be treated successfully with IVF, and the ability to fertilize enhanced by optimizing sperm preparation technologies. Another small series of cases was reported by the Monash group from patients seen between 1980 and 1983, indicating that the Australian team also attempted to fertilize oocytes and transfer embryos from male factor cases early on [25,26]. Their work will be described in some detail below.

Major questions that remained unanswered, at least for a while, were how to optimize the process of removing seminal plasma, micro-organisms and somatic cells, and how to determine the lowest threshold values for reduced sperm count, reduced motility and elevated frequency of abnormally shaped spermatozoa, a class of anomalies collectively referred to as oligo-astheno-teratozoospermia. It was clearly on the minds of reproductive specialists to follow up the pregnancies and children from IVF-related procedures and, most importantly, to collect evidence by performing prospective trials or indirectly through retrospective analysis and comparisons with untreated control groups. However, studies performed over the following 10–15 years showed that there was little impetus to follow and consult the couples with male factor infertility; many of the patients in those early years traveled over long distances to attend the first few clinics, and hence after discharge, many patients did not stay in contact with their clinics. Also, there may have been a lack of funding for follow-up studies. Short- and long-term safety of offspring, details about miscarriage and rare birth defects were only first published in the 1990s and 2000s [36], well after the new experimental procedures involving microsurgical fertilization had been introduced to enhance the chances of fertilization during IVF beyond just insemination and fertilization

in vitro. It was not until the publication of the work by the Brussels group that serious attempts at understanding the potential consequences of artificially forcing the process of fertilization were evaluated [37]. The debate regarding possible consequences in offspring from infertile men is still ongoing nearly 40 years after the first few pregnancies were established in the UK and Australia.

Mahadevan and co-workers from Alan Trounson's and Carl Wood's laboratory at Monash University described the use of IVF in five different groups of infertility patients [25]. Several teams had discovered earlier that IVF was not only a treatment for tubal infertility but also for other types of patients, such as those with unexplained and male factor infertility [24,35,38–40]. A separate paper by the Monash team described the successful application of IVF in men who had persistently low-quality semen, with 58% of the 45 patients studied having at least one successful fertilization [26]. Almost all of those embryos were transferred, with seven patients becoming pregnant in 63 cycles, and four babies born from three pregnancies (one was a twin birth). Fertilization was highly dependent on sperm motility and morphology, with no fertilization observed when motility was below 30%. It was stated that once embryos were obtained pregnancy did not seem to be affected, so the success of the method would be highly dependent on fertilization rate. During the 1981 Bourn Hall meeting, Edwards had assured his colleagues that motility was less a concern and that an effect was only seen when motility was less than 10%, but he did not provide details of the sperm preparation. At least a quarter of the male factor patients treated at Bourn Hall before 1982 had total fertilization failure, but success rates very much varied according to etiology.

The first broad prospective case series of treating infertile men using IVF were published in relatively quick succession ([26,38,41]. The confidence of the Bourn Hall team was reflected in the title of their publication: "In vitro fertilization, a treatment for male factor infertility" [41], which suggested that the usefulness of IVF for cases of male factor was no longer in question. This was a limited series, reporting on 122 couples over a period of 20 months, rather than the entire experience between 1980 and 1985. Four groups were included: patients with clear fertility in the female partners and infertility in the men; couples in which both partners were considered infertile; a small group of 13 couples with normal semen analyses before IVF but a clearly abnormal semen analysis during their IVF cycles; and seven couples with very high concentrations of spermatozoa (polyzoospermia), a now outdated and unlikely clinical condition.

New sperm preparation techniques were aimed at both removing seminal plasma, as it was considered toxic to gametes as well as the fertilization process [42], and also obtaining a high proportion of motile spermatozoa. Several sperm preparation methods were developed at Bourn Hall, partly based on prior work. The first of these was a fairly labor-intensive method of sample aggregation used in cases of extreme oligoasthenozoospermia, which relied on the collection of multiple samples over a one or two-week period [40]. For each sample, spermatozoa were prepared in a droplet of seminal plasma-free medium and stored at room temperature, as the loss of motility was lower than for storage at 37°C. Aggregated samples were then used for small volume insemination. The system for semen collection was considerably diverse during those days with the use of split ejaculates and collection directly into culture medium [41]. Collection in a single dry container in cases of male factor infertility was rare. Another preparation technique was the so-called sedimentation method, which involved the standard method of minimally two-step mild centrifugation and resuspension in 1–2 mL of fresh medium. The sample was then placed in a flat Petri dish covered with paraffin oil and left to sediment for 1–24 hours at room temperature under a 5% O_2, 5% CO_2 and 90% N_2 gas atmosphere in a glass desiccator. Cells and debris would fall to the bottom of the large droplet and spermatozoa would be removed from the top layer. These first two techniques were not reported in the early Monash work, but it is unknown if that would have made a difference. Another method involved swim-up and migration of motile spermatozoa into culture medium developed in the 1950s, according to Mortimer [43]. This technique was also described by the Monash team. It must be kept in mind that until the second half of the 1980s, sperm density gradients such as Percoll had not been tested clinically for sperm preparation [44]. Within a few years after the introduction of IVF for male factor infertility, density gradients would become a common type of sperm preparation and by 1990 many samples were treated that way. This may explain some of the rapid improvement seen with widescale micromanipulation in the early 1990s. Again, we do not know the extent of improvement, because comparative studies were not performed or published until very recently [45]. This study showed that swim-up techniques are either equivalent or better for embryo quality than density gradients, but that retrospective trial though multicenter was not randomized and seemed underpowered, increasing the chance of bias. Even after nearly 30 years of using ICSI, the efficacy and optimization of adjunct technology remains unclear.

Why was IVF not powerful enough for treating all cases of male factor? Which group benefitted and which did not? Without micromanipulation, fertilization rates were considerably lower than the results from ICSI as practiced nowadays, probably by a factor 2 or 3. In addition, with ICSI, samples from men with extremely low counts can still be used and azoospermic men can usually be treated using testicular or epidydimal biopsy. Samples with abnormal sperm morphology probably had the highest level of success, but reduced motility seemed particularly limiting as described by some groups [26]. This effect of motility was not seen by other teams [41], indicating that there may have been qualitative differences in sperm isolation and removal of seminal plasma. Rates of complete fertilization failure in obviously male factor couples were high, at 39% per cycle as reported by the Bourn Hall group [41], yet pregnancy rates after embryo transfer were comparable or better to those patients with other etiologies [46]. The worst results were seen when there was a combination of asthenozoospermia and oligozoospermia with a total fertilization failure rate of 60%, although deliveries of ongoing pregnancies were described for seven couples with extreme asthenozoospermia (< 3% motility) and sperm concentrations less than 1 million/mL, for whom the sample aggregation method of sperm preparation had been used. The major drawbacks of the IVF method were clearly the high incidence of complete fertilization failure and the labor-intensity of the sperm preparation procedures. The results quickly led to a realization that the methodology of IVF was not optimal for male factor infertility treatment, even though implantation rates were allegedly higher than in other groups of patients as many of the female partners were young and fertile. Micromanipulation of the fertilization process by direct injection of a spermatozoon into the ooplasm in the mouse was performed before publications of the first male factor

IVF series (Cohen and Zeilmaker, unpublished experiments; Trounson, personal communication), but progress in this area and live birth after assisted fertilization in the mouse was only first published by Gordon and Talansky in 1986 [15].

How Micromanipulation Became a Revolution for Male Factor Infertility Treatment

The micromanipulator, a device which aids in the microdissection and surgery of the living cell, was developed by Robert Chambers while at NYU (New York, USA) in 1912. His invention allowed dissection of the cell and separation of the chromosomes for the first time. Micromanipulation has been used in experimental cell biology for more than 100 years (https://utsic.org/2013/01/10/165/), and in experimental embryology and veterinary medicine for at least 50 years. The device and sub-components hook onto a microscope stage giving the observer a chance to precisely control small glass needles in three-dimensional space while visualizing the process through an inverted microscope. Combining the apparatus with an inverted microscope allowed free access to the slide, dish or setup containing the specimen above an array of changeable lenses. During the 1970s, this setup was a familiar tool in many experimental embryology laboratories and could also be equipped with real-time video and a monitor. These interphases gave biologists a system to fine-tune movements, removing or reducing the effects of normal hand tremor and permitting simple as well as complicated cell surgical interventions.

During the first years after the birth of Louise Brown, several embryologists suggested that the egg could be micromanipulated to come into very close contact with spermatozoa to promote fertilization, even when few spermatozoa were retrieved from seminal plasma. The initial experiments were rarely shared, but several investigators attempted to fertilize mouse oocytes microsurgically, using micromanipulation to directly inject spermatozoa into the ooplasm [47,48], although others did not publish their findings (Trounson, personal communication; Zeilmaker and Cohen, unpublished observations). There was very limited success in the mouse because of invasive membrane breakage and high rates of oocyte degeneration caused by piercing the egg with the relatively blunt glass needles used at the time. The reasons for

these failures are easy to determine in hindsight: the needles were not sharp enough, the glass relatively thick, an aperture/glass thickness ratio that remained the same after pulling (miniaturization of the capillary dimension), and the mouse oocyte membrane was a poor model as its oolemma is relatively fragile. The mature mouse oolemma breaks easily upon piercing with any instrument larger than a simple fluid injection needle such as those used in early gene injection experiments. Those very thin injection needles were made by pulling thin capillaries and gently breaking the closed tip on a holding pipette [49]. However, a larger diameter needle was necessary to accommodate the fairly large mouse spermatozoon. The first successful penetration of the oolemma and formation of a male pronucleus was demonstrated by early procedures in Yanagimachi's pioneering laboratory in Honolulu, following the injection of human and hamster spermatozoa into hamster oocytes [47]. This work was performed at the same time as the zona-free hamster egg test for human sperm function was being developed in the same laboratory [50]. Hamster oocytes are still a model for testing and training in the ICSI procedure, but other than demonstrating male pronucleus formation, the zygotes do not develop in vitro.

A pre-clinical model for microsurgical fertilization was required and the mouse oocyte was considered to be the most obvious system, as mouse in vitro fertilization and development to full-term had been established years earlier [51]. However, mouse oocytes are not easily microinjected with spermatozoa and often degenerate upon injection. Experimental embryologist Clement Markert (1983) [48] commented ironically when showing that fertilization could be established after single sperm microinjection *"The principal problem encountered in injecting sperm directly into the egg is that most of the eggs die at once from the microsurgical injury."* Nevertheless, Markert showed that even phenotypically challenged spermatozoa could fertilize a denuded mouse egg after injection. He also demonstrated, as did Yanagimachi before him, that all outer investments such as cumulus cells and zona pellucida were apparently unnecessary for fertilization once the sperm cell was directly exposed to the ooplasm. The fertilized eggs rarely developed to blastocysts and presumably because of this, embryos were not transferred to recipient foster females. Survival, fertilization and development rates were not provided in

Markert's 1983 paper, and it would take another decade before it became technically feasible for microinjected mouse eggs to routinely survive. The problem was related to the structure and behavior of the mouse oolemma during mechanical injection, and Kimura and Yanagimachi (1995) showed that a high rate of success with ICSI was only possible using a piezo-mediated drive of the needle into the ooplasm [52]. This was the first time that offspring was obtained after ICSI-derived technology in the mouse. Microsurgical fertilization is a rare example of embryology research where the clinical experiment usually preceded animal work [15–18,21].

The concept of sub-zonal sperm insertion – deposition of one or more motile spermatozoa into the perivitelline space – was first introduced by Alan Trounson's team at Monash University [53,16], but it was Jon Gordon and Beth Talansky at Mt. Sinai University in New York City who popularized preclinical microsurgical fertilization in the mouse, with the concept of allowing spermatozoa to naturally traverse the zona pellucida through an artificial hole, a process they referred to as zona drilling [15]. The artificial opening was made using very small amounts of acidified Tyrode's solution (ATS) released immediately adjacent to the zona pellucida, and this approach was often used to open or remove the zona pellucida until the early 1990s. The first non-contact non-toxic laser for opening the zona pellucida in the mouse was developed in 1993 during a collaboration between the Beckham Laser Institute at UC-Irvine and the IVF team at Cornell University Medical Center [54]. The earlier ATS procedure used a holding pipette on one of the micromanipulators to firmly grip the oocyte, with a small-bore injection pipette containing ATS on the opposite micromanipulator. The fine tools were made out of glass capillaries and prepared in the laboratory using a forge to shape the glass, a glass-puller to break the capillary, and a small grinding instrument to create an angled tip, if needed. Microtools, including holding pipettes, were not commercially available until the 1990s and had to be produced by each clinical laboratory that set up a microsurgical fertilization program. This may have been one of the aspects causing technical differences between laboratories and limiting some clinical embryologists from participating in the early research.

The first paper on zona drilling was not just a presentation of pioneering technology or proof that oocytes could survive after micromanipulation, fertilize and develop in vitro, but also showed that the procedure was compatible with implantation and live birth after the embryos were transferred using a surgical intra-uterine transplantation procedure [15]. The authors also demonstrated that with zona drilling the concentration of spermatozoa could be diluted to 100 times below the threshold required for normal in vitro fertilization in the mouse, although fertilization diminished from 75% to 15%. Polyspermy in zona-drilled mouse oocytes was not greater than in zona-intact controls, demonstrating that the block to polyspermy was active on the oolemma. Earlier experiments showed that rat and mouse oocytes from which the zona pellucida were removed could be fertilized resulting in monospermic fertilization [50]. Mouse oocytes fertilized with a significantly higher rate (75%) after the zona drilling procedure compared to zona-intact controls (22%), and when embryos were transplanted into recipient-foster females, term development was at the same rate (36.7%) as mouse IVF zona-intact controls (44.3%) [15].

The first detailed pre-clinical experiments with microsurgical fertilization by sub-zonal insertion of a single human spermatozoon were reported by Alan Trounson's laboratory from Monash University in Australia [53] after the first pilot experiment had been reported a few years earlier [55]. Jeff Mann, also from Monash University (Trounson Laboratory) subsequently reported on the first birth in the mouse after sub-zonal injection of a single spermatozoon [16]. It was not surprising that those who were interested in achieving live human offspring in cases of male factor infertility investigated less invasive technologies first, given the poor outcomes from animal models with ICSI-like procedures [48,56]. Even though the first offspring from mammalian ICSI in the rabbit were born in Japan in Dr. Iritani's laboratory in 1988, only 2/72 transfers leading to live births were reported in the first few papers [57]. This and early clinical work performed at the Jones Institute [58] resulting in poor fertilization outcomes, discouraged most fertilization specialists from performing ICSI clinically and transferring embryos for a few years. When considering the body of work from the pioneering microsurgical fertilization groups, it is not surprising that both zona drilling and sub-zonal insertion were the leading procedures pursued in clinical assisted fertilization during the first years, even though their application in the mouse led to unacceptable fertilization outcomes. It is perhaps a prime example of how the mouse model can elude clinical decisions.

The first babies born after microsurgical fertilization were conceived using an alternative method of zona drilling, as the acidified solution which was so successful in the zona drilling of mouse oocytes was found to be detrimental in the human [59,60]. Despite the relatively successful and routine use of acidified solution in human embryos for zona drilling, assisted hatching and biopsy procedures, the unfertilized egg clearly demonstrated a particular vulnerability [61,62]. Once there was a technical change in zona drilling from chemical to mechanical dissection, the partial zona dissection procedure became clinically successful and the first healthy babies were born [17]. Babies born from sub-zonal insertion were reported in quick succession [18,20], but both methods yielded modest monospermic fertilization rates. It was also determined that even at modest sperm concentrations outside the zona pellucida the use of partial zona dissection increased polyspermy. Unlike in the mouse, the block to polyspermy of human oocytes is regulated by the zona pellucida and not the oolemma [63]. In the human, polyspermy mechanisms resemble those seen in bovine and hamster eggs. This fundamental finding demonstrated the modest suitability of partial zona dissection and sub-zonal insertion for treating infertile men. What was needed was a method using a single spermatozoon directly inserted into the human ooplasm. Although the method of direct mouse egg injection existed, fertilization rates were modest and degeneration occurred frequently. The reasons for the disappointing observations made between 1988 and 1992 can be debated, although it seems likely that major technical differences existed in the micro-tool-making processes. The standard injection microtool developed for sub-zonal insertion (Monash University, Fishel and Antinori's team in Rome and Cornell University Medical Center) differed considerably from a much sharper, thinner enhanced model separately developed by Hubert Joris in Palermo, DeVroey and Van Steirteghem's laboratory (DeVroey, personal communication). The enhanced model tool could easily break the human oolemma with minimal indentation of the zona pellucida. The Belgian team also optimized suction control and visualization of membrane breakage as well as a meticulous setup process aligning the tools at high magnification and using some of the standards developed by Lanzendorf

et al. (1989) such as reducing sperm motility and applying tail breakage to each spermatozoon [58]. The highly technical aspects are what separated the first attempts at ICSI from those developed later in Brussels. The fertilization rates reported by the Brussels team were two to three times higher than seen with the prior approaches. The comparisons were so obvious that no further evidence appeared to be needed and within a year, ICSI became the dominant methodology for treating male factor infertility, and this has remained so for almost 30 years. The prospect of sterility for most men diagnosed with male infertility turned for the better in a timespan of 12 years. It was a remarkable and swift medical revolution. A feat accomplished by several groups publishing their technology and findings in a few dozen papers.

Acknowledgments Dr. Sharon Mortimer is gratefully acknowledged for critical reading of the manuscript.

References

[1] Von Baer KE. De Ovi Mammalium et Hominis Genesi ("On the Mammalian Egg and the Origin of Man"). Leipzig,Germany: Leopold Voss; 1827.

[2] Clift D, Schuh M. Restarting life: fertilization and the transition from meiosis to mitosis. Nat Rev Mol Cell Biol. 2013;**14**:549–562.

[3] Macomber D, Sanders MB. The spermatozoa count. Its value in the diagnosis, prognosis and treatment of sterility. N Engl J Med. 1929;**200**:981–984.

[4] Andrade-Rocha FT. On the origins of the semen analysis: a close relationship with the history of the reproductive medicine. J Hum Reprod Sci. 2017;**10**:242–255.

[5] Hotchkiss, RS. Fertility in Men. Philadelphia: JB Lippincott Company; 1944.

[6] MacLeod J. Semen quality in one thousand men of known fertility and in eight hundred cases of infertile marriage. Fertil Steril. 1951;**2**:115–139.

[7] Tyler ET, Singher HO. Male infertility; status of treatment, prevention and current research. J Am Med Assoc. 1956;**160**:91–97.

[8] Polge C, Smith AU, Parkes AS. Revival of spermatozoa after vitrification and dehydration at low temperatures. Nature 1949;**15**:666.

[9] Bunge Rg, Sherman JK. Fertilizing capacity of frozen human spermatozoa. Nature. 1953;**172**:767–768.

[10] Austin CR. Observation on the penetration of sperm into the mammalian egg. Aust J Sci Res B. 1951;**4**:581–596.

[11] Chang MC. Fertilizing capacity of spermatozoa deposited in the fallopian tubes. Nature. 1951;**168**:697–698.

[12] Sigman M, Baazeem A, Zini A. Semen analysis and sperm function assays: what do they mean? Semin Reprod Med. 2009;**27**:115–123.

[13] DeJonge C. Semen analysis: looking for an upgrade in class. Fertil Steril. 2012;**97**:260–266.

[14] Edwards RG, Steptoe PC. Birth after the reimplantation of a human embryo. Lancet. 1978;**312**:366.

[15] Gordon JW, Talansky BE. Assisted fertilization by zona drilling: a mouse model for correction of oligospermia. J Exp Zool. 1986;**239**:347–354.

[16] Mann JR. Full term development of mouse eggs fertilized by a spermatozoon microinjected under the zona pellucida. Biol Reprod. 1988;**38**:1077–1083.

[17] Cohen J, Malter H, Fehilly C, Wright G, Elsner C, Kort H, Massey J. Implantation of embryos after partial opening of oocyte zona pellucida to facilitate sperm penetration. Lancet. 1988;**2**:162.

[18] Ng SC, Bongso A, Ratnam SS, Sathananthan H, Chan CL, Wong PC, Hagglund L, Anandakumar C, Wong YC, Goh VH. Pregnancy after transfer of sperm under zona. Lancet. 1988;**2**:790.

[20] Fishel S, Antinori S, Jackson P, Johnson J, Lisi F, Chiariello F, Versaci C. Twin birth after subzonal insemination. Lancet. 1990;**335**:722–723.

[21] Palermo G, Joris H, Devroey P, Van Steirteghem AC. Pregnancies after intracytoplasmic injection of single spermatozoon into an oocyte. Lancet. 1992;**340**:17–18.

[22] Sennert D : Practical Physick. 4th Book. Published by Cole P Cornhill printing press. England, 1664.

[23] Kumar N, Singh AK. Trends of male factor infertility, an important cause of infertility: a review of literature. J Hum Reprod Sci. 2015;**8**:191–196.

[24] Edwards RG, Purdy JM (eds). Human Conception in Vitro. London: Academic Press; 1982.

[25] Mahadevan MM, Trounson AO, Leeton JF. The relationship of tubal blockage, infertility of unknown cause, suspected male infertility, and endometriosis to success of in vitro fertilization and embryo transfer. Fertil Steril. 1983;**40**:755–762.

[26] Mahadevan MM, Leeton JF, Trounson AO, Wood C. Successful use of in vitro fertilization for patients with persisting low-quality semen. Ann N Y Acad Sci. 1985;**442**:293–300.

[27] Aafjes JH, van der Vijver JC, Schenck PE. The duration of infertility: an important datum for the fertility prognosis of men with semen abnormalities. Fertil Steril. 1978;**30**:423–425.

[28] Cohen J, Malter H, Elsner C, Kort H, Massey J, Mayer MP. Immunosuppression supports implantation of zona pellucida dissected human embryos. Fertil Steril. 1990;**53**:662–665.

[29] Cohen J, Alikani M, Trowbridge J, Rosenwaks Z. Implantation enhancement by selective assisted hatching using zona drilling of human embryos with poor prognosis. Hum Reprod. 1992;**7**:685–691.

[30] Vandekerckhove P, O'Donovan PA, Lilford RJ, Harada TW. Infertility treatment: from cookery to science. The epidemiology of randomised controlled trials. Br J Obstet Gynaecol. 1993;**100**:1005–1036.

[31] Haldane JBS. Daedalus, or Science and the Future. A Paper read to the Heretics, Cambridge, on February 4, 1923. Pp. vii + 93. London: Kegan Paul and Co., Ltd.; 1924.

[32] Rock J, Menkin MF. In vitro fertilization and cleavage of human ovarian eggs. Science. 1944;**100**:105–107.

[33] Edwards RG, Steptoe PC. A Matter of Life: The Story of IVF: A Medical Breakthrough. London, UK: Finestride and Crownchime; 1980.

[34] Edwards RG. Maturation in vitro of human ovarian oocytes. Lancet. 1965;**286**:926–929.

[35] Edwards RG, Steptoe PC, Purdy JM. Establishing full-term human pregnancies using cleaving embryos grown in vitro. Br J Obstet Gynaecol. 1980;**87**:737–756.

[36] Catford SR, McLachlan RI, O'Bryan MK, Halliday JL. Long-term follow-up of intra-cytoplasmic sperm injection-conceived offspring compared with in vitro fertilization-conceived offspring: a systematic review of health outcomes beyond the neonatal period. Andrology. 2017;**5**:610–621.

[37] Wisanto A, Magnus M, Bonduelle M, Liu J, Camus M, Tournaye H, Liebaers I, Van Steirteghem AC, Devroey P. Obstetric outcome of 424 pregnancies after intracytoplasmic sperm injection. Hum Reprod. 1995;**10**:2713–2718.

[38] Cohen J, Fehilly CB, Fishel SB, Edwards RG, Hewitt J, Rowland GF, Steptoe PC, Webster J. Male infertility successfully treated by in-vitro fertilisation. Lancet. 1984;**1**:1239–1240.

[39] Lopata A. Successes and failures in human in vitro fertilization. Nature. 1980;**288**:642–643.

[40] Trounson AO, Leeton JF, Wood C, Webb J, Kovacs G. The investigation of idiopathic infertility by in vitro fertilization. Fertil Steril. 1980;**34**:431–438.

[41] Cohen J, Edwards R, Fehilly C, Fishel S, Hewitt J, Purdy J, Rowland G, Steptoe P, Webster J. In vitro

fertilization: a treatment for male infertility. Fertil Steril. 1985 **43**:422–432.

[42] Kanwar KC, Yanagimachi R, Lopata A. Effects of human seminal plasma on fertilizing capacity of human spermatozoa. Fertil Steril. 1979;**31**:321–327.

[43] Mortimer D. Sperm preparation methods. J Androl. 2000;**21**:357–366.

[44] Hyne RV, Stojanoff A, Clarke GN, Lopata A, Johnston WI. Pregnancy from in vitro fertilization of human eggs after separation of motile spermatozoa by density gradient centrifugation. Fertil Steril. 1986;**45**:93–96.

[45] Palini S, Stefani S, Primiterra M, Benedetti S, Barone S, Carli L, Vaccari E, Murat U, Feichtinger W. Comparison of in vitro fertilization outcomes in ICSI cycles after human sperm preparation by density gradient centrifugation and direct micro swim-up without centrifugation. JBRA Assist Reprod. 2017;**21**:89–93.

[46] Matson PL, Turner SR, Yovich JM, Tuvik AI, Yovich JL. Oligospermic infertility treated by in-vitro fertilization. Aust N Z J Obstet Gynaecol. 1986;**26**:84–87.

[47] Uehara T, Yanagimachi R. Microsurgical injection of spermatozoa into hamster eggs with subsequent transformation of sperm nuclei into male pronuclei. Biol Reprod. 1976;**15**:467–470.

[48] Markert CL. Fertilization of mammalian eggs by sperm injection. J Exp Zool. 1983;**228**:195–201.

[49] Gordon JW, Ruddle FH. Integration and stable germ line transmission of genes injected into mouse pronuclei. Science. 1981;**214**:1244–1246.

[50] Yanagimachi R, Yanagimachi H, Rogers BJ. The use of zona-free animal ova as a test-system for the assessment of the fertilizing capacity of human spermatozoa. Biol Reprod. 1976;**15**:471–476.

[51] Whittingham DG. Fertilization of mouse eggs in vitro. Nature. 1968;**220**:592–593.

[52] Kimura Y, Yanagimachi R. Intracytoplasmic sperm injection in the mouse. Biol Reprod. 1995;**52**:709–720.

[53] Laws-King A, Trounson A, Sathananthan H, Kola I. Fertilization of human oocytes by microinjection of a single spermatozoon under the zona pellucida. Fertil Steril. 1987;**48**:637–642.

[54] Neev J, Gonzalez A, Licciardi F, Licciardi F, Alikani M, Tadir Y, Berns M, Cohen J. Opening of the mouse zona pellucida by laser without a micromanipulator. Hum Reprod. 1993;**8**: 939–944.

[55] Metka M, Haromy T, Huber J, Schurz B. Apparative Insemination mit Hilfe des Mikromanipulators ("Artificial insemination using a micromanipulator"). Fertilität 1985;**1**:41–44.

[56] Keefer CL. Fertilization by sperm injection in the rabbit. Gamete Res. 1989;**22**:59–69.

[57] Iritani A, Utsumi K, Miyake M, Hosoi Y, Saeki K. In vitro fertilization by a routine method and micromanipulation. Ann New York Acad Sci 1988;**541**:583–590.

[58] Lanzendorf SE, Maloney MK, Veeck LL, Slusser J, Hodgen GD, Rosenwaks Z. A preclinical evaluation of pronuclear formation by microinjection of human spermatozoa into human oocytes. Fertil Steril. 1988;**49** 835–842.

[59] Malter HE, Cohen J. Partial zona dissection of the human oocyte: a nontraumatic method using micromanipulation to assist zona pellucida penetration. Fertil Steril. 1989;**51**:139–148.

[60] Malter HE. Micromanipulation in assisted reproductive technology. Reprod Biomed Online. 2016;**32**:339–347.

[61] Handyside AH, Kontogianni EH, Hardy K, Winston RM. Pregnancies from biopsied human preimplantation embryos sexed by Y-specific DNA amplification. Nature. 1990;**344**:768–770.

[62] Cohen J, Elsner C, Kort H, Malter H, Massey J, Mayer MP, Wiemer K. Impairment of the hatching process following IVF in the human and improvement of implantation by assisting hatching using micromanipulation. Hum Reprod. 1990;**5**:7–13.

[63] Gordon JW, Grunfeld L, Talansky BE, Garrisi GJ, Richards C, Wiczyk H, Rappaport D, Navot D, Laufer N. The human oocyte blocks polyspermy at the zona pellucida. Presented at the Forty-Fourth Annual Meeting of The American Fertility Society. Atlanta, GA, American Fertility Society, Birmingham;1988:10–13 (AL, in the Program Supplement, 1988).

Development of ICSI in Human Assisted Reproduction

Stephanie Cheung, Alessandra Parrella, Philip Xie, Sherina Lawrence, Mounia Haddad, Derek Keating, Zev Rosenwaks, and Gianpiero D. Palermo

Background

In 1934, Gregory Pincus and E. V. Enzmann demonstrated normal development of mammalian oocytes cultured in vitro [1]. Ten years later, a study reported on the initial stages of in vitro fertilization (IVF) [2]. These early achievements made the delivery of the world's first IVF baby possible [3]. Through efforts to enhance the efficiency of IVF, and particularly to expand this indication to the most severe form of male factor infertility, intracytoplasmic sperm injection (ICSI) was clinically applied in 1991 [4]. This evolution of assisted reproductive technology (ART), starting from IVF in the 1970s to micromanipulation in the 1990s, delineates the rapid progress of the reproductive medicine field. ART has become a panacea for couples struggling with infertility. ART procedures have evolved over time and have contributed to the increasing number of births by IVF throughout the decades [5]. Nevertheless, scientists continue to strive to develop new forms of treatment for infertility.

Early Micromanipulation

The proof that IVF was a viable option to infertile couples arrived in 1978, when the first live birth was achieved in a woman with bilateral tubal occlusion [3, 6]. From there onward, conventional IVF has been applied to treat infertile couples, particularly women with tubal indications. However, other forms of infertility did not benefit from standard in vitro insemination. Indeed, suboptimal spermatozoa with compromised kinetic or morphologic characteristics were unable to penetrate the glycoprotein layer surrounding the oocyte, and therefore failed to fertilize by standard IVF [7, 8].

Even with the adoption of microdroplet insemination, an IVF technique [9] in which a higher sperm concentration is incubated with oocytes in microdroplets under oil, the number of oocytes that were fertilized was still low. The need to treat men with impaired spermatogenesis led reproductive scientists to explore more radical alternatives to accomplish better fertilization results.

It was initially believed that the main barrier hindering the penetration of the spermatozoa into the oocyte was the zona pellucida (ZP). Therefore, an early proposal was removal of the ZP to facilitate fusion of the spermatozoa to the oolemma. However, as the ZP serves as a scaffold to support embryo growth, this led to polyspermia and decreased embryo developmental competence. A subsequent approach was to soften the ZP with trypsin or pronase to yield some fertilization; however, the embryos were unable to cleave [10]. In a separate study, zona drilling (ZD), a procedure in which the oocyte is exposed to acid (Tyrode's medium) to create a hole in the ZP, was used to facilitate the entrance of the sperm to the oocyte [11]. Although a fertilization rate of 32% was achieved, chemical damage from the 2.3 pH of the medium and the collateral issue of polyspermia limited the use of this application. As a result, partial zona dissection (PZD), requiring use of a mechanical measure to produce a virtual opening in the ZP, was developed. Although the fertilization rate improved to 45%, the rate of polyspermia was about 48%, and severely asthenozoospermic and teratozoospermic patients still reported total fertilization failure [12].

To facilitate penetration through the ZP while reining in polyspermia, a technique was developed to overcome male factor issues and improve clinical results. Subzonal insertion (SUZI) was developed to facilitate sperm–egg interactions bypassing the ZP and placing the sperm directly into the perivitelline space [13]. The fertilization rate increased and even couples with complete fertilization failure (CFF) obtained embryos for transfer. In a study including 43 couples with a history of CFF with IVF, the fertilization rate increased to 30.9% with an 80% cleavage rate, although the pregnancy rate remained low, ranging between 2.9% and 16.3% [14]. These early gamete manipulation techniques were capable of addressing only mild forms of male infertility, mostly as a result of semen parameters, but were virtually powerless in cases of male gamete dysfunction [15].

In the late 1980s, more radical attempts were carried out by injecting the spermatozoon directly into the oocyte. This approach was more effective, especially in cases with severe oligo- or teratozoospermia. The earliest experiments were performed in the sea urchin [16, 17] and the Chinese hamster [18, 19], although most of the mammalian oocytes did not survive. In a later study, however, the first pregnancy was achieved in the rabbit, followed by an unexpected, isolated birth in a bovine species [20, 21]. In 1987, human oocytes were used for this technique, but no embryos were replaced [22]. Although this technique was promising to alleviate male factor infertility, its routine application was very difficult because refined tools were needed and the key steps of the injection were poorly understood. It was only in 1992 that the correct procedure and proper tools were established (Figure 2.1), giving rise to the revolutionary technique now known as intracytoplasmic sperm injection, or ICSI [23].

The Dawn of ICSI

Since the initial attempts at gamete micromanipulation in the 1940s and early breakthroughs in the murine model in the 1960s [24], micromanipulation strategies in human ART remained challenging because of technological limitations resulting in oocyte damage and poor embryo implantation [22]. Inspired by early gamete micromanipulation procedures such as PZD and SUZI, a more direct and efficient approach was advanced to overcome spermatozoa abnormalities. To limit the amount of damage to the oocyte during micromanipulation, a more delicate and precise injector was required. Refinements of the micromanipulator included modification of the microinjector tubing to deliver consistent output to a 5-micron diameter needle, as well as modified holding and microinjection pipettes [25].

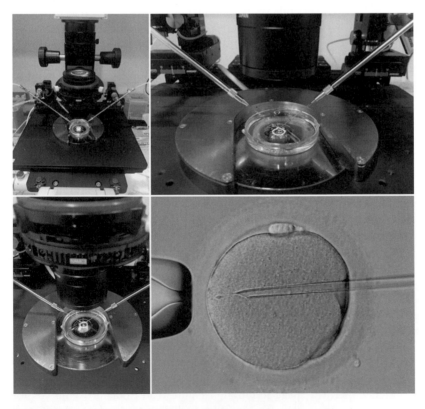

Figure 2.1 Micromanipulation station setup for ICSI. (A black and white version of this figure will appear in some formats. For the color version, please refer to the plate section.)

The first ICSI occurred during a SUZI procedure in which the oolemma was unintentionally penetrated by the microinjection pipette, and a single spermatozoon slipped inside the ooplasm. This first oocyte was not damaged by the injection, and two pronuclei observed the next morning confirmed successful fertilization [25]. The first live birth following ICSI reported in 1992 sparked the field's interest, and ICSI has since revolutionized the practice of reproductive medicine [23]. This effective method ensured the precise introduction of a single spermatozoon into the oocyte, preventing polyspermy, and also demonstrated the possibility of fertilizing any mature oocyte despite abnormal sperm morphology [15, 26, 27]. In terms of effectiveness in fertilization, ICSI was immediately able to yield a fertilization rate of 44% compared to its preceding technology, SUZI, which was able to achieve a fertilization rate of 18% [26]. The emergence of ICSI allowed a better understanding of the timing between sperm penetration and pronuclei appearance [28, 29], including one and three pronuclei fertilization. These findings demonstrated that the first zygotic mitosis is controlled by the sperm centrosome (Figure 2.2) [15, 30].

The early development of ICSI involved a great deal of fine-tuning and several protocol improvements. One important refinement was the aggressive immobilization of spermatozoa by creasing the flagellum firmly prior to injection. A study published in 1996 demonstrated that aggressive sperm immobilization improved fertilization and pregnancy rates compared to standard sperm immobilization [31]. After several upgrades and technical revisions, ICSI

became a reliable method to treat severe male factor infertility cases such as hypospermatogenesis or extreme teratozoospermia [15], and soon thereafter, azoospermic men [27]. Indications for ICSI were not limited to male factors, but also benefited non-male factor couples, including those with oocyte dysmorphism, low numbers of mature oocytes, and HIV/hepatitis C-discordant couples [32].

ICSI Applications for Male Factor Infertility

ICSI Utilizing Ejaculated Spermatozoa

The original indication for ICSI was to treat mainly male factor infertility such as suboptimal sperm concentration, severely impaired sperm kinetics, and poor sperm morphology (Figure 2.3). During its development, ICSI became a versatile treatment for most types of infertility. Currently, 90% of all ICSI cycles performed at our center utilize ejaculated specimens. ICSI was developed to enable the male gamete to bypass natural barriers surrounding the oocyte, such as cumulus cells, the ZP, as well as the oolemma, and it has been proven to be the most effective method to treat couples presenting with oligo-, astheno-, and/or teratozoospermia [33]. In addition, ICSI is the only viable method to treat cryptozoospermia, a condition in which spermatozoa are extremely scarce. In these cases, an extensive sperm search is required to identify all spermatozoa needed to inseminate the oocytes retrieved [27].

ICSI with Surgically Retrieved Spermatozoa

Because ICSI requires only one spermatozoon to fertilize an oocyte regardless of the morphological, kinetical, and maturational status of the male gamete, it represents the sole insemination approach for azoospermic men for whom spermatozoa can only be retrieved by surgical intervention. Epididymal aspiration has become an effective way to retrieve relatively mature spermatozoa for ICSI in men with obstructive azoospermia (OA), whether it is acquired (i.e., vasectomy) or results from genetic defects such as congenital bilateral absence of the vas deferens [34, 35]. Non-obstructive azoospermia (NOA), whether caused by hypogametogenesis, maturational arrest, or germ cell aplasia, requires surgical retrieval directly from the testicular seminiferous tubule [35, 36]). At our center, ICSI has allowed testicular spermatozoa to achieve a 48.4%

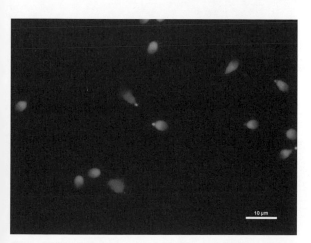

Figure 2.2 Pericentrin staining on spermatozoa assessing paternal centrosome. (A black and white version of this figure will appear in some formats. For the color version, please refer to the plate section.)

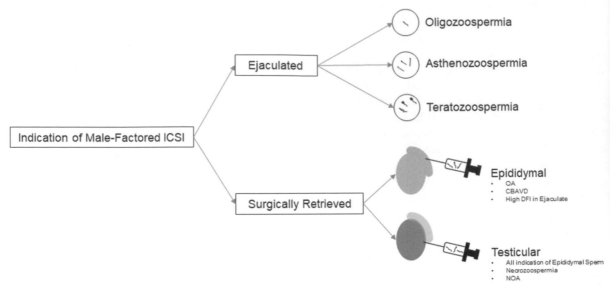

Figure 2.3 Male factor ICSI indications. (A black and white version of this figure will appear in some formats. For the color version, please refer to the plate section.)

fertilization rate and a 35.9% clinical pregnancy rate. Even in cases with Klinefelter's syndrome, ICSI has helped men with a non-mosaic XXY genotype to father offspring with a normal karyotype [37].

High DNA Fragmentation of the Male Gamete

While some male infertility etiologies are straightforward, unexplained infertility because of a subtle male factor remains challenging. To understand the etiology of these peculiar cases, supplementary tests may be needed prior to ICSI treatment [38]. Even though the sperm genome is highly compacted, oxidative damage during the transit through the male genital tract can result in DNA breakage (Figure 2.4). Moreover, sperm chromatin fragmentation (SCF) has been shown to be negatively correlated with sperm motility [27]. High SCF, resulting in recurrent pregnancy loss, can therefore be prevented by ICSI, as only the most motile spermatozoa are selected for insemination. In conjunction with ICSI, surgical retrieval of spermatozoa provided another approach to ameliorate the effect of high SCF [39].

Assisted Oocyte Activation

Although ICSI has been able to greatly alleviate male factor infertility, rare cases of fertilization failure after ICSI can still occur. While this can result from

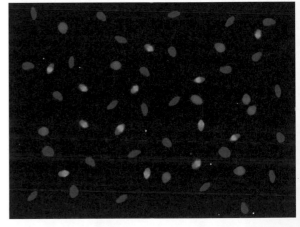

Figure 2.4 TUNEL assay depicting spermatozoa with fragmented DNA (green fluorescent signal). (A black and white version of this figure will appear in some formats. For the color version, please refer to the plate section.)

asynchronous oocyte maturation, it may also be attributed to a lack of a specific oocyte-activating factor in the spermatozoa. Assisted oocyte activation (AOA) can therefore be used to achieve successful fertilization and even clinical pregnancy. AOA can be carried out by exposing the oocytes, post-ICSI, to either a chemical agent or an electrical pulse [40]. Moreover, sperm-derived activating extracts or calcium-releasing compounds can be used to further enhance fertilization in these problematic cases. Oocyte activation agents include electroactivation, calcium ionophore, and strontium chloride [40–42]. During fertilization, a series of distinct Ca^{2+} oscillation spikes occurs in the oocyte. These cytosolic Ca^{2+} spikes release waves from the endoplasmic reticulum, initiated by a sperm-bound labile protein that has been shown to settle onto a sperm-specific phospholipase C zeta (PLCζ) [44] (Figure 2.5). Treatment with an oocyte-activating agent enhances

this process by increasing Ca^{2+} permeability at the cell membrane, allowing an influx of extracellular Ca^{2+} into the ooplasm and thereby inducing Ca^{2+} release from intracellular calcium stores (Figure 2.6).

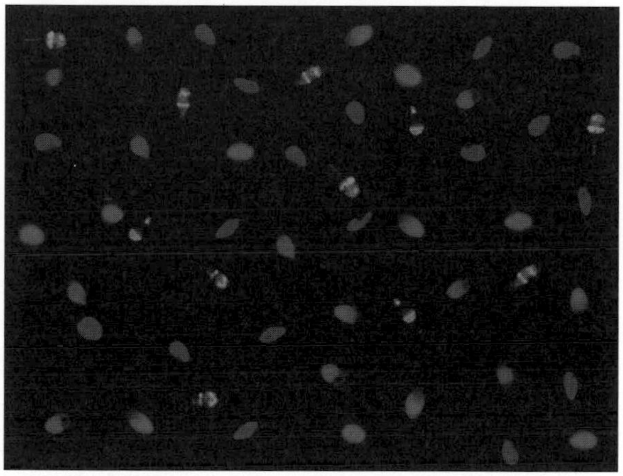

One pioneering study on AOA reported 17 couples with previously failed fertilization following ICSI. For these patients' subsequent ICSI cycles, AOA was carried out by injecting the spermatozoon with medium containing a high concentration of $CaCl_2$, followed by exposing the oocyte to calcium ionophore. As a result, couples with this peculiar defect were able to achieve an overall fertilization rate of over 70% [45]. While this treatment can effectively trigger oocyte activation, allowing concurrent sperm nuclear decondensation and thereby promoting zygote development, it is important to document a clear sperm-dependent oocyte activation deficiency (OAD), as is typical for globozoospermic cases (Figure 2.7). The demonstration of a specific sperm disturbance serves as a proper indication for AOA, identified in couples with a history of fertilization failure with ICSI and confirmed with the mouse oocyte activation test (MOAT) to measure the oocyte activation capacity of the spermatozoon. Couples with a history of failed fertilization caused by OAD were categorized as *suspected*, *somewhat related*, or *clearly related* to the spermatozoon. ICSI fertilization and pregnancy outcomes after AOA were then compared to the same

Figure 2.5 PLCζ, the putative soluble cytosolic factor, required for fertilization examined by immunofluorescence microscopy. (A black and white version of this figure will appear in some formats. For the color version, please refer to the plate section.)

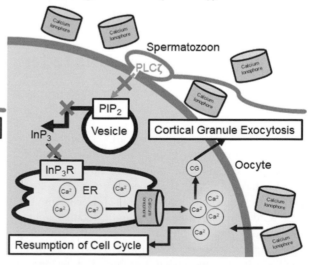

Figure 2.6 Mechanism of assisted oocyte activation. (A black and white version of this figure will appear in some formats. For the color version, please refer to the plate section.)

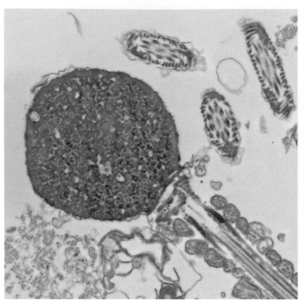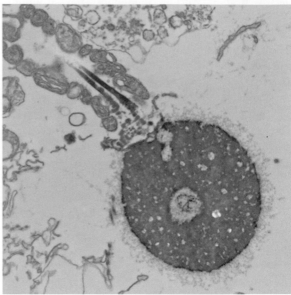

Figure 2.7 Transmission electron micrograph of globozoospermic specimen.

patients' previous cycles serving as controls. AOA consistently obtained higher fertilization and clinical pregnancy rates than those achieved from cycles of the same couples serving as controls [46].

Despite its demonstrated safety and effectiveness, it is imperative to remember that prior to using AOA treatment, the culpable gamete must first be identified. Therefore, AOA should be reserved only for those cases where a clear sperm-linked OAD has been diagnosed, and it should not simply be regarded as a remedy whenever unexplained fertilization failure occurs.

ICSI Applications for Non-Male Factor Infertility

Oocyte Dysmorphism

ICSI is a reliable technique that can also benefit non-male factor infertility. Using oocyte morphology to predict clinical outcome is questionable, but several studies have shown that oocyte quality reflects embryo developmental potential [47]. In conjunction with ICSI, it is possible to evaluate detailed oocyte morphology immediately after decoronization using high-magnification microscopy. This would not be feasible with standard IVF, in which the evaluation is limited to observation of the cumulus–oocyte

complex with limited information on the oocyte itself. Indeed, with standard in vitro insemination, the oocyte can be properly evaluated once the cumulus corona cells have been dispersed by the inseminating spermatozoa.

The normal metaphase II (MII) oocyte morphology is defined as an oocyte with a spherical structure surrounded by a homogenous ZP, with a cytoplasm free of inclusions and with a uniform polar body (PB). However, not all MII oocytes display this perfect morphology (Figure 2.8).

Oocyte dysmorphism can be characterized by an abnormal cytoplasm (dark or granular), cytoplasmic inclusions (vacuoles, refractile bodies, or smooth endoplasmic reticulum), non-spherical shapes, abnormal ZP, abnormal perivitelline space, and/or abnormal PB (fragment, giant, smooth, duplicated). Several studies have attempted to investigate the clinical outcomes of dysmorphic oocytes. Indeed, one such study showed that when these abnormal oocytes were inseminated via standard IVF, no fertilization was achieved, whereas the use of ICSI in these particular cases not only improved their fertilizing ability, but also provided a more satisfactory clinical outcome [48]. This success proved that sperm decondensation and pronuclear formation/migration are not influenced by cytoplasmic features when ICSI is applied. Another study showed that oocytes with cytoplasmic defects did not influence

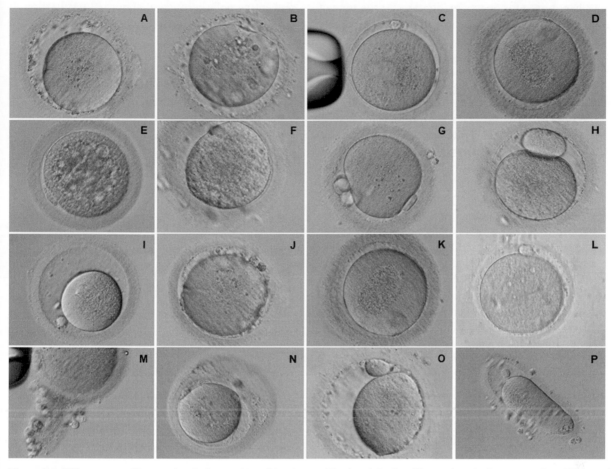

Figure 2.8 Different types of intraooplasmic dysmorphism: (A) inclusions, (B) refractile bodies, (C) smooth endoplasmic reticulum, (D) central granulation/dark center, (E) vacuoles, (F) granular ooplasm. Different types of extraooplasmic abnormalities: (G) fragmented PB, (H) large PB, (I) expanse of perivitelline space (PVS), (J) perivitelline debris. Different types of zona pellucida (ZP) deformities: (K) dark ZP, (L) thin ZP, (M) abnormal ZP, (N) bilayered ZP. Other types of oocyte dysmorphism: (O) irregular shape, (P) oval oocyte. (A black and white version of this figure will appear in some formats. For the color version, please refer to the plate section.)

fertilization and cleavage rates, although implantation and clinical pregnancy rates were compromised [49]. Furthermore, a similar study reported that some defects such as refractile bodies or granular cytoplasm could decrease fertilization and embryo developmental competence [50]. These findings were supported by the results of ICSI on oocytes with centered granularity, which achieved a 4.2% implantation rate [51, 52]].

Lastly, a few studies also demonstrated that although fertilization is not compromised, increased pregnancy loss may result from embryo aneuploidy that is possibly caused by dysmorphic oocytes [48, 53]. For example, an assessment concluded that fertilization and embryo developmental competence could not be attributed to oocyte characteristics [54].

In conclusion, while many oocyte anomalies have been described that may influence embryo selection, particularly with the advent of time-lapse observation, it is still not clear what impact these morphological traits have on clinical outcome.

Low Oocyte Maturity

To achieve normal fertilization and adequate embryo developmental competence, an oocyte undergoes certain modifications and completes essential processes involving the nucleus and cytoplasm [55]. During follicular antral formation, granulosa cells differentiate into two specialized subpopulations of cumulus complex (CC), in which the innermost layer consists of the corona radiata and the parietal granulosa cells. Communication between the oocyte and the corona cells is required for oocyte maturation. At the time of ovulation, resumption of meiosis along with an LH surge stimulates active secretion of hyaluronic acid, inducing the expansion of the cumulus corona mass, and the formation of the corona radiata, which is essential for proper spermatozoa capacitation and subsequent fertilization.

While germinal vesicles retrieved from smaller follicles are typically characterized by an unexpanded cumulus with multiple layers of granulosa cells, metaphase-I oocytes have a more subtle appearance with a well-dispersed surrounding cumulous cell. Oocyte nuclear maturity can only be assessed properly after removal of cumulus cells, and is confirmed by the extrusion of the first polar body in the perivitelline space, indicating successful completion of meiosis I and arrest at the MII stage of development. In standard IVF, the CC is retained prior to insemination; hence, oocyte morphology and, most importantly, maturity cannot be assessed. In contrast, removal of the CC is essential for ICSI and simultaneously allows for proper evaluation of oocyte maturity. MII oocytes are the optimal and sole maturational stage for ICSI. The number of MII oocytes retrieved at each cycle can be affected by follicle size, certain ovarian stimulation protocols, or the surgeon's ability to retrieve the smallest antral follicles [56]. ICSI offers an advantage in terms of "reading" oocytes following cumulus removal and enhances fertilization chances by direct spermatozoon injection [28].

Cryopreserved Oocytes

Oocyte cryopreservation provides several advantages in ART, including the ability to preserve fertility for cancer patients or for women who choose to postpone motherhood. The survival rate for cancer patients has dramatically improved in the last two decades, increasing the need for fertility preservation. Cryopreserving "young" oocytes also maintains fertility potential and improves outcomes for older women who have delayed childbearing.

Oocyte morphology prior to cryopreservation impacts the cell integrity during thawing. If the oocyte quality is suboptimal, the post-thaw survivability will be compromised [50]. It is important that the thawed oocytes maintain developmental competence without any major alterations, particularly of the ZP.

The cortical reaction is triggered when a single spermatozoon binds to glycoproteins on the oolemma, leading to hardening of the ZP, thus preventing polyspermy and abnormal fertilization. It has been shown that cryostress may cause an increase in intracellular calcium concentration, inducing a cortical reaction and a premature release of cortical granules, and consequently modifications of the ZP, hindering physiologic sperm–oocyte fusion by IVF. The ability to bypass natural obstacles represented by a modified ZP, and the receptivity of the oolemma during cryopreservation, make ICSI the optimal methodology to inseminate oocytes that have been frozen and thawed [57].

In Vitro Maturation (IVM)

In vitro maturation (IVM) is conducted on immature oocytes retrieved from small follicles of about 10 mm diameter, and it is usually considered an optional treatment mainly for patients with polycystic ovaries (PCOs) or a history of severe ovarian hyperstimulation syndrome (OHSS). It can also be extended to many other indications mainly related to defective oocyte maturation following a standard superovulation protocol [58]. Nonetheless, ultrastructural changes and altered properties of ZP have been observed in IVM oocytes [59]. In addition, the cumulus cells surrounding IVM oocytes have shown to carry a high apoptotic potential, requiring premature removal [60]. All these requirements may affect the ability of IVM oocytes to be fertilized by standard in vitro insemination. Thus, ICSI is the preferred insemination method for these cases, as it allows the hardened ZP of a denuded IVM oocyte to be bypassed.

Preimplantation Genetic Testing

Preimplantation genetic testing (PGT) is the primary method for detecting multiple types of genetic embryo anomalies. For instance, numerical chromosomal anomalies within the embryo can be detected by PGT for aneuploidy screening (PGT-A), common in women of advanced reproductive age. While the presence of structural anomalies such as translocation or deletions can be identified by PGT for structural rearrangement (PGT-SR), PGT for monogenic disorders (PGT-M) can screen embryos for genetic mutations, providing valuable information on conceptuses regarding a particular heritable genetic disorder (PGT-M) or aneuploidy (PGT-A).

Initially, PGT was performed on individual blastomeres of day-3 embryos at the six- to eight-cell stage. However, at this phase of development, the embryo has not completed its self-selection in terms of its ability to implant. Moreover, the removal of one or two blastomeres with a high level of pluripotency may affect the embryo's developmental competence [61]. Therefore, the need to assess a larger number of cells by trophectoderm biopsies has become the standard, as this does not appear to have any negative effect on the implantation rate.

Aside from the embryo stage, the genetic assessment has evolved as well. While FISH was the earliest technique used for genetic testing, followed by comparative genome hybridization (CGH) and comprehensive chromosome screening (CCS), PGT is now primarily performed by next-generation sequencing [62].

While both PGT-A and PGT-M have become increasingly common [63, 64], PGT-M is utilized by couples, often fertile, to identify the risk of a conceptus carrying a heritable defect. Conversely, PGT-A has been performed for approximately 31% of all ART cycles in 2016 alone [65]. Although PGT can be used with standard in vitro insemination, it has been strongly recommended that PGT be used in conjunction with ICSI for several reasons [32]. As ICSI requires the removal of cumulus cells from the oocyte, there would be no maternal genetic material remaining in the culture media or the trophectoderm biopsy sample that could alter test results. As ICSI requires only a single spermatozoon to inseminate the oocyte, there is no risk of paternal DNA contamination, as is the case with in vitro insemination where multiple spermatozoa attach to the ZP and may contaminate the molecular genetic technique. This was demonstrated by a recent study that reported a higher incidence of mosaicism in embryos inseminated by standard IVF cycles in comparison to ICSI [65]. In addition, the higher fertilization rate achieved by ICSI would provide more embryos available for genetic assessment [66].

While the universal adoption of PGT remains a matter of debate – concerns remain about putative embryo injury and genetic technical error contributing to embryo "wastage" for the above-mentioned reasons – ICSI is the preferable insemination method to use with PGT to avoid DNA contaminants that may contribute to the misinterpretation of results.

Popularity of ICSI

Infertility is defined as the inability to achieve pregnancy after 12 months of regular, unprotected sexual intercourse [67]. Indeed, the development of ART is correlated with the increasing awareness of infertility [5].

From 2002 to 2015, the percentage of impaired fecundity rose from 11.8% to 12.1% [68]. However, infertility afflicted approximately 7.4% of couples in 2002, and decreased to 6.7% from 2011 to 2015 [68]. In spite of decreasing infertility in the United States, the total number of ART cycles reported per year is steadily rising [5].

In 2003, the Society for Assisted Reproductive Technology (SART) reported a total of 112,988 annual ART cycles in the United States, which steadily grew to 237,385 cycles by 2016. Moreover, patients are opting for additional methods to enhance their chances of having a successful pregnancy, such as oocyte cryopreservation and PGT. From 2005 to 2013, the number of PGT cycles increased from 4928 to 10,497 per year [5]. Oocyte cryopreservation cycles in the United States rose from 575 cycles in 2009 to 8929 cycles in 2016 [5].

The popularity of ICSI can be attributed to multiple factors, including male factor infertility, patients conceiving at a later age, cancer treatment, and the desire to minimize risk of hereditary or sexually transmitted diseases [69]. The growth in PGT-A utilization may be a result of patients increasingly wanting to know the genetic profile of their embryos and enhance their chances of implantation.

Utilization of ICSI with Emerging Technologies

Stem Cells

Stem cell research in the field of reproductive medicine has made limited but steady advances. The pluripotency of stem cells gives rise to the possibility of reproducing oogenesis and spermatogenesis in patients whose reproductive functions are impaired [70]. The regenerative potential of stem cells is seen as promising, as their use may provide patients who are undergoing cancer therapy and/or have genetic conditions affecting gonadal function with the ability to generate their own gametes.

Scientists have successfully differentiated stem cells into male gametes [71, 72]. There are three methods to replicate spermatogenesis using stem cells to allow them to differentiate into primordial germ cells. The first method is to culture stem cells using induced pluripotent (iPS) cells or embryonic stem cells (ESC) into primordial germ cells (PGC). The second method is to use an individual's own bone marrow cells to repopulate the seminiferous tubules in the testis [73]. The third method is through therapeutic cloning to produce an individual's own genotype embryonic stem cells. This would be done by performing somatic cell nuclear transfer (SCNT) using the patient's somatic cell (e.g., a skin biopsy into an enucleated donor egg). Successful SCNT would then produce a blastocyst from which embryonic stem cells can be isolated and differentiated into pseudo sperm cells in vitro [74].

To emulate a complete in vitro spermatogenetic process from stem cells through PGC into a sperm-like cell, these cells need to be assessed for their function and genomic integrity. The functionality of these stem cell-derived spermatozoa can be tested for fertilization, embryo development, and implantation. Even once these steps are completed, the maturation and concentration of the pseudo sperm cell would be somewhat impaired and would therefore need to be injected into an oocyte by ICSI [75].

Indeed, several studies have used ICSI to prove the developmental competence of the sperm-like cell produced from stem cells to generate healthy offspring [76]. A study in animal models demonstrated the successful production of viable male gametes [72] and female gametes in vitro [77] derived from stem cells. Even the successful generation of these egg-like cells through differentiation of stem cells benefits from ICSI because of the verisimilar development of the ZP and deficient polyspermia-inhibiting mechanisms. This understanding favors the current and distant future of the utilization of ICSI as the optimal insemination method for in vitro gametogenesis (IVG).

Heritable Genome Editing

More than 10,000 monogenic disorders have been identified thus far, and many are dominant mutations in which one copy of a defective gene can lead to serious health consequences. For instance, a single mutation in the BRCA1 or BRCA2 genes can significantly increase the risk of breast, ovarian, and prostate cancers in men and women. PGT can prevent the transmission of genetic diseases to offspring by identifying euploid embryos that are free of mutations, but in some cases, the chance of obtaining a normal embryo is very low, even with multiple IVF attempts. To overcome this, scientists are researching the possibility of editing the genome of embryos, beginning with cases of monogenic disorders. Several approaches have been taken to accomplish this, but the most recent and simplest is with the clustered regularly interspaced short palindromic repeats technique (CRISPR).

In 2005, three different studies demonstrated that certain spacer regions in the bacterial genome contain sequences from bacteriophage DNA [78]. A subsequent study showed that the spacers generate short pieces of RNA that combine with endonucleases encoded in adjacent genes to degrade the DNA of an infecting virus [79]. These findings led to the two-part CRISPR-Cas9 system. A guide RNA (gRNA) containing a target sequence of approximately 20 nucleotides brings the Cas9 endonuclease to the DNA. Then, Cas9 creates a double-stranded break at the specified target site. Microinjection was an obvious choice for a convenient and effective method of delivering CRISPR-Cas9 components into embryos.

Once the DNA is successfully cleaved, the host cell recognizes the DNA as damaged and can repair it using two mechanisms: non-homologous end joining (NHEJ) or homology directed repair (HDR). The NHEJ pathway attempts to rejoin the broken strands but is often imprecise and responsible for frameshift mutations with consequent knockout of gene activity. The HDR mechanism uses another strand of DNA as a template to precisely repair the break via homologous recombination. This can be leveraged for genome editing by providing a donor DNA template to knock-in desired sequences at the break site.

Although heritable genome editing appears to offer a revolutionary solution, it carries several limitations. Mosaicism occurs when only some cells of the embryo gain the desired modifications while others do not. Mosaic embryos are unsuitable for clinical applications and are also difficult to detect with PGT. In a recent experiment correcting for a paternal mutation in the MYBPC3 gene causing hypertrophic cardiomyopathy, researchers proposed injecting the CRISPR-Cas9 solution by ICSI into the oocyte rather than at the zygote or blastocyst stage to reduce the rate of mosaicism, achieving 72.4% (42/58) uniformly corrected embryos [80].

While these results are promising, a more effective option for heritable editing may be to target the genome of gametes before fertilization. This approach would address the issue of mosaicism; additionally, it would be more palatable from a regulatory and ethical standpoint [81]. Our current research is focused on editing the DNA of spermatozoa. We are studying techniques that may allow successful gene editing after direct transfection of CRISPR components into mature spermatozoa. One of these is targeting linker regions, the exposed areas of DNA between histone- and toroid-bound regions. We are also exploring the editing efficiency in sperm DNA that has been remodeled by enucleated oocytes in a mouse model [82], a venture that forays into the field of IVG.

Despite the numerous technical, political, and ethical challenges, scientists are working to find solutions to improve the efficacy of genome editing in human embryos, which will certainly involve ICSI [83].

Conclusions

Based on early attempts to manipulate gametes such as PZD and SUZI, ICSI is indeed the most groundbreaking technique that has been developed to overcome extreme male infertility. ICSI in conjunction with surgical sperm retrieval has allowed men with even the most extreme male factor infertility to father their own children. While most of the clinical indications of ICSI are related to male infertility, the emergence of PGT and other embryo-screening techniques would not be as effective and concise without ICSI as a prerequisite. In addition, ICSI has proven to be the only effective method of fertilizing cryopreserved oocytes, which is helpful to patients who have undergone fertility preservation.

Since the first successful IVF in the 1970s to the early pioneering studies on gamete manipulation in the 1980s, advanced ART techniques have been adopted in the majority of infertility clinics, with ICSI considered the ultimate method to achieve fertilization.

References

[1] Pincus G, Enzmann EV. Can mammalian eggs undergo normal development in vitro? *Proceedings of the National Academy of Sciences of the United States of America* 1934;**20**:121–122.

[2] Menkin MF, Rock J. In vitro fertilization and cleavage of human ovarian eggs. *American Journal of Obstetrics and Gynecology* 1948;**55**:440–452.

[3] Steptoe PC, Edwards RG. Birth after the reimplantation of a human embryo. *Lancet* 1978;**2**: 366.

[4] Palermo G, Van Steirteghem A. Enhancement of acrosome reaction and subzonal insemination of a single spermatozoon in mouse eggs. *Molecular Reproduction and Development* 1991;**30**:339–345.

[5] Society for Assisted Reproductive Technology. *National Summary Report, 2018,* www .sartcorsonline.com/rptCSR_PublicMultYear.aspx.

[6] Steptoe PC, Edwards RG. Reimplantation of a human embryo with subsequent tubal pregnancy. *Lancet* 1976;**307**:880–882.

[7] Cohen J, Edwards R, Fehilly C, Fishel S, Hewitt J, Purdy J, Rowland G, Steptoe P, Webster J. In vitro fertilization: a treatment for male infertility. *Fertility and Sterility* 1985;**43**:422–432.

[8] Cohen J, Malter H, Wright G, Kort H, Massey J, Mitchell D. Partial zona dissection of human oocytes when failure of zona pellucida penetration is anticipated. *Human Reproduction* 1989; **4**:435–442.

[9] Svalander P, Wikland M, Jakobsson A-H, Forsberg A-S. Subzonal insemination (SUZI) or in vitro fertilization (IVF) in microdroplets for the treatment of male-factor infertility. *Journal of Assisted Reproduction and Genetics* 1994;**11**:149–155.

[10] Kiessling AA, Loutradis D, McShane PM, Jackson KV. Fertilization in trypsin-treated oocytes. *Annals of the New York Academy of Sciences* 1988;**541**:614–620.

[11] Gordon JW, Talansky BE. Assisted fertilization by zona drilling: A mouse model for correction of oligospermia. *Journal of Experimental Zoology* 1986;**239**:347–354.

[12] Tucker MJ, Bishop FM, Cohen J, Wiker SR, Wright G. Routine application of partial zona dissection for male factor infertility. *Human Reproduction* 1991;**6**:676–681.

[13] Ng SC, Bongso A, Ratnam SS, Sathananthan H, Chan CL, Wong PC, Hagglund L, Anandakumar C, Wong YC, Goh VH. Pregnancy after transfer of sperm under zona. *Lancet* 1988;**2**:790.

[14] Palermo G, Joris H, Devroey P, Van Steirteghem AC. Pregnancies after intracytoplasmic injection of single spermatozoon into an oocyte. *Lancet* 1992;**340**:17–18.

[15] Palermo G, Rosenwaks Z. Assisted fertilization for male-factor infertility. *Seminars in Reproductive Medicine* 1995;**13**(01):39–52.

[16] Hiramoto Y. An analysis of the mechanism of fertilization by means of enucleation of sea urchin eggs. *Experimental Cell Research* 1962;**28**:323–334.

[17] Hiramoto Y. Microinjection of the live spermatozoa into sea urchin eggs. *Experimental Cell Research* 1962;**27**:416–426.

[18] Uehara T, Yanagimachi R. Activation of hamster eggs by pricking. *Journal of Experimental Zoology* 1977;**199**:269–274.

[19] Uehara T, Yanagimachi R. Behavior of nuclei of testicular, caput and cauda epididymal spermatozoa injected into hamster eggs. *Biology of Reproduction* 1977;**16**:315–321.

[20] Goto K, Kinoshita A, Takuma Y, Ogawa K. Fertilisation of bovine oocytes by the injection of immobilised, killed spermatozoa. *The Veterinary Record* 1990;**127**:517–520.

[21] Iritani A, Utsumi K, Miyake M, Hosoi Y, Saeki K. In vitro fertilization by a routine method and by micromanipulation. *Annals of the New York Academy of Sciences* 1988;**541**:583–590.

[22] Lanzendorf SE, Maloney MK, Veeck LL, Slusser J, Hodgen GD, Rosenwaks Z. A preclinical evaluation of pronuclear formation by microinjection of human spermatozoa into human oocytes. *Fertility and Sterility* 1988;**49**:835–842.

[23] Palermo G, Joris H, Devroey P, Van Steirteghem AC. Induction of acrosome reaction in human spermatozoa used for subzonal insemination. *Human Reproduction* 1992;**7**:248–254.

[24] Lin TP. Microinjection of mouse eggs. *Science* 1966;**151**:333–337.

[25] Pereira N, Cozzubbo T, Cheung S, Palermo GD. Lessons learned in andrology: from intracytoplasmic sperm injection and beyond. *Andrology* 2016;**4**:757–760.

[26] Palermo G, Joris H, Derde MP, Camus M, Devroey P, Van Steirteghem A. Sperm characteristics and outcome of human assisted fertilization by subzonal insemination and intracytoplasmic sperm injection. *Fertility and Sterility* 1993;**59**:826–835.

[27] Palermo GD, Neri QV, Schlegel PN, Rosenwaks Z. Intracytoplasmic sperm injection (ICSI) in extreme cases of male infertility. *PLoS One* 2014;**9**:e113671.

[28] Palermo GD, Neri QV, Rosenwaks Z. To ICSI or not to ICSI. *Seminars in Reproductive Medicine* 2015;**33**:92–102.

[29] Palermo GD, Neri QV, Takeuchi T, Rosenwaks Z. ICSI: where we have been and where we are going. *Seminars in Reproductive Medicine* 2009;**27**:191–201.

[30] Palermo G, Munne S, Cohen J. The human zygote inherits its mitotic potential from the male gamete. *Human Reproduction* 1994;**9**:1220–1225.

[31] Palermo GD, Colombero LT, Schattman GL, Davis OK, Rosenwaks Z. Evolution of pregnancies and initial follow-up of newborns delivered after intracytoplasmic sperm injection. *JAMA* 1996;**276**:1893–1897.

[32] Practice Committees of the American Society for Reproductive Medicine, Society for Assisted Reproductive Technology. Intracytoplasmic sperm injection (ICSI) for non-male factor infertility: a committee opinion. *Fertility and Sterility* 2012;**98**:1395–1399.

[33] Palermo GD, Cohen J, Alikani M, Adler A, Rosenwaks Z. Intracytoplasmic sperm injection: a novel treatment for all forms of male factor infertility. *Fertility and Sterility* 1995;**63**:1231–1240.

[34] Schlegel PN, Cohen J, Goldstein M, Alikani M, Adler A, Gilbert BR, Palermo GD, Rosenwaks Z. Cystic fibrosis gene mutations do not affect sperm function during in vitro fertilization with micromanipulation for men with bilateral congenital absence of vas deferens. *Fertility and Sterility* 1995;**64**:421–426.

[35] Schlegel PN, Palermo GD, Alikani M, Adler A, Reing AM, Cohen J, Rosenwaks Z. Micropuncture retrieval of epididymal sperm with in vitro fertilization: importance of in vitro micromanipulation techniques. *Urology* 1995;**46**:238–241.

[36] Chan PT, Palermo GD, Veeck LL, Rosenwaks Z, Schlegel PN. Testicular sperm extraction combined with intracytoplasmic sperm injection in the treatment of men with persistent azoospermia postchemotherapy. *Cancer* 2001;**92**:1632–1637.

[37] Palermo GD, Schlegel PN, Sills ES, Veeck LL, Zaninovic N, Menendez S, Rosenwaks Z. Births after intracytoplasmic injection of sperm obtained by testicular extraction from men with nonmosaic Klinefelter's syndrome. *The New England Journal of Medicine* 1998;**338**:588–590.

[38] O'Neill CL, Parrella A, Keating D, Cheung S, Rosenwaks Z, Palermo GD. A treatment algorithm for couples with unexplained infertility based on sperm chromatin assessment. *Journal of Assisted Reproduction and Genetics* 2018;**35**:1911–1917.

[39] Xie P, Keating D, Parrella A, Cheung S, Rosenwaks Z, Goldstein M, Palermo GD. Sperm genomic integrity by TUNEL varies throughout the male genital tract. *Journal of Urology* 2020;**203**:802–808.

[40] Yanagida K, Katayose H, Yazawa H, Kimura Y, Sato A, Yanagimachi H, Yanagimachi R. Successful fertilization and pregnancy following ICSI and electrical oocyte activation. *Human Reproduction* 1999;**14**:1307–1311.

[41] Hoshi K, Yanagida K, Sato A. Pretreatment of hamster oocytes with Ca2+ ionophore to facilitate fertilization by ooplasmic micro-injection. *Human Reproduction* 1992;**7**:871–875.

[42] Yanagida K, Morozumi K, Katayose H, Hayashi S, Sato A. Successful pregnancy after ICSI with strontium oocyte activation in low rates of

fertilization. *Reproductive Biomedicine Online* 2006;**13**:801–806.

[43] Tavalaee M, Nomikos M, Lai FA, Nasr-Esfahani MH. Expression of sperm PLCzeta and clinical outcomes of ICSI-AOA in men affected by globozoospermia due to DPY19L2 deletion. *Reproductive Biomedicine Online* 2018;**36**:348–355.

[44] Wolny YM, Fissore RA, Wu H, Reis MM, Colombero LT, Ergun B, Rosenwaks Z, Palermo GD. Human glucosamine-6-phosphate isomerase, a homologue of hamster oscillin, does not appear to be involved in Ca2+ release in mammalian oocytes. *Molecular Reproduction and Development* 1999;**52**:277–287.

[45] Heindryckx B, Van der Elst J, De Sutter P, Dhont M. Treatment option for sperm- or oocyte-related fertilization failure: assisted oocyte activation following diagnostic heterologous ICSI. *Human Reproduction* 2005;**20**:2237–2241.

[46] Bonte D, Ferrer-Buitrago M, Dhaenens L, Popovic M, Thys V, De Croo I, De Gheselle S, Steyaert N, Boel A, Vanden Meerschaut F *et al.* Assisted oocyte activation significantly increases fertilization and pregnancy outcome in patients with low and total failed fertilization after intracytoplasmic sperm injection: a 17-year retrospective study. *Fertility and Sterility* 2019;**112**:266–274.

[47] Gilchrist RB, Lane M, Thompson JG. Oocyte-secreted factors: regulators of cumulus cell function and oocyte quality. *Human Reproduction Update* 2008;**14**:159–177.

[48] Alikani M, Palermo G, Adler A, Bertoil M, Blake M, Cohen J. Intracytoplasmic sperm injection in dysmorphic human oocytes. *Zygote* 1995;**3**:283–288.

[49] Serhal PF, Ranieri DM, Kinis A, Marchant S, Davies M, Khadum IM. Oocyte morphology predicts outcome of intracytoplasmic sperm injection. *Human Reproduction* 1997;**12**:1267–1270.

[50] Xia P. Intracytoplasmic sperm injection: correlation of oocyte grade based on polar body, perivitelline space and cytoplasmic inclusions with fertilization rate and embryo quality. *Human Reproduction* 1997;**12**:1750–1755.

[51] Kahraman S, Yakin K, Donmez E, Samli H, Bahce M, Cengiz G, Sertyel S, Samli M, Imirzalioglu N. Relationship between granular cytoplasm of oocytes and pregnancy outcome following intracytoplasmic sperm injection. *Human Reproduction* 2000;**15**:2390–2393.

[52] Meriano JS, Alexis J, Visram-Zaver S, Cruz M, Casper RF. Tracking of oocyte dysmorphisms for ICSI patients may prove relevant to the outcome in subsequent patient cycles. *Human Reproduction* 2001;**16**:2118–2123.

[53] Yakin K, Balaban B, Isiklar A, Urman B. Oocyte dysmorphism is not associated with aneuploidy in the developing embryo. *Fertility and Sterility* 2007;**88**:811–816.

[54] Swain JE, Pool TB. ART failure: oocyte contributions to unsuccessful fertilization. *Human Reproduction Update* 2008;**14**:431–446.

[55] Eichenlaub-Ritter U, Schmiady H, Kentenich H, Soewarto D. Recurrent failure in polar body formation and premature chromosome condensation in oocytes from a human patient: indicators of asynchrony in nuclear and cytoplasmic maturation. *Human Reproduction* 1995;**10**:2343–2349.

[56] Parrella A, Irani M, Keating D, Chow S, Rosenwaks Z, Palermo GD. High proportion of immature oocytes in a cohort reduces fertilization, embryo development, pregnancy and live birth rates following ICSI. *Reproductive Biomedicine Online* 2019;**39**:580–587.

[57] Kazem R, Thompson LA, Srikantharajah A, Laing MA, Hamilton MP, Templeton A. Cryopreservation of human oocytes and fertilization by two techniques: in-vitro fertilization and intracytoplasmic sperm injection. *Human Reproduction* 1995;**10**:2650–2654.

[58] Walls ML, Ryan JP, Keelan JA, Hart R. In vitro maturation is associated with increased early embryo arrest without impairing morphokinetic development of useable embryos progressing to blastocysts. *Human Reproduction* 2015;**30**:1842–1849.

[59] Hatirnaz S, Ata B, Hatirnaz ES, Dahan MH, Tannus S, Tan J, Tan SL. Oocyte in vitro maturation: A systematic review. *Turkish Journal of Obstetrics and Gynecology* 2018;**15**:112–125.

[60] Shu YM, Zeng HT, Ren Z, Zhuang GL, Liang XY, Shen HW, Yao SZ, Ke PQ, Wang NN. Effects of cilostamide and forskolin on the meiotic resumption and embryonic development of immature human oocytes. *Human Reproduction* 2008;**23**:504–513.

[61] Kirkegaard K, Hindkjaer JJ, Ingerslev HJ. Human embryonic development after blastomere removal: a time-lapse analysis. *Human Reproduction* 2012;**27**:97–105.

[62] Fragouli E. Next generation sequencing for preimplantation genetic testing for aneuploidy: friend or foe? *Fertility and Sterility* 2018;**109**:606–607.

[63] Coates A, Kung A, Mounts E, Hesla J, Bankowski B, Barbieri E, Ata B, Cohen J, Munne S. Optimal

euploid embryo transfer strategy, fresh versus frozen, after preimplantation genetic screening with next generation sequencing: a randomized controlled trial. *Fertility and Sterility* 2017;**107**:723–730.e723.

[64] Forman EJ, Hong KH, Ferry KM, Tao X, Taylor D, Levy B, Treff NR, Scott RT, Jr. In vitro fertilization with single euploid blastocyst transfer: a randomized controlled trial. *Fertility and Sterility* 2013;**100**:100–107.e101.

[65] Palmerola K, Vitez S, Amrane S, Fischer C, Forman E. Minimizing mosaicism: assessing the impact of fertilization method on rate of mosaicism after next-generation sequencing (NGS) preimplantation genetic testing for aneuploidy (PGT-A). *Journal of Assisted Reproduction and Genetics* 2018;**36**.

[66] Jun SH, O'Leary T, Jackson KV, Racowsky C. Benefit of intracytoplasmic sperm injection in patients with a high incidence of triploidy in a prior in vitro fertilization cycle. *Fertility and Sterility* 2006;**86**:825–829.

[67] Zegers-Hochschild F, Adamson GD, de Mouzon J, Ishihara O, Mansour R, Nygren K, Sullivan E, van der Poel S, International Committee for Monitoring Assisted Reproductive Technology, World Health Organization. The International Committee for Monitoring Assisted Reproductive Technology (ICMART) and the World Health Organization (WHO) Revised Glossary on ART Terminology, 2009. *Human reproduction* 2009;**24**:2683–2687.

[68] Centers for Disease Control and Prevention. *Key Statistics from the National Survey of Family Growth*. 20 June 2017, www.cdc.gov/nchs/nsfg/key_statistics/i.htm.

[69] World Health Organization. *WHO Laboratory Manual for the Examination and Processing of Human Semen*. 5th ed., 2010. World Health Organization, Geneva.

[70] Vassena R, Eguizabal C, Heindryckx B, Sermon K, Simon C, van Pelt AM, Veiga A, Zambelli F, ESHRE special interest group Stem Cells. Stem cells in reproductive medicine: ready for the patient? *Human Reproduction* 2015;**30**:2014–2021.

[71] Hayashi K, Ogushi S, Kurimoto K, Shimamoto S, Ohta H, Saitou M. Offspring from oocytes derived from in vitro primordial germ cell-like cells in mice. *Science* 2012;**338**:971–975.

[72] Hayashi K, Ohta H, Kurimoto K, Aramaki S, Saitou M. Reconstitution of the mouse germ cell specification pathway in culture by pluripotent stem cells. *Cell* 2011;**146**:519–532.

[73] Neuhaus N, Schlatt S. Stem cell-based options to preserve male fertility. *Science* 2019;**363**:1283–1284.

[74] Matoba S, Zhang Y. Somatic Cell Nuclear Transfer Reprogramming: Mechanisms and Applications. *Cell Stem Cell* 2018;**23**:471–485.

[75] Pelosi E, Forabosco A, Schlessinger D. Germ cell formation from embryonic stem cells and the use of somatic cell nuclei in oocytes. *Annals of the New York Academy of Sciences* 2011;**1221**:18–26.

[76] Sato T, Katagiri K, Gohbara A, Inoue K, Ogonuki N, Ogura A, Kubota Y, Ogawa T. In vitro production of functional sperm in cultured neonatal mouse testes. *Nature* 2011;**471**:504–507.

[77] Hayashi K, Hikabe O, Obata Y, Hirao Y. Reconstitution of mouse oogenesis in a dish from pluripotent stem cells. *Nature Protocols* 2017;**12**:1733–1744.

[78] Christin JR, Beckert MV. Origins and applications of CRISPR-mediated genome editing. *The Einstein Journal of Biology and Medicine* 2016;**31**:2–5.

[79] Makarova KS, Grishin NV, Shabalina SA, Wolf YI, Koonin EV. A putative RNA-interference-based immune system in prokaryotes: computational analysis of the predicted enzymatic machinery, functional analogies with eukaryotic RNAi, and hypothetical mechanisms of action. *Biology Direct* 2006;**1**:7.

[80] Ma H, Marti-Gutierrez N, Park S-W, Wu J, Lee Y, Suzuki K, Koski A, Ji D, Hayama T, Ahmed R *et al.* Correction of a pathogenic gene mutation in human embryos. *Nature* 2017;**548**:413.

[81] Adashi E, Cohen IG. Heritable genome editing—edited eggs and sperm to the rescue? *JAMA* 2019;**322**:1754–1755.

[82] Wang J, Parrella A, Xie P, Rosenwaks Z, Palermo GD. A step toward gene remodeling of mammalian spermatozoa by CRISPR-Cas9. *Fertility and Sterility* 2019;**112**:e262.

[83] Stein R. *Scientists attempt controversial experiment to edit DNA in human sperm using CRISPR*. Npr.org. 2019. www.npr.org/sections/health-shots/2019/08/22/746321083/scientists-attempt-controversial-experiment-to-edit-dna-in-human-sperm-using-cri.

Current ICSI Applications and Clinical Outcomes

Derek Keating, Stephanie Cheung, Philip Xie, June Wang, Zev Rosenwaks, and Gianpiero D. Palermo

Introduction

Since its inception in 1992, the use of ICSI has become more prevalent as the number of indications for the technique continues to rise [1]. The advantages of ICSI in cases of male factor infertility are well documented; however, the rapid increase in ICSI use has not been counterbalanced by an equal rise in male infertility diagnoses, leading some to question whether ICSI is being misused or even abused [2–4].

The supreme benefit of ICSI is that it enables the insemination of one oocyte with one spermatozoon. This is particularly important for patients with severe oligozoospermia, cryptozoospermia, and azoospermia. In these cases, ICSI is the only treatment option available to the couple once spermatozoa are retrieved from the proximal part of the genital tract, such as the vas deferens, epididymis, or testis.

In this chapter, we will elaborate on the expansion of ICSI as the primary ART option and the clinical outcomes with the use of this sophisticated treatment, at our center in New York City and throughout the world.

ICSI Utilization and Outcome at Weill Cornell Medicine

At Weill Cornell Medicine, 54,864 ART cycles were performed between January 1, 1993, and July 1, 2019. Over the last two decades, the proportion of couples treated by ICSI insemination compared to standard in vitro insemination has risen dramatically. In 1993, the allocation of ICSI was just 32.2% of ART cycles, with 397 cases reported in that year. This allocation rose to 48.8% just 2 years later. By 2002, ICSI accounted for nearly three-quarters of all ART cycles performed at our center at 73.6%, and by then, 12,723 ICSI cycles had been performed. The utilization has continued to increase, with over 95.4% of ART cycles performed at Weill Cornell utilizing ICSI insemination in 2018.

In total, we have performed over 39,500 ICSI cycles in these 26 years, with 90.3% of cases using an ejaculated sperm source and 9.7% using spermatozoa retrieved directly from the male genital tract. To date, we have achieved a cumulative clinical pregnancy rate per embryo transfer of 38.5% with ICSI (12,878/ 33,489), which has led to the birth of 14,418 newborns from 11,069 deliveries.

Ejaculated Spermatozoa

Ejaculated spermatozoa have been utilized in 36,275 ICSI cycles at our center between 1993 and 2019. A total of 309,501 oocytes have been injected in these cases, with 301,237 oocytes surviving the initial injection. Of those that survived, 78.2% fertilized normally with 2-pronuclei (2PN), while 2.5% and 3.5% displayed abnormal fertilization with 1- or 3-pronuclei (1PN, 3PN), respectively. No fertilization was observed in 15.8% of the injected oocytes.

When we consider ICSI cycles that included a fresh embryo transfer, over 29,000 utilized fresh ejaculate, with 61 utilizing electroejaculate, or spermatozoa obtained after electrically stimulating the prostate, and 51 utilizing fresh retrograde ejaculate samples. The fertilization rate for cycles utilizing fresh and frozen ejaculated samples was 186,328/247,627 (75.4%) and 25,500/33,652 (75.8%), respectively. For electroejaculate, fresh samples had a fertilization rate of 470/ 616 (76.3%), while frozen electroejaculate had a rate of 180/262 (68.7%). Lastly, fresh retrograde ejaculate had a fertilization rate of 377/483 (78.1%), while frozen retrograde had a rate of only 27/45 (60.0%). The fertilization results are depicted in Figure 3.1. The resulting clinical pregnancy rate was 11,814/ 29,121 (40.6%) with fresh ejaculate and 1,415/3,880 (36.5%) with frozen ejaculate, a significant decrease from fresh samples (P<0.0001). For electroejaculate, fresh samples yielded a clinical pregnancy rate of 29/ 61 (47.5%), while frozen resulted in a clinical

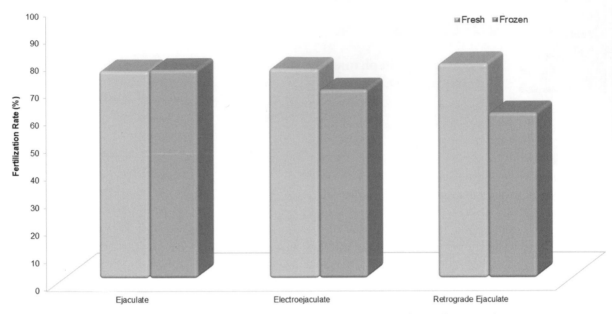

Figure 3.1 Comparison of ICSI fertilization rates with different sperm sources and whether fresh or frozen. Fertilization rates remain comparable throughout the different specimen origins and utilization conditions. (A black and white version of this figure will appear in some formats. For the color version, please refer to the plate section.)

pregnancy rate of 11/26 (42.3%). Fresh retrograde samples had a pregnancy rate of 20/51 (39.2%), and frozen had a pregnancy rate of only 1/8 (12.5%). These clinical pregnancy rates are depicted in Figure 3.2. While fertilization is comparable between fresh and frozen sources, there is a clear statistical advantage for the utilization of a fresh ejaculate as opposed to frozen in terms of clinical pregnancy rate at 40.6% and 36.5%, respectively ($P<0.0001$).

In 2,313 ICSI cycles, the ejaculate sperm concentration was $\leq 1 \times 10^6$/mL, which is defined as severe oligozoospermia. These patients also suffered from an abnormal motility of 19.6% and abnormal morphology of 1.5% normal forms. These patients had lower fertilization than patients without severe oligozoospermia at 62.3%; however, 45.9% (n=1,062) of these cycles led to a clinical pregnancy, defined as the presence of at least one fetal heartbeat.

An additional 364 patients presented with cryptozoospermia, where no spermatozoa were visualized in the initial sample in a Makler chamber, requiring their ejaculates to be centrifuged at 3,000g to be reevaluated. In these cases, there was a final concentration of 0.3×10^6/mL with 32.6±36% motility. These cases

resulted in a fertilization rate of 54.5%, providing a mean of 1.1 embryos replaced per treatment cycle, yielding a satisfactory clinical pregnancy rate of 44.8%.

Surgically Retrieved Spermatozoa

In azoospermic cases, spermatozoa can be surgically extracted from the male genital tract and used for ICSI. In 3,123 cases, spermatozoa were aspirated from the epididymis or retrieved by microdissecting the seminiferous tubules within the testis.

Patients presenting with obstructive azoospermia (OA), with either congenital (congenital bilateral absence of the vas deferens) or acquired (trauma, infection, or prior operations, among other causes) etiology, were treated by microsurgical epididymal sperm aspiration (MESA). A comparison of ICSI outcomes for couples with male partners with either congenital or acquired OA is shown in Table 3.1. To summarize, patients who presented with congenital causes of OA had a more favorable ICSI prognosis than those who had acquired their obstruction.

In terms of fertilization potential, fresh and frozen spermatozoa perform very similarly with a fertilization rate of 71.8% for fresh MESA sperm and 70.9% for frozen MESA specimens. However, we have demonstrated a lower clinical pregnancy rate when using frozen

Table 3.1 Specimen characteristics and ICSI clinical outcome of couples who utilized a MESA specimen in men with obstructive azoospermia, according to either congenital or acquired diagnoses. Congenital causes of azoospermia yield higher fertilization ($P<0.01$) and clinical pregnancy rates ($P<0.001$).

	Congenital	Acquired
Cycles	601	617
Density ($\times 10^6$/mL ± SD)	27.6 ± 45	19.9 ± 26
Motility (M ± SD)	8.2 ± 12	11.2 ± 15
Morphology (M ± SD)	1.2 ± 2	1.0 ± 2
Fertilization (%)	4,389/6,084 (72.1)[*]	3,824/5,470 (69.9)[*]
Clinical pregnancies (%)	317 (52.7)[†]	264 (42.8)[†]

[*] χ^2, 2x2, 1 df, effect of obstructive etiology on fertilization rates, $P<0.01$

[†] χ^2, 2x2, 1 df, effect of obstructive etiology on clinical pregnancy rates, $P<0.001$

epididymal spermatozoa in comparison to fresh (Figure 3.3).

The majority of couples with male factor infertility incapable of producing ejaculated spermatozoa are characterized by non-obstructive azoospermia (NOA). Our reproductive urologists have been able to recover rare spermatozoa directly from the seminiferous tubule using microTESE in 62.1% of cases. We have also performed ICSI in 296 cycles in which the male partner suffers from OA as opposed to NOA. The sample characteristics and performance of these spermatozoa extracted directly from the germinal epithelium in obstructive and non-obstructive cases are presented in Table 3.2. Testicular spermatozoa from couples with OA have higher fertilization ($P<0.00001$) and clinical pregnancy rates ($P<0.05$).

We have also had success with testicular sperm extraction and subsequent ICSI cycles for couples in which the male partner is afflicted with Klinefelter's syndrome. Klinefelter's syndrome is the result of the presence of an extra X chromosome, leading to (47, XXY), and men with non-mosaic Klinefelter's are often azoospermic by early adulthood as a result of spermatogenic arrest. From 1992 to 2019, 328

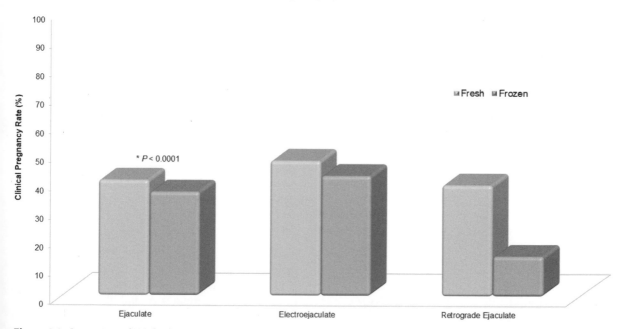

Figure 3.2 Comparison of ICSI fertilization rates with different sperm sources and whether fresh or frozen. Among the three groups, the clinical pregnancy rate appears higher when a fresh specimen is used, reaching significance ($P<0.0001$) in the ejaculated source.

[*]χ^2, 2x2, 1 df, effect of ejaculated sample status on clinical pregnancy rates, $P<0.0001$. (A black and white version of this figure will appear in some formats. For the color version, please refer to the plate section.)

Table 3.2 Sample characteristics and ICSI outcome for couples who utilized TESE specimen in cases of azoospermia, according to either obstructive (OA) or non-obstructive (NOA) diagnoses. The obstructive indications for testicular sperm extraction provided higher fertilization (P<0.00001) and clinical pregnancy rates (P<0.05).

	Obstructive	Non-obstructive
Cycles	296	1,609
Density (× 10^6/mL ± SD)	1.8 ± 7	0.8 ± 7
Motility (M ± SD)	3.3 ± 8	3.0 ± 13
Morphology (M ± SD)	0	0
Fertilization (%)	1,771/2,660 (66.6)[*]	7,984/16,478 (48.5)[*]
Clinical pregnancies (%)	126 (42.6)[†]	578 (35.9)[†]

[*] χ^2, 2x2, 1 df, effect of azoospermic etiology on fertilization rates, P<0.00001

[†] χ^2, 2x2, 1 df, effect of azoospermic etiology on clinical pregnancy rates, P<0.05

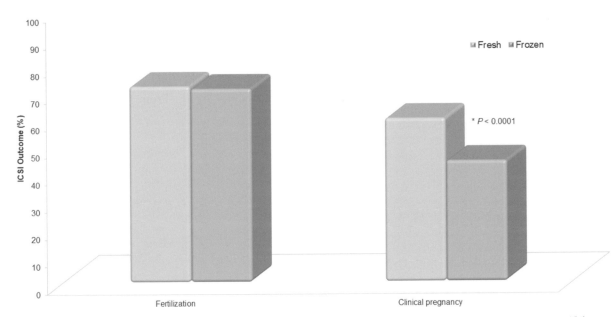

Figure 3.3 Comparison of ICSI fertilization and clinical pregnancy rates when utilizing fresh or frozen epididymal spermatozoa. While fertilization rates remain comparable, the utilization of a freshly retrieved epididymal specimen provides a higher clinical pregnancy rate.

[*]χ^2, 2x2, 1 df, effect of epididymal specimen status on clinical pregnancy rates, P<0.0001. (A black and white version of this figure will appear in some formats. For the color version, please refer to the plate section.)

testicular biopsies have been performed on the male partners of 238 couples, with spermatozoa identified in 206 (62.8%) of these testicular retrievals. This has led to a fertilization rate of 47.8% and a delivery rate of 39.1%, resulting in 49 boys and 44 girls [5].

Similar to spermatozoa retrieved from the epididymis, testicular spermatozoa yielded a similar fertilization rate regardless of whether the sample was fresh or frozen. There was a significantly higher clinical pregnancy rate when a fresh testicular specimen was used for ICSI. A fertilization rate of 49.7% was achieved with fresh testicular spermatozoa, and 48.7% was achieved with cryopreserved specimen. The utilization of fresh testicular spermatozoa led to a 40.2% clinical pregnancy rate, while cycles utilizing frozen specimens led to a clinical pregnancy rate of 35.1% (P<0.04; Figure 3.4).

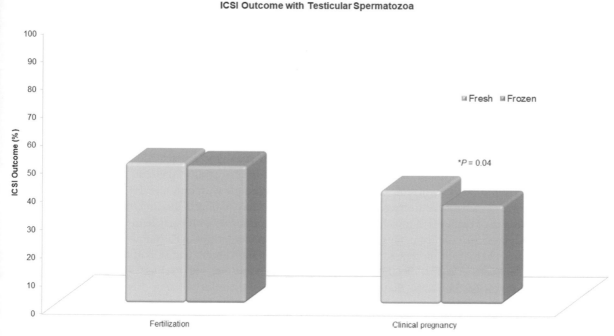

Figure 3.4 Comparison of ICSI fertilization and clinical pregnancy rates when utilizing fresh or frozen testicular spermatozoa. While fertilization rates remain comparable, the utilization of a freshly retrieved epididymal specimen provides a higher clinical pregnancy rate. $^*\chi^2$, 2x2, 1 df, effect of testicular specimen status on clinical pregnancy rates, P=0.04. (A black and white version of this figure will appear in some formats. For the color version, please refer to the plate section.)

Extreme ICSI

In some cases in which spermatozoa are not readily identified even after high-speed centrifugation, an extensive sperm search is required. At our center, we have had 986 ICSI cycles in which the search for injectable male gametes exceeded 30 minutes and lasted as long as 3.75 hours for ejaculated cases and 6.5 hours for cycles using surgically retrieved spermatozoa, and were carried out by as many as eight embryologists. When the extensive searches took more than 3 hours, only a range of 1–3 spermatozoa were able to be found in ejaculated samples, with a range of 0–2 motile. Extensive searches of surgically retrieved samples that lasted over 3 hours had a range of 1–7 spermatozoa identified, with a range of 0–1 motile. Despite this, searches for ejaculated sperm lasting more than 3 hours still yielded a fertilization rate of 40.4% and a clinical pregnancy rate of 25.0%. Similarly, searches lasting more than 3 hours for ICSI cycles utilizing surgically retrieved spermatozoa yielded a fertilization rate of 30.0% and a clinical pregnancy rate of 44.8%. For these cases, it was important to prioritize finding and injecting motile spermatozoa, but this was often not possible, or there were not enough spermatozoa to inject the entire oocyte cohort from a single case. Despite these issues, satisfactory clinical pregnancy rates were achieved. The study highlights the necessity to continue searching for a spermatozoon for injection, even when they are incredibly rare and/or extremely dysmorphic [6, 7].

Impact of Oocyte Cytoplasmic Maturity on ICSI Outcome

It has recently been proposed that cytoplasmic and membrane maturity are important factors to consider when injecting oocytes, which is not as manifest as the presence of a polar body indicating nuclear maturity. It has been observed that extending the in vivo and in vitro maturation times in couples with a history of complete and unexpected fertilization failure has led to proper fertilization. Indeed, patients with a history of complete fertilization failure can benefit by adjusting the in vivo maturation time by tweaking the timing between hCG administration and oocyte retrieval, as well as the in vitro maturation time by modulating the time between retrieval and cumulus removal, and the time between cumulus removal and ICSI, improving the fertilization rate to 77.7% in subsequent cycles [8].

To further evaluate the effect of cytoplasmic maturity, we grouped couples according to the level of the nuclear maturity of the oocytes retrieved. ICSI cycles with a female partner ≥35 years old were allocated according to the proportion of mature oocytes at the time of denudation: optimal (100–76%), adequate (75–51%), partial (50–25%), and minimal (25–1%). The outcomes of the cycles included in these groups were then assessed. Despite no differences in patient demographics, patient stimulation protocol, and semen parameters, there was a remarkable decrease in normal fertilization, availability of embryos to transfer on days 3 and 5, implantation rate, clinical pregnancy rate, and live birth rate as proportional maturity decreased ($P<0.0001$). Conversely, 3PN fertilization rose ($P=0.003$), as well as the proportion of unfertilized oocytes ($P<0.0001$) when the maturity worsened. Moreover, pregnancy loss increased inversely to nuclear maturity ($P=0.0001$). These findings highlight the necessity of not only nuclear but also cytoplasmic maturity to optimize clinical outcome for couples undergoing ART [9].

Microfluidic Sperm Sorting

At our center, we frequently test the male partner for the presence of DNA fragmentation in their ejaculate. DNA fragmentation assays, such as the sperm chromatin structure assay (SCSA), terminal deoxynucleotidyl dUTP transferase nick-end labeling (TUNEL), the comet assay, and the sperm chromatin dispersion (SCD) tests each assess whether the male gamete carries DNA damage, both single and double stranded, which could jeopardize a couple's chances of achieving reproductive success. Indeed, DNA fragmentation has been shown to hinder a couple's ability to conceive naturally [10], with intrauterine insemination [11], and with standard IVF [12]. Sperm DNA integrity has been previously shown to have an inverse correlation with motility [6]. Therefore, we have begun to utilize a commercial microfluidic device (ZyMōt™ Multi device; DxNow, Gaithersburg, Maryland) to allow the most motile spermatozoa to select themselves for ICSI. First, a semen specimen is loaded into an inlet where it enters a chamber separated by a porous filter. Then, during incubation, spermatozoa with the highest progressive motility and putatively superior genomic integrity pass through the chip and are collected after 30 minutes and subsequently utilized for ICSI.

DNA fragmentation of semen samples processed by microfluidics proved to be astonishingly low compared to the raw specimen, and to an aliquot of the same specimen processed by standard density gradient. In our pilot study, the ejaculates of 23 consenting men were screened for their sperm chromatin fragmentation (SCF) levels by TUNEL. The raw specimen presented with 20.7±10% SCF, which fell to 12.5±5% after density gradient selection ($P<0.001$). However, microfluidic sorting of the same raw specimen yielded a final sample with only 1.8±1% SCF ($P<0.0002$) [13].

We have utilized this microfluidic sperm sorting on four couples with persistently elevated SCF in their ejaculate and prior ART failure in conjunction with ICSI at our center. The SCF of the raw specimen was 34.1±9%, which fell to 1.6±0.7% after microfluidics ($P<0.02$). Couples utilizing this novel selection technique for their ICSI cycles after failure with density gradient cycles at our center demonstrated an increase in clinical pregnancy rates from 25.0% (1/4) to 50.0% (2/4) and a rise in implantation rates from 5.2% (1/19) to 25.0% (2/8). Moreover, one pregnancy obtained by density gradient centrifugation was lost, but both clinical pregnancies obtained by ICSI with microfluidics were ongoing or delivered at the time of the study [13].

Encouraged by these findings, 16 couples with elevated SCF in the male partners' ejaculate, ICSI failure with density gradient selection performed elsewhere, and a history of no euploid embryos underwent microfluidic sperm sorting with ICSI at our center. The SCF in the male partners' sample again showed a remarkable decrease, from 29.9±9% in the raw to 1.2±0.4% in the microfluidic-sorted samples. These couples had embryo euploidy rates that rose from 0% (0/12) after density gradient to 51% (19/37; $P<0.001$) after microfluidics. Furthermore, couples who underwent fresh embryo transfer achieved higher clinical pregnancy rates (0/7 vs. 6/12, $P<0.05$). Couples who underwent preimplantation genetic testing for aneuploidy prior to transfer achieved a remarkable implantation rate of 80% that remained at that level to the delivery (4/5; $P=0.01$); all had a more successful outcome compared with prior cycles. Microfluidic sperm sorting can enhance sperm genomic integrity, leading to improved clinical outcomes in couples unable to conceive because of subtle male factor infertility [13].

Assisted Oocyte Activation

The implementation of ICSI has been able to greatly alleviate male factor infertility by attenuating defects of the zona pellucida and sperm acrosomal dysfunction, making it a valuable technique for a variety of infertility indications. However, rare cases of total fertilization failure after ICSI can still occur when the spermatozoa partially or completely lack the specific oocyte activating factor [14].

The process of oocyte activation begins when a sperm protein, phospholipase C zeta (PLCζ), is delivered into the oocyte during sperm–egg fusion. At this time, cytosolic Ca^{2+} oscillations characterized by a series of distinct Ca^{2+} spikes take place within the oocyte and are required to resume meiosis, eventually leading to successful fertilization [15,16]. Furthermore, the oocyte must have a receptive mature cytoplasm to generate the correct Ca^{2+} oscillation patterns. When this prerequisite fails, assisted oocyte activation (AOA) can be used to artificially trigger the release of intracellular $Ca^{?+}$ to induce oocyte activation by the generation of calcium spikes within the oocyte [17].

Although it has been generally accepted that AOA would be beneficial for cases with a confirmed sperm-related oocyte activation deficiency [17], there is currently no clinical consensus on the optimal protocol. AOA has been carried out by exposing post-injection oocytes to an electrical pulse or a chemical agent such as strontium chloride or calcium ionophore. While earlier studies have suggested that electrical pulses successfully induce oocyte activation and improve fertilization rates following ICSI, activation using chemical agents has become increasingly popular in recent years [18,19]. A study comparing the effectiveness of ionomycin and calcimycin in AOA treatment cycles confirmed that higher fertilization rates in both mouse and human oocytes resulted from the use of ionomycin rather than calcimycin [20]. Another study comparing strontium chloride to ionomycin for the AOA of ICSI-inseminated oocytes concluded that while strontium chloride appeared to support better embryo development, ionomycin provided more consistent results in achieving oocyte activation [19].

At our center, we used AOA with calcium ionophore for 12 couples with a maternal age of 38.1 ± 3 years and a paternal age of 42.6 ± 5 years. Ejaculated spermatozoa were assessed by semen analysis, which yielded an average concentration of 57.8 ± 27×10^6/mL, 42.1 ± 17% motility, and an overall normal morphology of 1.1 ± 0.5% with >90% head defects. Prior to undergoing cycles with AOA treatment, these couples underwent a total of 13 ICSI cycles, resulting in a slim fertilization rate of 16.4% (18/110). Moreover, no couples received the replacement of a conceptus because of poor embryo development. All couples subsequently underwent a total of 24 ICSI cycles with AOA by exposing post-ICSI oocytes to calcium ionophore. These cycles resulted in a 46.0% (80/174) fertilization rate ($P<0.00001$) and a 21.1% (4/19) clinical pregnancy rate.

This procedure is now widespread. Indeed, an extensive multicenter study including data from IVF centers in Austria and Germany confirmed that 79 ICSI cycles with AOA treatment yielded significantly higher fertilization and clinical pregnancy rates than 88 ICSI cycles performed without the activating factor [21]. Regardless of the protocol used, the AOA procedure alters the physiological process of fertilization. This, as expected, has raised concerns regarding the procedure's safety. A similar prospective study of 57 couples revealed that, in comparison to their historical control ICSI cycles without AOA, subsequent cycles with AOA led to significantly improved cleavage, blastocyst formation, clinical pregnancy rates, and live birth rates. Reassuringly, all children born from these cycles were healthy [22]. This has been decisive in the compilation of a recent study assessing the health of children born from AOA ICSI cycles. Couples participating in this prospective follow-up study underwent a total of 237 AOA ICSI cycles that resulted in the birth of 31 singletons and 16 twin children. When these children were 2–3 months old, parents completed standardized questionnaires focusing on the health of the offspring. Additionally, pediatricians performed clinical examinations of the children. Only three children from the twin group were diagnosed with major malformations. Minor malformations were detected in seven singletons and one twin. Overall, birth characteristics and congenital malformations were within the expected range [23]. This multicenter observation indicates that, in addition to providing higher fertilization rates, AOA appears to be a safe and reliable treatment for couples with a history of failed fertilization with ART.

Assessing the Safety of ICSI

Despite the standardization of ICSI and the large number of babies born worldwide from this procedure, there are still concerns about its safety. These concerns primarily stem from the perception that as the injected spermatozoa are selected arbitrarily, the physiological steps of zona pellucida binding and oolemma fusion are completely bypassed [24]. Therefore, there is uncertainty about whether the use of suboptimal spermatozoa may transmit undesirable genetic traits and contribute to offspring abnormalities [24]. For instance, high sperm aneuploidy in infertile men with secretory azoospermia is expected to cause a higher frequency of gonosomal abnormalities in male offspring, because of possible meiotic defects that arise during the male germ line maturation [25]. An in-house genetic assessment of 5-year-olds revealed a 3.6% incidence of gonosomal abnormalities in ICSI children compared to 0.15% incidence in children who were naturally conceived. In addition, it appears that a deletion in the AZF region of the Y-chromosome as well as a compromised ability to produce spermatozoa can be found in male ICSI offspring [26,27].

Concerns regarding the safety of ICSI are not limited to the inheritance of specific fertility-related traits; they also include the development and postnatal well-being of ICSI offspring. Early studies on ICSI children have concluded that the rate of malformation from ICSI is no higher than that of naturally conceived offspring reported in New York State. In addition, a study of 14,211 ART children revealed that ICSI and standard IVF malformation rates were comparable [7]. Furthermore, while several studies on children born through ART demonstrated an increased rate of neonatal malformations and imprinting errors, they did not link these cases to the ICSI procedure itself [7]. It has also been observed by the CDC that children born by ART have a higher incidence of younger gestational age and lower birthweight [28]. These findings led to our study on the birth of ICSI-conceived children, which demonstrated that singleton neonates resulting from multiple embryo implantation retained the weight of offspring born from multiple gestations of the same order that progressed to term [29]. Studies on the perinatal outcomes and congenital malformations of ICSI offspring also found that preterm birth and low birthweight were related to multifetal gestation, and that perinatal outcomes of ICSI newborns were like those of newborns conceived via standard IVF. This finding was corroborated by several studies carried out in Denmark, Norway, Israel, and the Netherlands [24].

More recent studies on the reproductive health of young ICSI adults have been carried out assessing male and female offspring independently, compared to a naturally conceived cohort. A comparison of 54 men conceived via ICSI to 57 naturally conceived found that the mean levels of follicle-stimulating hormone (FSH), luteinizing hormone (LH), testosterone, and inhibin B were similar for both groups even after controlling for BMI and age [30]. However, by comparing semen parameters, they found that ICSI-conceived men had lower median sperm concentrations (17.7 vs. 37.0 million/mL), total sperm counts (31.9 vs. 86.8 million/mL), and total motile sperm counts (12.7 vs. 38.6 million) than their naturally conceived peers within the same age range [31]. Similarly, a follow-up study on 18- to 22-year-old women conceived from ICSI demonstrated a comparable hormonal profile to that of their naturally conceived peers [32]. Although reassuring, these are preliminary findings that remain to be confirmed by further multicenter studies.

With ICSI widely considered the most effective treatment option for male factor infertility, even enabling azoospermic men to father their own child, questions have also been raised about the use of surgically retrieved spermatozoa with ICSI. These qualms are related to the possibility of transmitting to offspring genetic defects related to male factor infertility. Additionally, the incidence of aneuploidy and Y chromosomal defects appears to have an inverse correlation with sperm concentration [33,34]. As it is important to obtain a chromosomally healthy embryo, assessment of the male gamete genome should be carried out. This is particularly useful in couples with implantation failure despite a young female partner and therefore at a low risk for oocyte aneuploidy. In azoospermic men, who are known to have a higher incidence of constitutional karyotypic abnormality [34], a higher incidence of testicular sperm aneuploidy has been suggested because of their impaired spermatogenesis [35]. The notion of testicular spermatozoa having higher aneuploidy is supported by a limited number of studies that compare ejaculated and surgical sperm aneuploidy, assessed by the fluorescence in situ hybridization (FISH) technique (Figure 3.5). One of the earliest of these reports, carried out on 34 men, claimed that testicular spermatozoa present a chromosomal aneuploidy as high as 19.6% compared to 13% in ejaculated spermatozoa [36]. This study was performed on 153 to 1,751 sperm cells, and used only three fluorescent probes for

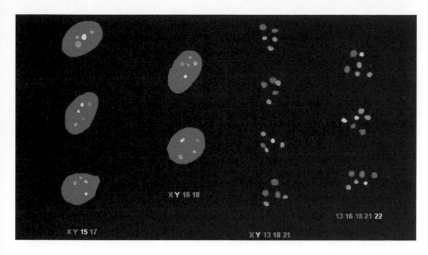

Figure 3.5 Fluorescent in situ hybridization assay depicting ploidy of spermatozoa. (A black and white version of this figure will appear in some formats. For the color version, please refer to the plate section.)

chromosomes X, Y, and 18. Another study, utilizing four chromosome probes, assessed 98 to 1,796 sperm cells from 27 men and revealed an incidence of 11.4% testicular sperm aneuploidy compared to 2.2% in the ejaculated spermatozoa [37]. A similar study carried out later by Rodrigo et al. concluded that testicular sperm aneuploidy was 8.8% compared to 0.5% aneuploidy in ejaculated spermatozoa [38]. This study included 35 men and assessed 480 to 638 sperm cells using five chromosome probes. More recently, Vozdova et al. conducted a study on 17 patients in whom eight chromosomes on at least 500 spermatozoa were screened, indicating a 4.9% incidence of aneuploidy in testicular spermatozoa compared to 0.9% in the ejaculated specimen [39]. Although a greater number of fluorescent probes were implemented compared to previous studies, the difference in aneuploidy between testicular and ejaculated spermatozoa did not reach statistical significance.

In spite of these findings, the reported higher prevalence of testicular sperm aneuploidy has not translated to higher incidences of pregnancy loss or aneuploid conceptuses. Moreover, ICSI offspring generated from surgically retrieved gametes also did not suffer from higher karyotypic aneuploidy than children generated from ejaculated specimens. The overall rate of congenital malformations was 2.6% in offspring generated from ejaculated spermatozoa, while for those conceived from testicular spermatozoa, it was 2.0% [40,41]. Furthermore, children born by surgically retrieved spermatozoa did not appear to demonstrate any concerning outcomes related to

psychological, motorial, or overall developmental characteristics [6].

These findings have led us to reassess aneuploidy in spermatozoa retrieved directly from the germinal epithelium, with the use of FISH followed by a confirmatory NGS assessment [42]. In this reassessment, 9-chromosome FISH was performed on at least 1,000 sperm cells per specimen for 87 ejaculated, two epididymal, and four testicular specimens, as well as a donor control. FISH revealed an overall sperm aneuploidy of 3.6% in the ejaculated specimen, 1.2% for the epididymal, and 1.1% in the testicular specimens compared to 0.9% in the donor control. In this cohort, cycles using ejaculated spermatozoa yielded a 22% clinical pregnancy rate that resulted in 62.5% miscarriages, while the cycles using surgical specimens yielded a 50% clinical pregnancy rate, all progressing to term. A subsequent copy number variant (CNV) assessment was carried out by NGS on 16 ejaculated, two epididymal, and four testicular specimens, as well as a donor control. This assessment yielded 11.1% aneuploidy in the ejaculated spermatozoa, while the epididymal and testicular groups had 1.8% and 1.5% sperm aneuploidy, respectively ($P<0.0001$). Cycles using ejaculated spermatozoa in this cohort yielded a pregnancy rate of 47.2% with 29.2% pregnancy loss, while the surgically retrieved group yielded a 50% clinical pregnancy rate, all progressing to term. Finally, an additional prospective analysis using FISH and NGS was performed for three men who had normal spermatogenesis but underwent testicular biopsies because of high DNA fragmentation in their ejaculated specimens. This assessment revealed 2.8%

FISH aneuploidy in the ejaculated spermatozoa compared to 1.2% aneuploidy for the testicular specimens. These findings were corroborated by an NGS assessment that yielded 8.4% ejaculated sperm aneuploidy compared to 1.3% aneuploidy in the testicular specimens (P=0.02). These men and their partners underwent ICSI cycles utilizing ejaculated spermatozoa, which did not yield any clinical pregnancies. These couples then underwent ICSI with testicular spermatozoa that resulted in a 100% clinical pregnancy rate, all to term, suggesting that the use of surgically retrieved spermatozoa in combination with ICSI is an effective and safe method of treatment for severe male factor infertility [42].

In summary, no significant long-term developmental differences have been found in connection with ICSI, although further follow-up on ICSI adults should be carried out to evaluate the reproductive capacity of these individuals. The most prevalent factor that can lead to adverse postnatal outcomes in children conceived by ART is that of high order gestation [7], which is a common occurrence in assisted reproduction. However, the adoption of single embryo transfer has considerably reduced this issue. In addition, recent preliminary findings have shown that ICSI offspring generated from surgically retrieved spermatozoa do not show a higher autosomal or gonosomal aneuploidy than children resulting from ejaculated spermatozoa, indicating that it is safe to use testicular spermatozoa for ICSI, at least in terms of their chromosomal content.

Global ICSI Results

Throughout the world, ICSI is frequently utilized because of its versatility and abundance of indications. The most recent report on ART data worldwide provided by the International Committee for Monitoring Assisted Reproductive Technology, compiling data from 2,560 clinics located in 65 countries for the year 2011, has found that ICSI was utilized in 66.5% of non-donor cycles, a slight decline from 67.4% in 2010. This study reported a 50.2% ICSI utilization rate in Asia, 68.9% in Europe, 85.5% in Latin America, 96.6% in the Middle East, 73.2% in North America, and 68.8% in the sub-Saharan Africa region. This utilization of ICSI has led to a reported 26.2% pregnancy rate and a 19.0% delivery rate compared to conventional in vitro insemination with reported pregnancy and delivery rates of 24.0% and 17.6%, respectively [2].

A 2018 study on ICSI in the United States, focusing on 10 distinct regions, found ICSI use rising from 39.2±3.8% to 42.5±2.5% ($P<0.001$), and live birth rate per cycle increasing from 34.3±3.6% to 37.0±2.6% (P=0.001). Moreover, the study found that this steady increase in ICSI utilization correlated with a twofold increase in couples presenting with male factor infertility, as a result of, as observed by the authors, the incorporation of the Kruger strict sperm morphology into the most recent WHO manual released in 2010 [4].

Europe has also seen a higher utilization of ICSI, although not quite to the level reported in the United States. In a study done by the European IVF-Monitoring Consortium (EIM) that considered 5,919,320 ART cycles performed between 1997 and 2011, there was a yearly increase in the proportion of ICSI used for 12 consecutive years beginning in 1997, although this proportion of ICSI compared to standard in vitro insemination stabilized beginning in 2008 at just below 70%. The authors of this study found that because of incomplete data, they were not able to accurately assess the per-cycle clinical pregnancy and delivery rates. Moreover, the data they were able to analyze indicated an annual pregnancy rate per embryo transfer that rose from just above 25% in 1999 to over 30% in 2011 [43]. The more recent study by the EIM focused on the year 2014 and reported that 362,285 ICSI cycles were performed in 1,279 institutions across 39 countries, with Italy, Germany, and Spain each performing over 40,000 ICSI cycles. In terms of fresh treatments, ICSI accounted for 71.3% of those reported. Across Europe, the per-transfer pregnancy rate was 32.9%, higher than the 27.8% achieved in 2013. This led to a delivery rate of 25.5% per embryo transfer in the continent [3].

Conclusions

The inception of ICSI has allowed couples with seemingly no chance at starting their own family the possibility of realizing that goal. Despite the changing landscape of reproductive medicine, ICSI has been able to endure because of its extreme versatility; in fact, it continues to be the most widely used ART technique worldwide [2,7].

An expanding focus on the function and role of the male gamete in the reproduction process has led to the development of many new assays to complement routine semen analysis, including assays for measuring sperm DNA fragmentation, aneuploidy, and centrosome assessment to measure the ability of the spermatozoa to generate a proper mitotic spindle and propel proper embryonic cleavage [6]. The pressing need to enhance pregnancy outcome has rendered more popular the utilization of PGT-A, carried out by DNA sequencing technology. This has contributed to favoring the utilization of ICSI combined with cryopreservation of the conceptus [7].

Because of the success achieved by ART worldwide, the expectation of the infertile population is that reproductive medicine practitioners will be able to overcome situations of spermatogenic arrest, germ cell aplasia, or exhaustion of ovarian reserve. Researchers are intently focusing on ways to create spermatozoa through in vitro spermatogenesis, and coaxing stem cell differentiation to generate neogametogenesis in men who lack spermatogenic ability [44,45]. Research is also being conducted on the utilization of pluripotent stem cells or organ culture systems to replicate oogenesis, which has been achieved in vitro in mouse models [44].

The quest to find the best spermatozoon for injection will be ever present, thus guaranteeing that the utilization of ICSI will continue to grow.

References

[1] Hamberger L, Lundin K, Sjogren A, Soderlund B. Indications for intracytoplasmic sperm injection. *Human Reproduction* 1998;**13** Suppl 1: 128–133.

[2] Adamson GD, de Mouzon J, Chambers GM, Zegers-Hochschild F, Mansour R, Ishihara O, Banker M, Dyer S. International Committee for Monitoring Assisted Reproductive Technology: world report on assisted reproductive technology, 2011. *Fertility and sterility* 2018;**110**:1067–1080.

[3] De Geyter C, Calhaz-Jorge C, Kupka MS, Wyns C, Mocanu E, Motrenko T, Scaravelli G, Smeenk J, Vidakovic S, Goossens V *et al*. ART in Europe, 2014: results generated from European registries by ESHRE: The European IVF-monitoring Consortium (EIM) for the European Society of Human Reproduction and Embryology (ESHRE). *Human Reproduction* 2018;**33**:1586–1601.

[4] Zagadailov P, Hsu A, Stern JE, Seifer DB. Temporal differences in utilization of intracytoplasmic sperm injection among U.S. regions. *Obstetrics and Gynecology* 2018;**132**:310–320.

[5] Palermo GD, Schlegel PN, Sills ES, Veeck LL, Zaninovic N, Menendez S, Rosenwaks Z. Births after intracytoplasmic injection of sperm obtained by testicular extraction from men with nonmosaic Klinefelter's syndrome. *The New England Journal of Medicine* 1998;**338**:588–590.

[6] Palermo GD, Neri QV, Schlegel PN, Rosenwaks Z. Intracytoplasmic sperm injection (ICSI) in extreme cases of male infertility. *PLoS One* 2014;**9**:e113671.

[7] Palermo GD, O'Neill CL, Chow S, Cheung S, Parrella A, Pereira N, Rosenwaks Z. Intracytoplasmic sperm injection: state of the art in humans. *Reproduction* 2017;**154**:F93–F110.

[8] Pereira N, Neri QV, Lekovich JP, Palermo GD, Rosenwaks Z. The role of in-vivo and in-vitro maturation time on ooplasmic dysmaturity. *Reproductive Biomedicine Online* 2016; **32**:401–406.

[9] Parrella A, Irani M, Keating D, Chow S, Rosenwaks Z, Palermo GD. High proportion of immature oocytes in a cohort reduces fertilization, embryo development, pregnancy and live birth rates following ICSI. *Reproductive Biomedicine Online* 2019;**39**:580–587.

[10] Oleszczuk K, Augustinsson L, Bayat N, Giwercman A, Bungum M. Prevalence of high DNA fragmentation index in male partners of unexplained infertile couples. *Andrology* 2013;**1**:357–360.

[11] Bungum M, Humaidan P, Spano M, Jepson K, Bungum L, Giwercman A. The predictive value of sperm chromatin structure assay (SCSA) parameters for the outcome of intrauterine insemination, IVF and ICSI. *Human Reproduction* 2004;**19**:1401–1408.

[12] Frydman N, Prisant N, Hesters L, Frydman R, Tachdjian G, Cohen-Bacrie P, Fanchin R. Adequate ovarian follicular status does not prevent the decrease in pregnancy rates associated with high sperm DNA fragmentation. *Fertility and Sterility* 2008;**89**:92–97.

[13] Parrella A, Keating D, Cheung S, Xie P, Stewart JD, Rosenwaks Z, Palermo GD. A treatment approach for couples with disrupted sperm DNA integrity and recurrent ART failure. *Journal of Assisted Reproduction and Genetics* 2019;**36**: 2057–2066.

[14] Neri QV, Lee B, Rosenwaks Z, Machaca K, Palermo GD. Understanding fertilization through intracytoplasmic sperm injection (ICSI). *Cell Calcium* 2014;**55**:24–37.

[15] Tavalaee M, Nomikos M, Lai FA, Nasr-Esfahani MH. Expression of sperm PLCzeta and clinical outcomes of ICSI-AOA in men affected by globozoospermia due to DPY19L2 deletion. *Reproductive Biomedicine Online* 2018;**36**: 348–355.

[16] Wolny YM, Fissore RA, Wu H, Reis MM, Colombero LT, Ergun B, Rosenwaks Z, Palermo GD.

Human glucosamine-6-phosphate isomerase, a homologue of hamster oscillin, does not appear to be involved in Ca2+ release in mammalian oocytes. *Molecular Reproduction and Development* 1999;**52**:277–287.

[17] Bonte D, Ferrer-Buitrago M, Dhaenens L, Popovic M, Thys V, De Croo I, De Gheselle S, Steyaert N, Boel A, Vanden Meerschaut F *et al.* Assisted oocyte activation significantly increases fertilization and pregnancy outcome in patients with low and total failed fertilization after intracytoplasmic sperm injection: a 17-year retrospective study. *Fertility and Sterility* 2019;**112**:266–274.

[18] Mansour R, Fahmy I, Tawab NA, Kamal A, El-Demery Y, Aboulghar M, Serour G. Electrical activation of oocytes after intracytoplasmic sperm injection: a controlled randomized study. *Fertility and Sterility* 2009;**91**:133–139.

[19] Norozi-Hafshejani M, Tavalaee M, Azadi L, Bahadorani M, Nasr-Esfahani MH. Effects of assisted oocyte activation with calcium-ionophore and strontium chloride on in vitro ICSI outcomes. *Iran Journal of Basic Medical Sciences* 2018;**21**:1109–1117.

[20] Nikiforaki D, Vanden Meerschaut F, de Roo C, Lu Y, Ferrer-Buitrago M, de Sutter P, Heindryckx B. Effect of two assisted oocyte activation protocols used to overcome fertilization failure on the activation potential and calcium releasing pattern. *Fertility and Sterility* 2016;**105**:798–806 e792.

[21] Ebner T, Koster M, Shebl O, Moser M, Van der Ven H, Tews G, Montag M. Application of a ready-to-use calcium ionophore increases rates of fertilization and pregnancy in severe male factor infertility. *Fertility and Sterility* 2012;**98**: 1432–1437.

[22] Ebner T, Oppelt P, Wober M, Staples P, Mayer RB, Sonnleitner U, Bulfon-Vogl S, Gruber I, Haid AE, Shebl O. Treatment with Ca2+ ionophore improves embryo development and outcome in cases with previous developmental problems: a prospective multicenter study. *Human Reproduction* 2015;**30**:97–102.

[23] Mateizel I, Verheyen G, Van de Velde H, Tournaye H, Belva F. Obstetric and neonatal outcome following ICSI with assisted oocyte activation by calcium ionophore treatment. *Journal of Assisted Reproduction and Genetics* 2018;**35**:1005–1010.

[24] Pereira N, O'Neill C, Lu V, Rosenwaks Z, Palermo GD. The safety of intracytoplasmic sperm injection and long-term outcomes. *Reproduction* 2017;**154**:F61-f70.

[25] Ferguson KA, Wong EC, Chow V, Nigro M, Ma S. Abnormal meiotic recombination in infertile men and its association with sperm aneuploidy. *Human Molecular Genetics* 2007;**16**:2870–2879.

[26] Katagiri Y, Neri QV, Takeuchi T, Schlegel PN, Megid WA, Kent-First M, Rosenwaks Z, Palermo GD. Y chromosome assessment and its implications for the development of ICSI children. *Reproductive Biomedicine Online* 2004;**8**:307–318.

[27] Kent-First MG, Kol S, Muallem A, Blazer S, Itskovitz-Eldor J. Infertility in intracytoplasmic-sperm-injection-derived sons. *Lancet* 1996;**348**:332.

[28] Schieve LA, Meikle SF, Ferre C, Peterson HB, Jeng G, Wilcox LS. Low and very low birth weight in infants conceived with use of assisted reproductive technology. *The New England Journal of Medicine* 2002;**346**:731–737.

[29] Pereira N, Cozzubbo T, Cheung S, Rosenwaks Z, Palermo GD, Neri QV. Identifying maternal constraints on fetal growth and subsequent perinatal outcomes using a multiple embryo implantation model. *PLoS One* 2016;**11**:e0166222.

[30] Belva F, Roelants M, De Schepper J, Van Steirteghem A, Tournaye H, Bonduelle M. Reproductive hormones of ICSI-conceived young adult men: the first results. *Human Reproduction* 2017;**32**:439–446.

[31] Belva F, Bonduelle M, Roelants M, Michielsen D, Van Steirteghem A, Verheyen G, Tournaye H. Semen quality of young adult ICSI offspring: the first results. *Human Reproduction* 2016;**31**:2811–2820.

[32] Belva F, Roelants M, Vloeberghs V, Schiettecatte J, Evenepoel J, Bonduelle M, de Vos M. Serum reproductive hormone levels and ultrasound findings in female offspring after intracytoplasmic sperm injection: first results. *Fertility and Sterility* 2017;**107**:934–939.

[33] Hopps CV, Mielnik A, Goldstein M, Palermo GD, Rosenwaks Z, Schlegel PN. Detection of sperm in men with Y chromosome microdeletions of the AZFa, AZFb and AZFc regions. *Human Reproduction* 2003;**18**:1660–1665.

[34] Nakamura Y, Kitamura M, Nishimura K, Koga M, Kondoh N, Takeyama M, Matsumiya K, Okuyama A. Chromosomal variants among 1790 infertile men. *International Journal of Urology* 2001;**8**:49–52.

[35] Oppedisano L, Haines G, Hrabchak C, Fimia G, Elliott R, Sassone-Corsi P, Varmuza S. The rate of aneuploidy is altered in spermatids from infertile mice. *Human Reproduction* 2002;**17**:710–717.

[36] Levron J, Aviram-Goldring A, Madgar I, Raviv G, Barkai G, Dor J. Sperm chromosome abnormalities in men with severe male factor infertility who are undergoing in vitro fertilization with intracytoplasmic sperm injection. *Fertility and Sterility* 2001;**76**:479–484.

[37] Palermo GD, Colombero LT, Hariprashad JJ, Schlegel PN, Rosenwaks Z. Chromosome analysis of epididymal and testicular sperm in azoospermic patients undergoing ICSI. *Human Reproduction* 2002;**17**:570–575.

[38] Rodrigo L, Rubio C, Peinado V, Villamon R, Al-Asmar N, Remohi J, Pellicer A, Simon C, Gil-Salom M. Testicular sperm from patients with obstructive and nonobstructive azoospermia: aneuploidy risk and reproductive prognosis using testicular sperm from fertile donors as control samples. *Fertility and Sterility* 2011;**95**:1005–1012.

[39] Vozdova M, Heracek J, Sobotka V, Rubes J. Testicular sperm aneuploidy in non-obstructive azoospermic patients. *Human Reproduction* 2012;**27**:2233–2239.

[40] Bonduelle M, Wilikens A, Buysse A, Van Assche E, Devroey P, Van Steirteghem AC, Liebaers I. A follow-up study of children born after intracytoplasmic sperm injection (ICSI) with epididymal and testicular spermatozoa and after replacement of cryopreserved embryos obtained after ICSI. *Human Reproduction* 1998;**13** Suppl1: 196–207.

[41] Halliday J. Outcomes for offspring of men having ICSI for male factor infertility. *Asian Journal of Andrology* 2012;**14**:116–120.

[42] Cheung S, Schlegel PN, Rosenwaks Z, Palermo GD. Revisiting aneuploidy profile of surgically retrieved spermatozoa by whole exome sequencing molecular karyotype. *PLoS One* 2019;**14**: e0210079.

[43] Ferraretti AP, Nygren K, Andersen AN, de Mouzon J, Kupka M, Calhaz-Jorge C, Wyns C, Gianaroli L, Goossens V, European IVF-Monitoring Consortium. Trends over 15 years in ART in Europe: an analysis of 6 million cycles. *Human Reproduction Open* 2017;2017:hox012.

[44] Hayashi M, Kawaguchi T, Durcova-Hills G, Imai H. Generation of germ cells from pluripotent stem cells in mammals. *Reproductive Medicine and Biology* 2018;**17**:107–114.

[45] Sosa E, Chen D, Rojas EJ, Hennebold JD, Peters KA, Wu Z, Lam TN, Mitchell JM, Sukhwani M, Tailor RC *et al.* Differentiation of primate primordial germ cell-like cells following transplantation into the adult gonadal niche. *Nature Communications* 2018;**9**:5339.

Chapter 4

Rescue ICSI of IVF Failed-Fertilized Oocytes

Carly Barber, Vivian Kimble, Alexandrea Ramsey, and Zsolt Peter Nagy

Introduction

Over time, assisted reproductive technology (ART) has quickly became the hope and "magic" to treat infertility [1]. Before intracytoplasmic sperm injection (ICSI [2]), conventional insemination was (and still is in many parts of the world) the method of inseminating oocytes. When semen parameters fall under what is considered "normal values," including concentration, motility and morphology, studies have shown that using conventional IVF leads to fertilization rates of 60–70%; however, unexpected low or total fertilization failure (TFF) can happen occasionally [3,4].

Total failure of fertilization in an ART cycle can cause additional stress for a couple, adding to the financial and emotional burden that infertility patients endure [5]. The percentage of patients that experience TFF varies between different clinics and has been reported to be as low as 3.5% to as high as 15–20% [6]. With knowledge on TFF, potentially poor semen parameters or repetitive experiences of low fertilization rates, embryologists have tested and brought into play rescue intracytoplasmic sperm injection (RICSI); the re-insemination of oocytes with ICSI after total or near TFF from conventional IVF.

The introduction of RICSI came with the new discovery and practice of ICSI. Prior to ICSI/RICSI, 1-day-old unfertilized oocytes were re-inseminated with conventional IVF. Embryologists eventually discovered that RICSI had a higher success rate and could better help patients overcome TFF [7]. To determine which oocytes are a candidate for RICSI, all of the cumulus and corona cells are removed so the oocytes can be examined carefully for evidence of fertilization and to check the morphology of oocytes, because only unfertilized mature oocytes should be re-inseminated [8]. In its early days, RICSI was performed on 1-day-old oocytes that did not fertilize; now, fertilization checks are typically performed at earlier stages. Depending on how and when fertilization is observed: early, late or via a polarization microscope, allows RICSI to be done at different times post conventional insemination. Late RICSI occurs when re-insemination is done the next day (18 hours after insemination), whereas early RICSI occurs the same day, usually 4–6 hours post initial insemination.

In 1993, Nagy et al. were the first to attempt RICSI on oocytes that failed to fertilize after conventional IVF [9]. They took 115 MII oocytes that failed to show signs of fertilization 24 hours after conventional insemination, injected a single sperm via ICSI and had a 38% success rate of two pronuclear fertilization; however, another 21% of oocytes were observed to have more than 2 pronuclei (2 PN). In 1996 Lundin et al. reported the first pregnancy via RICSI [10]. Lundin's clinic obtained a mean fertilization rate of 46.5% when performing RICSI on day old oocytes and two transfers resulted in pregnancies (6.9%) [10]. While RICSI can be performed routinely when needed, embryologists also have a conscious duty to consider each individual patient's history and the gametes that are involved to maximize the chance that the cycle will end in a pregnancy [11].

Contributing Factors to Fertilization Failure

There are several factors that contribute to why fertilization failure is seen in ART. RICSI can also be a useful diagnostic tool in determining which step of the fertilization process is contributing to the couple's infertility issues and can provide information on whether the issue lies with the ova or sperm. Studies have shown that successful fertilization with donor sperm following failed insemination with husband's spermatozoa indicates that the problem could be sperm quality, whereas failure of both to fertilize oocytes may indicate defects in the patient's ova [12]. Diagnosing the cause of infertility is important for clinics when deciding which ART procedure will be best for that individual patient.

Since the beginning of infertility diagnosis, male factors have been common diagnoses for couples seeking fertility treatment. Most of the failures of conventional IVF are caused by male factor infertility and issues such as sub-optimal semen parameters and dysfunction of sperm binding sites on the zona pellucida, could be avoided if ICSI were used instead [13].

Through bypass of the cumulus cells and zona and direct injection of the sperm into the cytoplasm, RICSI has the ability to increase fertilization of day-1 oocytes [11]. Studies have been done to compare the outcome of conventional IVF versus ICSI. One study by Yuzpe 2012 concluded that the IVF group was more efficient because it had better implantation rates, higher pregnancy rates and shorter procedure times than the ICSI group [14]. Because of this, many clinics prefer conventional IVF and choose to use ICSI only in cases of male factor infertility. Preferences for using conventional IVF can lead to TFF in some cases, and therefore increase the consideration and use of RICSI.

Aside from semen issues, patients who have fertilization failure post conventional insemination may have another concern such as oocyte quality and maturity. When doing conventional IVF, it is difficult to know if the oocytes being inseminated are mature or not. If a significant portion of the eggs are immature, then fertilization rates will be low.

Another way in which a patient's cycle can fail when using conventional IVF is if the egg and sperm fail to fuse properly, which can be caused by impairments of any of the gametes [5]. A failure in any of the essential steps of fertilization will cause infertility, and abnormalities in this part of the process can be hard to diagnose or predict. Thus, RICSI can be a great tool for saving these cycles.

Embryologists have limited options for TFF. The first is to cancel the present cycle and to offer ICSI directly in a subsequent cycle; however, this can be emotionally and financially costly to the patient [15]. The second is to use RICSI in the hopes of saving the cycle and also give embryologists a better understanding of what caused the cycle to fail. As mentioned, most conventional IVF cases fail because of male factor deficiencies, and, in contrast, ICSI failure is commonly caused by lack of oocyte activation, which could be caused by oocyte or sperm defects [5]. If RICSI is successful, then it is likely that the issue is the spermatozoa and that ICSI should be used for all future cycles. If RICSI fails in this circumstance, then this could indicate that the issue is the oocyte and subsequent ICSI cases will also have a higher chance of failure.

The Process of RICSI

There are different approaches for RICSI, with the choice of approach made on what is best in terms of patient outcome. The approaches include late RICSI, early RICSI, and/or with a polarization microscope. Figure 4.1 details these different techniques methodically laid out in various protocols, with each having its own advantages and disadvantages. Timing between retrieval (triggering ovulation) and re-insemination has a substantial impact on the success of RICSI [4]. When RICSI was performed 4–6 hours post insemination versus 6–8 hours there was an increase in the fertilization rate from 55.9% to 66.5% [16]. Another study found that shorter timing protocols also impacted pregnancy and implantation rates. Liu et al. divided their patient cohort into three groups: 6 hours (pregnancy rate: 64.71%, implantation rate: 57.58%), 6–8 hours (pregnancy rate: 58.33%, implantation rate: 40.07%) and 8 hours (pregnancy rate: 51.51%, implantation rate: 34.92%) [17]. One of the main reasons that the shorter protocol had better success is related to oocyte aging, which has a negative correlation to future success of fertilization and implantation [18]. Jin et al. compared implantation rates of RICSI 3 hours after insemination to a control group of ICSI oocytes; implantation rates were not significantly different between the two groups [19]. These studies provide guidance when finding the right protocol to follow using RICSI. As oocytes have critical stages in development and maturation (both nuclear and cytoplasmic), timing is a critical factor in the desire to increase fertilization of a RICSI case.

The earliest indication of fertilization in oocytes (by light microscope observation) is the extrusion of the second polar body. It has been shown that following ICSI, 65% of oocytes released the second polar body within 3 hours and 90% of fertilized eggs extruded a polar body by 6 hours [7,18,20,21]. Accurately timing fertilization and checking for polar bodies after insemination is crucial when separating fertilized and unfertilized oocytes [22]. One study found that 93.3% of the oocytes with a second

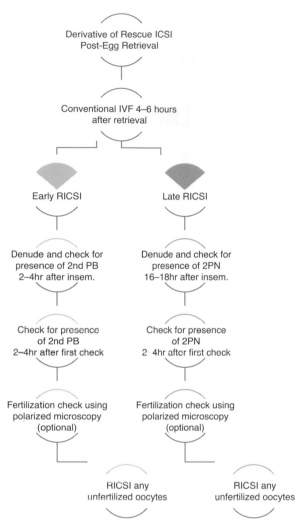

Derivative of Rescue ICSI
Post-Egg Retrieval

Conventional IVF 4–6 hours
after retrieval

Early RICSI

Late RICSI

Denude and check for
presence of 2nd PB
2–4hr after insem.

Denude and check for
presence of 2PN
16–18hr after insem.

Check for presence
of 2nd PB
2–4hr after first check

Check for presence
of 2PN
2–4hr after first check

Fertilization check using
polarized microscopy
(optional)

Fertilization check using
polarized microscopy
(optional)

RICSI any
unfertilized oocytes

RICSI any
unfertilized oocytes

Figure 4.1 Flow chart of RICSI with two different timing options. (A black and white version of this figure will appear in some formats. For the color version, please refer to the plate section.)

polar body 4 hours after insemination were confirmed to have normally fertilized 14–18 hours post insemination [19].

However, there is one potential concern when performing RICSI 6 hours after the retrieval: delayed oocyte maturation. An oocyte may not have extruded the second polar body at the time of assessment, but could still have been successfully penetrated by sperm. If the initial injected/inseminated spermatozoa successfully penetrates, but the timing of extrusion of the second polar body was delayed for the embryologist, the oocyte would then establish 3 pronuclei (3 PN) as a result of the latent spermatozoa chromatin

and the RICSI [23]. To overcome this problem, some studies checked for the presence of the second polar body at the time of stripping, separated the fertilized embryos and then waited 2 hours before doing a second check on the possibly unfertilized ones; again, separating any that presented a second polar body [20,24]. This method helps to reduce the number of oocytes that could be mistaken as unfertilized because of delayed maturation and therefore reduces (or avoids) the number of 3 PN embryos created. The downside to this method is increased timing before RICSI leading to oocyte aging. Moon and colleagues presented a method of identifying and re-inseminating only failed fertilized oocytes through use of polarized light microscopy to determine whether oocytes are still in metaphase I because of spindle appearance prior to cellular division [23]. The researchers assumed that oocytes showing a single (metaphase II) spindle had not been penetrated by spermatozoa while considering the presence of two spindles in other oocytes to be a sign of "silent" sperm penetration. In Moon et al.'s experience, this approach generated a higher rate of normal fertilization [23]. Using the presence of a second polar body, one study reported 11.36% polyploidy rates after RICSI [25], whereas another study using the polarization view reported only 4.5% polyploidy rates [23]. Hirabayashi et al. found that abnormal fertilization or delay could be caused by oocyte aberration, when comparing fertilization between RICSI and IVF+RICSI [26]. In that study, it was suggested that 3 PN fertilization was caused by lack of second polar body extrusion OR polyspermy. The IVF group presented a higher 3 PN rate than the RICSI group but the difference was not significant, and there was no significant difference in pregnancy rates between the groups. Overall, their study suggested that RICSI is an effective treatment for failed fertilization of IVF with considerations of the second polar body presence [26].

Another way to determine successful fertilization is to wait for the presence of 2 distinct pronuclei (2 PN) 16–18 hours after insemination. However, there has been a recorded pregnancy (twins) from three RICSI embryos that did not have distinct 2 PN 16 hours after RICSI, indicating that failure to observe 2 PN at the standard time (16–18 hours after insemination) of fertilization assessment may not be completely accurate when determining successful fertilization in the case of RICSI [27]. Pronuclei can appear as early as 3 hours after insemination [21] or as late as 25 hours after insemination [28]. It has been reported that 80% of oocytes have two visible pronuclei 8 hours post insemination [4] and 99% of oocytes have two visible pronuclei 16 hours post insemination [20,29].

There is a delicate balance when trying to achieve accurate determination of whether fertilization occurred with the least amount of oocyte aging. Because oocyte aging is crucial in the outcome of RICSI, studies have shown that it is important to perform RICSI as early as possible by shortening the IVF insemination time [30]. In assessment of timing, it is critical to consider the metabolites of cumulus cells that lead to over-maturation of oocytes and cause poor fertilization [19]. When performing RICSI, use of polarized microscopy will allow a spindle view assessment of fertilization while preventing double insemination and shorten the time needed before re-insemination, limiting oocyte aging [23]. In contrast, when conventional IVF insemination was performed with shorter timing of exposure between oocytes and spermatozoa, this led to higher fertilization rates and better quality embryos compared to those of oocytes derived following longer gamete co-incubation [17,31].

Outcomes After RICSI

The ultimate goal of ART is a healthy live birth for patients that come through treatment. Patients who experience TFF still have the chance at this, as there are many published studies that show success with use of RICSI for patients throughout their IVF journey. As standard protocols have changed and improved over time, RICSI pregnancy rates have increased. Although some protocols have been proven to be more successful, clinics have achieved live births from a variety of RICSI protocols. Huang et al. compared early RICSI to conventional IVF and ICSI, and found that the three groups had similar clinical pregnancy rates and similar numbers of healthy children delivered, with the early RICSI group achieving a total of 254 clinical pregnancies and 197 (33.67%) live births [15]. Overall, RICSI has been used in many different settings with the same goal in mind – successful implantation and live birth.

Many IVF labs have approached RICSI differently, resulting in various outcomes and success rates. When RICSI is done 16–18 hours after insemination (late RICSI) fertilization rates tend to be lower than with early RICSI (4–6 hours after insemination).

Kuczynski et al. reported a successful fertilization (2 PN) rate of 30.4 % for late RICSI, but no pregnancies occurred from this cohort [32]. In contrast, Moon et al. used a spindle view method during early RICSI that resulted in a fertilization rate of 68.7% [23]. Reviewing these studies, fertilization rates are much higher when RICSI is done within a closer time frame to the initial insemination time (closer to the trigger time). Further evidence of the optimal time window for RICSI comes from a study by Chen et al., who performed a comparison between oocytes that received RICSI 6 hours and 22 hours after conventional insemination [7]. The 6-hour group consisted of 226 MII oocytes, of which 70.3% fertilized. This was significantly higher than the fertilization rate obtained in the 22-hour group, wherein 167 MII oocytes had a fertilization rate of 48.5% [7]. In another study, RICSI was successful in all 43 patients when performed 4 hours after initial insemination, with a total fertilization rate of 93.3% for all oocytes re-inseminated [19]. As various studies state various times of RICSI post initial conventional insemination, timing proves to be a critical factor in RICSI fertilization outcomes and the sooner the embryologists are aware of any fertilization failure, the better chances they are able to give to the patients' cases once assessed.

Early RICSI has been shown to result in relatively high fertilization and in most studies seems to be comparable to other fertilization methods. Cleavage embryo quality of RICSI was also not found to be significantly different from that of conventionally inseminated embryos [8,9]. Recent improvements in embryo culture conditions have resulted in successful growth of cleavage embryos into blastocysts, allowing transfers to occur during this stage leading to higher pregnancy rates and lower rates of multiple gestations [33]. However, RICSI studies present lower pregnancy rates and live birth rates overall. Some clinics reported significantly lower implantation rates after transfer of embryos generated from late RICSI compared to early RICSI. One such study by Pourmasumi et al. achieved a late RICSI fertilization rate of 54.32%, although of the embryos transferred, no pregnancies were reported. The authors concluded that late RICSI might not be a good option for prevention of complete fertilization failure and for rescue of an IVF cycle [4]. In contrast, several studies reviewed achieved improved results when it came to early RICSI. One study achieved 254 clinical RICSI pregnancies

(43.42%), which corresponded closely with the clinical pregnancy rates of IVF (45.33%) and ICSI (44.39%) [15]. The early RICSI group in that study also resulted in 197 (33.67%) live births [15]. A retrospective study reviewed papers published between 2013 and 2016 and found that RICSI has led to a total of 248 pregnancies resulting in 177 births or ongoing pregnancies [34]. Another retrospective study by Chen et al. compared the neonatal outcomes of early RICSI (233 children) and ICSI (906 children) [6]. There were no increased risks of stillbirths, perinatal death or birth defects in the early RICSI group, and there were no differences found in gender rate, birthweight, gestational age or prematurity between the two groups [6]. Studies publishing outcomes after RICSI are summarized in Table 4.1.

Considerations on Access, Cost, Insurance and Resources

When planning ART treatment, patients and clinicians consider several factors, including the accessibility of the services. For mode of insemination a relevant question is: Are conventional insemination costs and outcome worth the time and effort or would intervention by ICSI be better? Many factors are taken into consideration in terms of where and how ART is available to infertile patients.

According to a review by Teoh et al., use of IVF is dependent on socio-economic class and education. IVF, per cycle, can cost between US$3,000 and US$9,000 around the world, including Canada, UK, Australia, Brazil and other countries [46]. In the USA costs can be even higher, posing a great financial burden that prevents many patients from accessing IVF treatment.

Patients considering ART treatment will look at what type of insemination is more affordable as well as potentially covered by insurance. When considering materials and resources, RICSI can be seen as an additional cost to extend a treatment cycle, instead of cancellation [25]. Based on a comparative study among four Dutch IVF centers in 2006, the cost of conventional insemination procedures was between $253 and $384 in the Netherlands, whereas the cost of ICSI was found to be between $483 and $678. Compared with conventional insemination, ICSI will always be more costly because of additional materials needed, such as advanced instruments and procedures, although the difference in price can be small

when looking at the overall cost of the cycle. Clinics across the board need to consider what is gained versus what is lost in terms of resources, time and outcome probability. Pricing is likely to vary over time and increase with the economy at hand.

The processes of ART are complex, requiring precision and experience to provide optimal outcomes for patients. Compared with conventional IVF, ICSI is a more invasive and time-consuming procedure; therefore, increasing the workload and hours worked for staff at fertility clinics [47]. The process of RICSI being performed on TFF cycles results in more IVF for patients to produce transferable embryos, with additional work for embryologists and additional hours required to perform the RICSI [17]. The process of RICSI comes at a cost to the staff and the clinic, but can lead to overall decreases in cost and stress for the patient. Shalom-Paz et al. calculated the cost of a RICSI cycle with a follow-up ICSI cycle for patients who did not get pregnant and compared that to a canceled IVF cycle and a follow-up ICSI cycle for all patients in that group [36]. The RICSI approach for 100 patients would, on average, result in 38 live births out of 189 cycles, whereas canceling would result in only 30 live births out of 200 cycles. The cost per one live birth using this model would be 25% less for the RICSI group and patients would experience less emotional distress, which accompanies cancellation of a cycle [36].

Even if a patient's cycle undergoes total/partial fertilization failure, the resources and outcomes of saving a cycle with RICSI would be more beneficial than canceling altogether. After RICSI, embryos created could then be vitrified and used later for frozen embryo transfer. Even with a lower pregnancy rate (8.53%), studies still show success with RICSI and there is potential for embryonic advancement and improved knowledge of factors that attribute to TFF and transfer cycles [38]. The major consensus of most studies is that RICSI post standard conventional insemination is a useful evaluation tool to reduce fertilization failure in future cycles. RICSI can be used to evaluate the compatibility of spermatozoa and oocytes giving clinics more information into what caused TFF in a particular patient, giving more data than can be provided by sperm analysis [9,35].

Moreover, whether health insurance fully or partially covers infertility treatment, providers typically have strict policies and restrictions for patients who desire ICSI and would prefer coverage than to spend the extra expenses if they are unable to afford extra

Table 4.1 Review of publications on RICSI timing and outcomes

Authors	Year	RICSI timing (hours after retrieval)	Number of patients / cycles in study	No. of injected oocytes	No. of. fertilized (%)	No. of ET	No. of pregnancies (%)	Outcome
Tsirigotis [35]	1995	Late 24 hours post CONV	Not mentioned	121	58 (48)	14 patients	1 (~7)	
Lundin [10]	1996	Day 2 ICSI	57 patients	167	44 (46.5)	29 patients	2 (~7)	
Palermo [2]	1992	6–18 hours after SUZI injection	8 cycles	47	31 (66)	7 patients	4 (57)	
Yuzpe [3]	2000	Late 19–22 hours	32 patients	234	141 (60.2)	29 patients	6 (20.7)	
Shalom-Paz [36]	2011	Late post 18 hours	92 patients	Not mentioned	Not mentioned (56.2)	92 patients	20 (21.7)	
Jarmuz [37]	2015	Late 20 hours	120 patients	1384	(57.1)	64 patients	3 (4.7)	
Ming [38]	2012	Late	534 cycles	4824	2170 (44.98)	607 patients	67 (11.03)	
Zhu [16]	2011	Early (4–6) Group A / Late (6–8) Group B	77 cycles / 16 cycles	579 / 98	365 (63) / 51 (52)	69 patients / 12	30 (43.5) / 0 (0)	
Eftekhar [4]	2013	Late 24 hours	15 cycles	Not mentioned	Not mentioned (54.32)	7 patients	0 (0)	
Nagy [18]	1995	Late	15 patients	93	45 (53)	No transfers	n/a	
Morton [39]	1997	Late	54 patients	439	215 (58)	48	8 (14.8)	
Park [40]	2000	Late	29 cycles	95	14 (14.7)	No transfers	n/a	
Kuczynski [32]	2002	Late 18–20 hours	120 cycles	Not mentioned	Not mentioned (30.4)	100	0 (0)	
Chen [7]	2003	Late 22 hours / Early 6 hours	20 patients / 25 patients	167 / 226	81 (48.5) / 159 (70.3)	20 patients / 25 patients	1 (5) / 12 (48)	
Nagy [30]	2006	Early 3–6 hours post insemination	30 patients	184	166 (90)	68	8 (12)	
Liu [17]	2014	Early	180 patients	1332	884 (66.37)	180 patients	104 (57.78)	
Huang [15]	2015	Early 4–6 hours	730 cycles	Not mentioned	Not mentioned	730 patients	254 (34.79)	
Jin [19]	2014	Early 4 hours	43 cycles	443	355 (80.1)	43 patients	16 (37.2)	

Table 4.1 (cont.)

Authors	Year	RICSI timing (hours after retrieval)	Number of patients / cycles in study	No. of injected oocytes	No. of. fertilized (%)	No. of ET	No. of pregnancies (%)	Outcome
Hirabayashi [26]	2006	Early 6 hours	128 patients	681	470 (69)	84 patients	25 (29.8)	
Yuxia [41]	2018	Early	102 patients	919	646 (70.29)	102 patients	62 (60.78)	
Lombardi [42]	2003	Case study late 20 hours	1 patient	12	9 (75)	1 patient	1 (100)	
Chian [27]	2003	Case study late 18 hours	1 patient	4	No signs of fert	1 patient	1 (100)	Twins 3 embryos transferred
Moon [43]	2015	2 case studies late	2 patients	19	12 (63)	2 patients	2 (100)	
Esfandiari [44]	2007	Case study late	1 patient	8	7 (87.5)	1 patient	1 (100)	7 embryos transferred
Singh [45]	2013	Case study late	1 patient	4	3 (75)	1 patient	1 (100)	3 embryos transferred

CONV, conventional insemination; ET, embryo transfer; Fert, fertilization; n/a, not applicable; SUZI, subzonal insemination.

costs for ICSI. Patients who do not qualify for ICSI coverage under their plans must rely on conventional insemination. Rescue insemination is a good back-up procedure for patients who do not qualify for ICSI, and still yields embryos viable for future use. Sheehan et al. report use of RICSI for patients who have failed or low fertilization rates [48].

When considering RICSI, the higher probability of chromosomal abnormalities and other risks should also be taken into account [10,36]. A case report by Pehlivan et al. compared results of FISH analysis on embryos created from RICSI 21 hours post initial insemination for a couple with unexpected fertilization failure [49]. They used FISH to give specific chromosomal outcomes and found that second-day ICSI typically yields a higher rate of aneuploid embryos [49]. Accordingly, preimplantation genetic testing options may be considered with RICSI cases, as well as cryopreservation rather than fresh transfer [38]. In addition to the extra resources needed, possible inconveniences to patients and staff, and higher rates of abnormalities, many studies also found that RICSI can have poor outcomes [37].

Because of the various risks and lower pregnancy rates, many studies concluded that RICSI insemination should not be considered as a routine protocol in IVF but instead used when considering ICSI for subsequent cycles [10]. On the other hand, many clinics have achieved live births from RICSI, saving cycles from TFF and giving patients hope when undergoing such a stressful and emotional process. Patients who seek ART treatment should be given all options that may lead to success, whether this be to completely follow conventional insemination, ICSI or, with lab discretion, RICSI.

Conclusions

In attempts to salvage total (or near total) fertilization failure experienced after conventional insemination, RICSI was introduced. While ICSI insemination is available for patients at most IVF clinics, conventional insemination is still more frequently performed as it is seen as a more "natural" and more cost-effective approach than ICSI. Also, the policies of clinics and/or those of insurance companies (where relevant) may mandate conventional insemination prior to the use of ICSI. Additionally, many clinics experience a slightly improved IVF outcome when conventional insemination is performed, compared to ICSI insemination. For all these reasons

conventional insemination remains an integral part of ART. Unfortunately, conventional IVF comes with the drawback of being associated with occasional total (or near total) fertilization failures, even in cases when traditional sperm parameters are adequate. In recent decades, several studies have demonstrated that performing ICSI on the failed fertilized oocytes can result in successful fertilization, embryo development and pregnancy, thus the IVF cycle can be rescued. It has also been demonstrated, that the sooner the RICSI is performed, the better the outcomes. While "early RICSI" poses both technical and logistical challenges for the IVF laboratory, it clearly provides several benefits to the patients. Relative to starting a new IVF cycle, RICSI also shortens time to pregnancy and is a more cost-effective approach. For all these reasons, RICSI should be a primary consideration in cases of TFF after conventional insemination.

References

[1] Steptoe PC, Edwards RG. Birth after the reimplantation of a human embryo. Lancet 1978;2:366. https://doi.org/10.1016/s0140-6736(78) 92957-4.

[2] Palermo G, Joris H, Devroey P, Lancet AVS. Pregnancies after intracytoplasmic injection of single spermatozoon into an oocyte. Lancet 1992;340:17–8. https://doi.org/10.1016/0140-6736(92)92425-F.

[3] Yuzpe AA, Liu Z, Fluker MR. Rescue intracytoplasmic sperm injection (ICSI) – salvaging in vitro fertilization (IVF) cycles after total or near-total fertilization failure. Fertil Steril 2000;73:1115–9. https://doi.org/10.1016/S0015-0282(00)00522-7.

[4] Eftekhar M, Pourmasumi S, Razi M-H. Efficacy of rescue ICSI after total fertilization failure in conventional IVF. J Infertil Reprod Biol 2013;1:58–62.

[5] Mahutte NG, Arici A, Williams L. Failed fertilization: is it predictable? Curr Opin Obstet Gynecol 2003;15:211–8. https://doi.org/10.1097/01 .gco.0000072858.73466.aa.

[6] Chen L, Xu Z, Zhang N, Wang B, Chen H, Wang S, et al. Neonatal outcome of early rescue ICSI and ICSI with ejaculated sperm. J Assist Reprod Genet 2014;31:823–8. https://doi.org/10.1007/s10815-014-0245-9.

[7] Chen C, Kattera S. Rescue ICSI of oocytes that failed to extrude the second polar body 6 h post-insemination in conventional IVF. Hum Reprod 2003;18:2118–21. https://doi.org/10.1093/humrep/deg325.

[8] Nagy ZP, Liu J, Joris H, Verheyen G, Tournaye H, Camus M, et al. Andrology: the result of intracytoplasmic sperm injection is not related to any of the three basic sperm parameters. Hum Reprod 1995;**10**:1123–9. https://doi.org/10.1093/oxfordjournals.humrep.a136104.

[9] Nagy ZP, Joris H, Liu J, Staessen C, Devroey P, Van Steirteghem AC. Fertilization and early embryology: Intracytoplasmic single sperm injection of 1-day-old unfertilized human oocytes. Hum Reprod 1993;**8**:2180–4. https://doi.org/10.1093/oxford journals.humrep.a138000.

[10] Lundin K, Sjögren A, Hamberger L. Reinsemination of one-day-old oocytes by use of intracytoplasmic sperm injection. Fertil Steril 1996;**66**:118–21. https://doi.org/10.1016/s0015-0282(16)58397-6.

[11] Swain JE, Pool TB. ART failure: oocyte contributions to unsuccessful fertilization. Hum Reprod Update 2008;**14**:431–46. https://doi.org/10.1093/humupd/dmn025.

[12] Trounson A, Webb J. Fertilization of human oocytes following reinsemination in vitro. Fertil Steril 1984;**41**:816–9. https://doi.org/10.1016/S0015-0282(16)47891-X.

[13] Tesarik J. Rescue ICSI revisited. Hum Reprod 2003;**18**:2122–3. https://doi.org/10.1093/humrep/deg425.

[14] Yuzpe AA. The ART Laboratory. n.d.

[15] Huang B, Qian K, Li Z, Yue J, Yang W, Zhu G, et al. Neonatal outcomes after early rescue intracytoplasmic sperm injection: an analysis of a 5-year period. Fertil Steril 2015;**103**:1432–1437.e1. https://doi.org/10.1016/j.fertnstert.2015.02.026.

[16] Zhu L-x, Ren X-l, Wu L, Hu J, Li Y-f, Zhang H-w, et al. Rescue ICSI: choose the optimal rescue window before oocyte aging. J Reprod Contracept 2011;**22**:29–36. https://doi.org/10.1016/S1001-7844(12)60004-2.

[17] Liu W, Liu J, Zhang X, Han W, Xiong S, Huang G. Short co-incubation of gametes combined with early rescue ICSI: an optimal strategy for complete fertilization failure after IVF. Hum Fertil 2014;**17**:50–5. https://doi.org/10.3109/14647273.2013.859746.

[18] Nagy ZP, Staessen C, Liu J, Joris H, Devroey P, Van Steirteghem AC. Prospective, auto-controlled study on reinsemination of failed-fertilized oocytes by intracytoplasmic sperm injection. Fertil Steril 1995;**64**:1130–5. https://doi.org/10.1016/s0015-0282(16)57973-4.

[19] Jin H, Shu Y, Dai S, Peng Z, Shi S, Sun Y. The value of second polar body detection 4 hours after insemination and early rescue ICSI in preventing complete fertilisation failure in patients with borderline semen. Reprod Fertil Dev 2014;**26**:346–50. https://doi.org/10.1071/RD12369.

[20] Nagy ZP, Janssenswillen C, Janssens R, De Vos A, Staessen C, Van de Velde H, et al. Timing of oocyte activation, pronucleus formation and cleavage in humans after intracytoplasmic sperm injection (ICSI) with testicular spermatozoa and after ICSI or in-vitro fertilization on sibling oocytes with ejaculated spermatozoa. Hum Reprod 1998;**13**:1606–12. https://doi.org/10.1093/humrep/13.6.1606.

[21] Payne D, Flaherty SP, Barry MF, Matthews CD. Preliminary observations on polar body extrusion and pronuclear formation in human oocytes using time-lapse video cinematography. Hum Reprod 1997;**12**:532–41. https://doi.org/10.1093/humrep/12.3.532.

[22] Van Den Bergh M, Bertrand E, Englert Y. Second polar body extrusion is highly predictive for oocyte fertilization as soon as 3 hr after intracytoplasmic sperm injection (ICSI). J Assist Reprod Genet 1995;**12**:258–62. https://doi.org/10.1007/BF02212928.

[23] Moon JH, Son WY, Henderson S, Mahfoudh A, Dahan M, Holzer H. Spindle examination in unfertilized eggs using the polarization microscope can assist rescue ICSI. Reprod Biomed Online 2013;**26**:280–5. https://doi.org/10.1016/j.rbmo.2012.10.019.

[24] Nagy ZP, Liu J, Joris H, Devroey P, Van Steirteghem A. Fertilization and early embryology: time-course of oocyte activation, pronucleus formation and cleavage in human oocytes fertilized by intracytoplasmic sperm injection. Hum Reprod 1994;**9**:1743–8. https://doi.org/10.1093/oxford journals.humrep.a138786.

[25] Cao S, Wu X, Zhao C, Zhou L, Zhang J, Ling X. Determining the need for rescue intracytoplasmic sperm injection in partial fertilisation failure during a conventional IVF cycle. Andrologia 2016;**48**:1138–44. https://doi.org/10.1111/and.12551.

[26] Hirabayashi Y, Tawara F, Ishii M, Muramatsu H, Kanayama N. Evaluation of rescue ICSI on oocytes without extrusion of the second polar body in cases of moderately disturbed fertilization. J Mamm Ova Res 2006;**23**:135–40. https://doi.org/10.1274/jmor.23.135.

[27] Chian R-C, Lapensée L, Phillips S, Tan S-L. Observation of pronuclei may not be an absolute indicator for fertilization in rescue intracytoplasmic sperm injection oocytes. Reprod Med Biol 2003;**2**:83–5. https://doi.org/10.1046/j.1445-5781.2003.00020.x.

[28] Balakier H. Fertilization and early embryology: tripronuclear human zygotes: The first cell cycle and subsequent development. Hum Reprod 1993;8:1892–7. https://doi.org/10.1093/oxford journals.humrep.a137955.

[29] Jiaen L, Zsolt N, Hubert J, Herman T, Johan S, Michel C, et al. Analysis of 76 total fertilization failure cycles out of 2732 intracytoplasmic sperm injection cycles. Hum Reprod 1995;10:2630–6. https://doi.org/10.1093/oxfordjournals .humrep.a135758.

[30] Nagy ZP, Rienzi LF, Ubaldi FM, Greco E, Massey JB, Kort HI. Effect of reduced oocyte aging on the outcome of rescue intracytoplasmic sperm injection. Fertil Steril 2006;85:901–6. https://doi.org/10.1016/j .fertnstert.2005.09.029.

[31] Gianaroli L, Fiorentino A, Magli MC, Ferraretti AP, Montanaro N. Prolonged sperm-oocyte exposure and high sperm concentration affect human embryo viability and pregnancy rate. Hum Reprod 1996;11:2507–11. https://doi.org/10.1093/oxford journals.humrep.a019149.

[32] Kuczynski W. Rescue ICSI of unfertilized oocytes after IVF. Hum Reprod 2002;17:2423–7. https://doi .org/10.1093/humrep/17.9.2423.

[33] Jones GM, Trounson AO, Lolatgis N, Wood C. Factors affecting the success of human blastocyst development and pregnancy following in vitro fertilization and embryo transfer. Fertil Steril 1998;70:1022–9. https://doi.org/10.1016/S0015-028 2(98)00342-2.

[34] Simopoulou M, Giannelou P, Bakas P, Gkoles L, Kalampokas T, Pantos K, et al. Making ICSI safer and more effective: a review of the human oocyte and ICSI practice. In Vivo 2016;30:387–400.

[35] Tsirigotis M, Nicholson N, Taranissi M, Bennett V, Pelekanos M, Craft I. Late intracytoplasmic sperm injection in unexpected failed fertilization in vitro: diagnostic or therapeutic? Fertil Steril 1995;63:816–9. https://doi.org/10.1016/S0015-028 2(16)57487-1.

[36] Shalom-Paz E, Alshalati J, Shehata F, Jimenez L, Son WY, Holzer H, et al. Clinical and economic analysis of rescue intracytoplasmic sperm injection cycles. Gynecol Endocrinol 2011;27:993–6. https:// doi.org/10.3109/09513590.2011.579655.

[37] Jarmuz P, Ocali O, Baldwin M, Sakkas D, Barrett C. Success rates of rescue ICSI and analysis of embryo cleavage rates by real time video imaging. Fertil Steril 2015;104:E301. https://doi.org/10.1016/j .fertnstert.2015.07.943.

[38] Ming L, Liu P, Qiao J, Lian Y, Zheng X, Ren X, et al. Synchronization between embryo development and endometrium is a contributing factor

for rescue ICSI outcome. Reprod Biomed Online 2012;24:527–31. https://doi.org/10.1016/j .rbmo.2012.02.001.

[39] Morton PC, Wright G, Yoder CS, Brockman WDW, Tucker MJ, Kort HI. Reinsemination by intracytoplasmic sperm injection of 1-day-old oocytes after complete conventional fertilization failure. Fertil Steril 1997;68:488–91. https://doi.org/ 10.1016/S0015-0282(97)00223-9.

[40] Park KS, Song HB, Chun SS. Late fertilization of unfertilized human oocytes in in vitro fertilization and intracytoplasmic sperm injection cycles: Conventional insemination versus ICSI. J Assist Reprod Genet 2000;17:419–24. https://doi.org/10 .1023/A:1009409100941.

[41] He Y, Liu H, Zheng H, Li L, Fu X, Liu J. Effect of early cumulus cells removal and early rescue ICSI on pregnancy outcomes in high-risk patients of fertilization failure. Gynecol Endocrinol 2018;34:689–93. https://doi.org/10.1080/09513590 .2018.1433159.

[42] Lombardi E, Tiverón M, Inza R, Valcárcel A, Young E, Bisioli C. Live birth and normal 1-year follow-up of a baby born after transfer of cryopreserved embryos from rescue intracytoplasmic sperm injection of 1-day-old oocytes. Fertil Steril 2003;80:646–8. https://doi.org/ 10.1016/S0015-0282(03)00996-8.

[43] Moon JH, Henderson S, Garcia-Cerrudo E, Mahfoudh A, Reinblatt S, Son WY. Successful live birth after transfer of blastocyst and frozen blastocyst from rescue ICSI with application of polarized light microscopy for spindle examination on unfertilized eggs. J Ovarian Res 2015;8. https://doi.org/10.1186/ s13048-015-0150-6.

[44] Esfandiari N, Claessens EA, Burjaq H, Gotlieb L, Casper RF. Ongoing twin pregnancy after rescue intracytoplasmic sperm injection of unfertilized abnormal oocytes. Fertil Steril 2008;90:199.e5-199.e7. https://doi.org/10.1016/ j.fertnstert.2007.07.1299.

[45] Singh N, Malhotra N, Shende U, Tiwari A. Successful live birth after rescue ICSI following failed fertilization. J Hum Reprod Sci 2013;6:77–8. https://doi.org/10.4103/0974-1208 .112388.

[46] Teoh PJ, Maheshwari A. Low-cost in vitro fertilization: current insights. Int J Womens Health 2014;6:817–27. https://doi.org/10.2147/IJWH .S51288.

[47] Xi QS, Zhu LX, Hu J, Wu L, Zhang HW. Should few retrieved oocytes be as an indication for intracytoplasmic sperm injection? J Zhejiang Univ

47

Sci B 2012;**13**:717–22. https://doi.org/10.1631/jzus.B1100370.

[48] Sheehan DA, Patel JC, Pauli SA, Pang SC, Go KJ. "Rescue" ICSI: saving a treatment cycle from fertilization failure. Fertil Steril 2013;**100**:S531. https://doi.org/10.1016/j.fertnstert.2013.07.290.

[49] Pehlivan T, Rubio C, Ruiz A, Navarro J, Remohí J, Pellicer A, et al. Embryonic chromosomal abnormalities obtained after rescue intracytoplasmic sperm injection of 1-day-old unfertilized oocytes. J Assist Reprod Genet 2004;**21**:55–7. https://doi.org/10.1023/B:JARG.0000025939.26834.93.

Chapter

5

Morphological Sperm Selection Before ICSI

Pierre Vanderzwalmen, Barbara Wirleitner, Guy Cassuto, Romain Imbert, and Maximillian Murtinger

Introduction

Of all semen parameters, sperm morphology, assessed by Kruger's strict criteria, is the best predictor of a man's fertilizing potential. A strong link between sperm morphological characteristics and male fertility has been shown by many investigators [1]. Morphologically abnormal spermatozoa have reduced capability to fertilize because of impairment of one or more of the following steps: binding to the receptors of the zona pellucida (ZP), fusion with the oolemma or decondensation and release of the oocyte activation protein phospholipase C (PLCzeta) hindering resumption of the MII oocyte meiosis. Natural selection of spermatozoa is thought to prevent entrance of spermatozoa with defective function, which may be considered as a natural way to prevent adverse outcome.

The introduction of the intracytoplasmic sperm injection (ICSI), considered a tremendously helpful tool to overcome the infertility of couples when conventional IVF treatment has failed, has transgressed the natural process of spermatozoa selection and fertilization [2]. Since the introduction of ICSI, little attention has been given to spermatozoa because it was thought that the oocyte contributes most to embryo development and that the spermatozoon is only tagging along its DNA. Nevertheless, there is still debate regarding the consequences of injecting spermatozoa with morphological defects as it becomes more and more accepted that such spermatozoa show defective intracellular sperm function and molecular defects that contribute to early embryonic development disturbance, failure of blastocyst formation, miscarriages, and congenital birth defects [3]. Observing that such non-physiological fertilization carries a risk of transferring putative negative effects to the offspring [4], it might be reasonable to develop optimized selection techniques based, i.e., on the biochemical ability of the spermatozoa to bind to

solid hyaluronic acid or on improved morphological spermatozoa selection [5].

Almost 20 years ago, Bartoov et al. [5] introduced a non-invasive technique for more precise morphological evaluation of motile spermatozoa named "motile-sperm organelle-morphology examination" (MSOME). Replacement of the standard bright field or the Hoffman modulation contrast optics by the Nomarski differential interference contrast optics (DIC) allowed a better three-dimensional view of the head and midpiece. Examination with the DIC optics at 1000× magnification changed the perception of how a spermatozoon selected for injection should appear. With this meticulous approach permitting examination in real time of the fine morphology of motile spermatozoa, we became aware of the presence of abnormalities presenting as concavities (also called "craters," "hollows," or "lacunae") of different depth and location on the head that we define as vacuole-like structures (VLS), which were found to be related to DNA integrity and to provide an indirect reflection of the pathological situation [6,7].

The aim of the first part of this chapter is to provide information on which defects to deselect among a multitude of abnormalities, respectively spermatozoa with nuclear and asymmetrical insertion of the neck. The technical procedures combining MSOME spermatozoa evaluation and ICSI named IMSI will be described in the second part of the chapter.

Which Morphological Defects to Deselect and Why?

Pathological Character of Nuclear VLS: Abnormal Chromatin Condensation and Potential Epigenetic Mechanism Defects

During the late stage of spermiogenesis, elongation and progressive condensation of the chromatin takes place, which, with simultaneous acrosome attachment, results in the typical shape of the sperm head. The high degree of chromatin condensation protects the mature spermatozoa against physical and chemical damage and it is only within the ooplasm of an activated oocyte that the sperm chromatin becomes decondensed, resulting in substitution of its protamine by oocyte-derived histones [8]. The aim of these unique cellular reconstruction processes that involve chromosomal packaging and require 600–1000 spermatid-specific genes [9], is to protect the paternal genome during the transit from the male to the oocyte prior to fertilization. During a normal spermiogenesis process, chromatin condensation is associated with biochemical changes such as replacement of about 85% of histones by arginine-rich protamines and the formation of chromatin-stabilizing disulfide bonds. The spermatozoon delivers a novel epigenetic signature to the egg that is required in early embryogenesis and is crucial for normal embryo development and the offspring [10]. As a consequence, distribution of the remaining 15% of histones is not random but concerns gene regions involved in epigenetic control [11,12].

A first key question to investigate concerns the significance of VLS and whether they are the morphological manifestation of histone-protamine transition dysfunction. A clear consensus showing a negative correlation between the incidence of VLS and abnormally condensed chromatin was observed in several studies [13,14]. Boitrelle et al. [6,14] and Cassuto et al. [7] observed negative chromatin condensation at the site of the VLS and Boitrelle et al. [6] concluded that a large VLS appears to be a nuclear "thumbprint" linked to failure of chromatin condensation. By analyzing sperm DNA methylation and RNA transcripts in spermatozoa, a recent study showed the paternal contribution and the crucial role of sperm epigenetics in embryonic development. Epigenetic modifications in mature spermatozoa play an important role and are the consequence of altered methylation profiles that may increase the risk of fertilization failure, dysfunction of embryogenesis, preterm birth, low birthweight, congenital anomalies, and autism perinatal mortality [15,16]. In men with impaired spermatogenesis, the sperm epigenetic landscape (DNA methylation errors and gene expression defects) is frequently altered compared to normozoospermic sperm [17].

A second fundamental question to address is whether VLS are related to alteration in the methylation pattern and whether potential epigenetic mechanism defects could be the consequence of chromatin condensation failures? Cassuto et al. [18] detected different levels of DNA methylation after morphological sperm selection using the MSOME approach. Sperm DNA methylation level was significantly lower in the normal morphological group compared with the group of abnormal spermatozoa carrying VLS. Previously, the same authors observed a strong correlation between presence of nuclear VLS and chromatin defects [6,7]. Out of these preliminary studies, we may assume that hypermethylation, a source of epigenetic defects, is related to abnormal sperm morphology and presence of VLS.

Taken together, these data support the idea that erroneous condensation of sperm DNA has a great impact on male fertility. All these potential epigenetic pattern disturbances may represent the basis of numerous human disorders. As a consequence, the pathological character of nuclear VLS must not be underestimated. In light of their higher frequency of abnormal decondensation and incorrect methylation pattern compared to morphologically normal spermatozoa, there is a tangible and strong argument to deselect sperm carrying VLS.

Which Midpiece to Select?

As in most mammals, human centrioles and centrosomes are inherited paternally. According to Van Blerkom and Davis [19], the centriole is, after the nucleus, the most important sperm organelle for initiation of the intra-ooplasmic fertilization process, being responsible for the formation of the sperm aster. The sperm centrosome plays a central role in establishment of the first and subsequent embryonic mitotic spindles. The proximal centriole plays a crucial role in fertilization and its dysfunction may cause fertilization failure through lack of a sperm aster.

A tapering-shaped midpiece is related to abnormal centrosomal function as a consequence of aberrant microtubule organization [20]. The MSOME selection of spermatozoa with a morphologically straight midpiece rather than a tapering one may result in choosing sperm with functional centrosomes, positively influencing fertilization rates and embryo development after ICSI [20]. According to Cassuto et al. [21], an asymmetrical insertion of the neck (connecting piece just behind the nucleus and the proximal centriole) negatively influences embryo development.

Application of IMSI, Indications and Outcome of IMSI in an IVF Program

Randomized trials comparing ICSI and IMSI are scarce and results inconsistent, probably because of the different inclusion criteria used. The superiority of IMSI over ICSI is still a matter of debate, and for some, IMSI did not provide any significant improvement in clinical outcomes compared with ICSI in terms of oocyte fertilization rates, early embryo development, implantation, clinical pregnancy, or live birth rates [22]. Moreover, application of IMSI is, in the first instance, not beneficial [22].

On the other hand, several studies have assessed the efficiency of IMSI and provided reassuring evidence for its use in specific indications [23]. Patients with very poor sperm [24], or with repeated implantation failures after ICSI [25,26] and with absence of blastocysts [27], benefited the most in terms of increasing pregnancy rate and decreasing miscarriage rates.

One of the main benefits of IMSI is the improvement in embryo quality and the higher rate of blastocysts obtained per cycle when morphologically good-quality spermatozoa are selected [28]. It is well reported that sperm selection with DIC optics provides higher fertilization and blastulation rates. More blastocysts provide a higher chance of the patient achieving a pregnancy in successive vitrified embryo transfer cycle(s), thus increasing the cumulative pregnancy rate. Poor responders or patients of advanced maternal age could benefit from such a procedure if one more blastocyst per cycle can be produced.

Regardless of whether ICSI or IMSI is used to select a normal spermatozoon and produce a blastocyst, the capacity to implant will be similar. This is one reason why some do not perceive the advantage of IMSI, particularly in cases of normal male infertility. But if we consider severe teratozoospermia, and moreover when there are few oocytes to inject originating from a woman of advanced age, with ICSI the probability of selecting a normal spermatozoon decreases, with a consequence of few or absent blastocysts.

To date, there are not sufficient published studies concerning the health of children born after ICSI from which to draw any firm conclusions about the long-term safety of this procedure. However, it is important to emphasize that animal data are absolutely unequivocal on this point and clearly indicate that DNA damage in the male germ line is potentially hazardous for the embryo and therefore for the resulting offspring [4]. According to recently published papers, sperm nucleus morphological normalcy, assessed at high magnification, could decrease the prevalence of major fetal malformations in ICSI children [10,29].

Technique and Procedure to Perform IMSI

Practical and technical aspects of morphologically normal sperm selection [30] must be considered to facilitate workflow while performing IMSI and avoid damage to the oocytes.

General Equipment, Reagents, and Supplies

Several companies offer complete equipment to perform IMSI, so we make no mention of specific brand names.

Morphological observation or sperm selection is performed on an inverted light microscope equipped with DIC/Nomarski differential interference contrast optics, with dry or immersion objective lenses at 63× or 100× magnification. The use of a dry objective allows easy handling of the dishes. This is particularly true when few oocytes are placed in the dish for injection, resulting in frequent changes.

Sperm Preparation Before IMSI

The sperm preparation consists of discontinuous density gradient centrifugation. In cases of severe oligo-astheno-teratozoospermia, and according to the concentrations of round cells, debris, and tissue, several gradient columns are prepared, each with one layer of 90% or two layers of 70% and 90%. With several gradient columns, the round cells, debris, and tissue (in case of surgical retrieval) are dilute, preventing entrapment of the spermatozoa in the upper layers [31]. Following gradient centrifugation (20–30 minutes at 600 up to 1800 g), a small aliquot of washed sperm is deposited in the IMSI dish. The prepared sperm suspension will swim-out in a long "snake" shape drop (Figures 5.1 and 5.2) before selection and oocyte injection.

Classification

Although our classification of the spermatozoa into four groups (normal form and presence of VLS) improved the results in terms of blastocyst rate after selection of

(a)

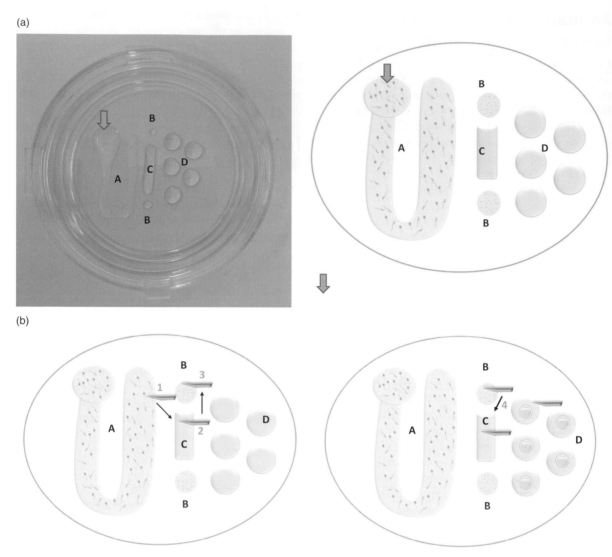

(b)

Figure 5.1 (a) Sperm selection under DIC optics followed by oocyte injection on a microscope equipped with HMC or bright field optics. (b) Left: sperm selection under DIC optics; right: oocyte injection with HMC or bright field optics. A: Swim out "snake" drop (HTF-HEPES-HSA); B: host-selected spermatozoa micro drops (HTF-HEPES-HSA); C: sperm immobilization drop (10% PVP); D: oocyte injection drops (HTF-HEPES-HSA); Arrow: position to deposit an aliquot of sperm suspension. (A black and white version of this figure will appear in some formats. For the color version, please refer to the plate section.)

class I spermatozoa [27], we have adapted the classification according to a recent manuscript by Berkovitz et al. [32]. They analyzed the genomic stability of spermatozoa and found an association with the deepness of VLS and their location in the cellular compartment, that is, the nucleus and equatorial region.

Our new classification discriminates between a group with abnormal shape without LNV and a group with abnormal shape with LNV, and different locations (Table 5.1, Figures 5.3 and 5.4).

Table 5.2 gives an example of a chart in which the percentages of different classes of spermatozoa (MSOME evaluation) from fresh semen or after preparation and washing can be reported (in the column "%"). When performing IMSI, the number of oocytes injected with the different classes of spermatozoa can be indicated in the column "# Oocytes injected." With such an approach, it is possible to follow exactly the development of embryos according to the type of injected spermatozoa.

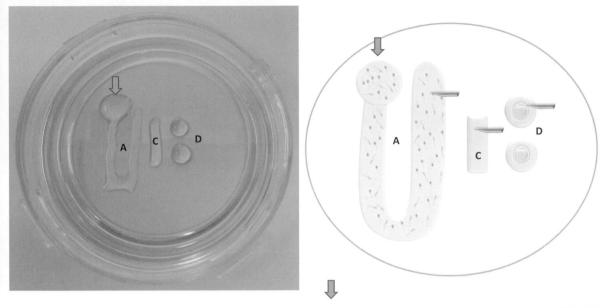

Figure 5.2 Sperm selection followed by oocyte injection on a microscope equipped with DIC optics. A: Swim out "snake" drop (HTF-HEPES-HSA); C: sperm immobilization drop (10% PVP); D: oocyte injection drops (HTF-HEPES-HSA); Arrow: position to deposit an aliquot of sperm suspension. (A black and white version of this figure will appear in some formats. For the color version, please refer to the plate section.)

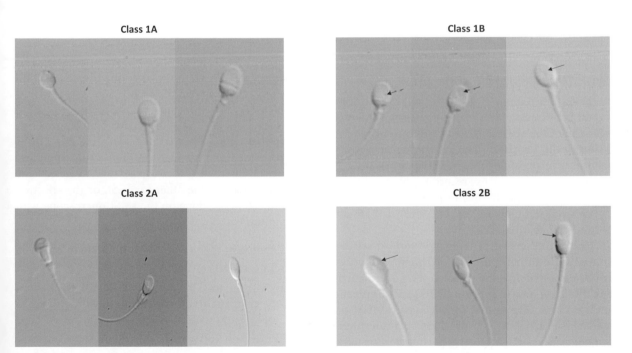

Figure 5.3 Class 1 and class 2 spermatozoa. Arrows indicate the presence of small, smooth VLS. (A black and white version of this figure will appear in some formats. For the color version, please refer to the plate section.)

Table 5.1 Classification according to the general shape, location, and depth of VLS

Class	Morphology	VLS		
1	Normal shape	Max. 2 small smooth VLS	1 A	1 B
2	Abnormal *Shape, Acrosome, Midpiece, Tail*	Max. 2 small smooth VLS	2 A	2 B
3	Normal	Deep VLS Acrosomal Vac.	3 A	
	Abnormal	Deep VLS Acrosomal Vac.		3 B
4	Normal	Deep Equatorial – Nuclear Vac.	4 A	
	Abnormal	Deep Equatorial – Nuclear Vac.		4 B

Two Strategies to Perform IMSI

We have adjusted our strategy for IMSI according to several criticisms. The first concerns prolonged exposure of the spermatozoa to a temperature of 37° C during the selection process, with negative consequences in terms of an increase in the rate of VLS [33]. However, using time-lapse recording, Neyer et al. [34] observed no changes in the morphology of the spermatozoa and no increase in the rate of VLS after 24 hours incubation at 37°C.

The second criticism is that prolonged selection time of male gametes may be detrimental to oocytes by promoting their aging with resulting overmaturity. The timing of oocyte pick-up (OPU) and preparation for IMSI is similar to that for the classical ICSI procedure. Nevertheless, if a previous spermocytogram diagnostic revealed cryptozoospermia and/or teratozoospermia, we may expect more time to be needed for sperm selection if we detect similar parameters on the day of the OPU. To avoid aging of the oocytes, it is advised to organize the OPU for after the sperm preparation. Following such a policy, oocyte injection can be done in the interval time between 36 hours and 40 hours post HCG, thus preventing overmaturation (ageing) of the oocytes.

The third criticism concerns the prolonged period of time for oocytes out of the incubator during spermatozoa selection. To avoid this, two strategies can be implemented: (i) a standard IMSI procedure employing two different microscopes, one to select the spermatozoa and the other for ICSI, or (ii) selection and injection are done on the IMSI microscope with maximum two oocytes at a time.

First Approach: Sperm Selection and Oocyte Injection on Two Different Microscopes

To reduce the time for the oocytes out of the incubator, spermatozoa are first selected using the Nomarski DIC optic and then injected on the ICSI microscope equipped with HMC optics.

Preparation of IMSI Dishes

Under sterile conditions, several drops are deposited on glass bottom dishes (Figure 5.1).

Sperm selection PVP drops (drop A) –– On the left side of the dish, one drop with a "snake" shape is deposited.

Table 5.2 Routine workflow chart for morphological evaluation (%) or quantitative assessment during IMSI (# oocytes injected)

Class	%	# Oocytes injected	Class	%	# Oocytes injected
1 A			1 B		
2 A			2 B		
3 A					
			3 B		
4 A					
			4 B		

Host-selected spermatozoa micro drops (B) –– Adjacent to the elongated drops of PVP (C), very small drops (< ~1 μL) of HTF-HEPES-HSA are deposited with a small stripper pipette. The micro drops will host the spermatozoa that will be selected in drop A until oocyte injection.

Sperm immobilization drops (C) –– A small drop of 10% PVP in which sperm immobilization will take place is deposited in the dish.

Oocyte injection drops (D) –– The right side of the dish contains five drops of HTF-HEPES-HSA in which oocyte injection will take place.

All drops are covered with sterile mineral oil.

Spermatozoa Selection and Injection

The procedure is performed at 37°C. An aliquot of prepared sperm is deposited in the upper part of drop A (volume depends on the concentration and motility). In case of severe asthenozoospermia, the sperm aliquot is deposited at least 1 hour before starting selection to allow time for the spermatozoa to swim out in the "snake" drop.

Motile spermatozoa are aspirated on the right edge of drop A (Figure 5.1(b): A) and placed in drop C for selection (Figure 5.1(b): B). The normal looking ones are then transferred in the host-selected spermatozoa micro drop (Figure 5.1 (b): C). The spermatozoa in drop B are released carefully to keep them motile until performing ICSI.

After collecting spermatozoa (if possible, 1.5 times the number of oocytes to inject), the dish is removed from the IMSI station and placed on a 37°C heating stage for 30 minutes.

After this period of incubation at 37°C, the oocytes are placed into the culture media (D) and ICSI is performed using a conventional Hoffman microscope at 400× magnification. Motile spermatozoa are aspirated from the pre-selected host drop (B), (Figure 5.1 (b): D) immobilized in the PVP drop (C) before injection.

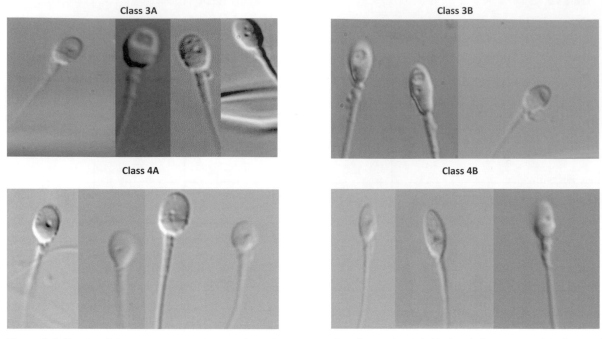

Figure 5.4 Class 3 and class 4 spermatozoa. Arrows indicate the presence of small, smooth VLS. (A black and white version of this figure will appear in some formats. For the color version, please refer to the plate section.)

Second Approach: Sperm Selection and Oocyte Injection on the IMSI Station

An aliquot of prepared sperm is deposited in the upper part of drop A (volume depends on the concentration and motility). In case of severe asthenozoospermia, the sperm aliquot is deposited at least 1 hour before starting selection to allow time for the spermatozoa to swim out in the "snake" drop.

When selection and injection are performed on the same microscope, a maximum of two oocytes are placed directly in the IMSI dish (drop D). According to the number of metaphase 2 oocytes, a minimum of two dishes are prepared (Figure 5.2). Before starting such an approach, the quality of the spermatozoa should be assessed to ensure that the time taken to select one class 1 or 2 spermatozoa (Table 5.1) will not exceed 2–3 minutes per oocyte. Sperm aspiration from drop A, immobilization and selection in drop C and injection in drop D are similar to that for classical ICSI. After injection, the two oocytes are deposited in culture medium and put in an incubator. The next two oocytes are placed in a new IMSI dish pre-warmed on the heating stage. After removal of the two injected oocytes, the first IMSI dish is placed on

a heating stage at 37°C until the next selection and injection step.

Conclusions

One of the most essential questions is not under which technical conditions the selection of spermatozoa should be recommended but rather whether we have to consider selecting the best spermatozoa and, if possible, exclude those carrying defects. Among a large panel of morphological abnormalities, this chapter considered abnormal spermatozoa carrying defects such as LNV or neck insertion defects.

Sperm quality is one of the main factors determining the fate of the embryo and sperm epigenetic signature plays a large role in deciding embryonic development [35]. The literature reveals a clear significant correlation between presence of LNV on the head and higher risk of DNA hypermethylation, but selection with improved optics (DIC) gives us an opportunity to identify and deselect this before oocyte injection. Such an approach would ultimately improve ART outcomes by decreasing the risk of birth defects, major malformations, and epigenetic diseases in the offspring as well for future generations through ICSI.

The introduction of IMSI has raised awareness among embryologists that, for ICSI, selection of sperm must be given proper attention. The application of IMSI leads to more blastocysts of higher quality, increasing the chance to transfer an embryo with high implantation potential and to achieve the birth of a healthy baby. But without optimal optics the probability of selecting a normal spermatozoon decreases as the severity of the teratozoospermia increases. Therefore, a combination of low responder and advanced maternal age (women >38 years, and reduced correction and reparation capacity) together with severe teratozoospermia is the first candidate for accurate sperm selection to increase the chances of obtaining one embryo with potentiality to further develop.

As the sperm proximal centriole plays a central role in establishment of the first and subsequent embryonic mitotic spindles, deselection of asymmetrical insertion of the neck is also mandatory.

There is now a trend to perform molecular diagnostics of the sperm (DNA fragmentation, chromatin decondensation, methylation pattern, aneuploidy). Why, therefore, would we deny IMSI, knowing that morphologically abnormal spermatozoa indirectly reflect the picture of their molecular status?

References

[1] Nikolettos N, Kiipker W, Demirel C, Schopper B, Blasig C, Sturm R, et al. Fertilization potential of spermatozoa with abnormal morphology. Hum Reprod. 1999; **14** (Suppl. 1), 47–70.

[2] Palermo G, Joris H, Devroey P, Van Steirteghem A. Pregnancies after intracytoplasmic injection of single spermatozoon into an oocyte. Lancet. 1992; **340**, 17–18.

[3] Schagdarsurengin U, Paradowska A, Steger K. Analysing the sperm epigenome: roles in early embryogenesis and assisted reproduction. Nat Rev Urol. 2012; **9**, 609–19.

[4] Cassuto NG, Hazout A, Bouret D, Balet R, Larue L, Benifla JL, et al. Low birth defects by deselecting abnormal spermatozoa before ICSI. Reprod Biomed Online. 2014; **28**, 47–53.

[5] Bartoov B, Berkovitz A, Eltes F. Selection of spermatozoa with normal nuclei to improve the pregnancy rate with intracytoplasmic sperm injection. N Engl J Med. 2001; **345**, 1067–8.

[6] Boitrelle F, Ferfouri F, Petit JM, Segretain D, Tourain C, Bergere M, et al. Large human sperm vacuoles observed in motile spermatozoa under high magnification: nuclear thumbprints linked to failure of chromatin condensation. Hum Reprod. 2011; **26**, 1650–8.

[7] Cassuto NG, Hazout A, Hammoud I, Balet R, Bouret D, Barak Y, et al. Correlation between DNA defect and sperm-head morphology. Reprod Biomed Online. 2012; **24**, 211–18.

[8] Vanderzwalmen P, Imbert R, Jareno-Martinez D, Stecher A, Vansteenbrugge A, Vanderzwalmen S, et al. Intracytoplasmic morphologically selected sperm injection. Nagy ZP et al., (eds), In Vitro Fertilization: A Textbook of Current and Emerging Methods and Devices (Second ed.) Springer Nature, Switzerland 2019; 415–428.

[9] Zheng H, Stratton C, Morozumi K, Jin J, Yanagimachi R, Yan W. Lack of Spem1 causes aberrant cytoplasm removal, sperm deformation, and male infertility. PNAS. 2007; **104**:6852–7.

[10] Gaspard O, Vanderzwalmen P, Wirleitner B, Ravet S, Wenders F, Eichel V, et al. Impact of high magnification sperm selection on neonatal outcomes: a retrospective study. J Assist Reprod Genet. 2018; **35**: 1113–21.

[11] Tavalaee M, Razavi S, Nasr-Esfahani MH. Influence of sperm chromatin anomalies on assisted reproductive technology outcome. Fertil Steril. 2009; **91**, 1119–26.

[12] Oliva R, Ballesca JL. Altered histone retention and epigenetic modifications in the sperm of infertile men. Asian J Androl. 2012; **14**, 239–240.

[13] Franco JG Jr, Mauri AL, Petersen CG, Massaro FC, Silva LF, Felipe V, et al. Large nuclear vacuoles are indicative of abnormal chromatin packaging in human spermatozoa. Int J Androl. 2012; **35**, 46–51.

[14] Boitrelle F, Albert M, Petit J-M, Ferfouri F, Wainer R, Bergere M, et al. Small human sperm vacuoles observed under high magnification are pocket-like nuclear concavities linked to chromatin condensation failure. Reprod Biomed Online. 2013; **27**, 201–11.

[15] Shaoqin G, Zhenghui Z, Xueqian Z, Yuan H. [Epigenetic modifications in human spermatozoon and its potential role in embryonic development.] Yi Chuan. 2014; **36**, 439–46.

[16] Schagdarsurengin U., Paradowska A., Steger K. Analysing the sperm epigenome: roles in early embryogenesis and assisted reproduction. Nat Rev Urol. 2012; **9**, 609–19.

[17] Marques CJ, Carvalho F, Sousa M, Barros A. Genomic imprinting in disruptive spermatogenesis. Lancet. 2004; **363**, 1700–2.

[18] Cassuto, G, Montjean D, Siffroi JP, Bouret D, Marzouk F, Copin H, Benkhalifa M. Different levels of DNA methylation detected in human sperms after

morphological selection using high magnification microscopy. BioMed Res Int. 2016; 1–7 http://dx .doi.org/10.1155/2016/6372171.

[19]   Van Blerkom J, Davis P. Evolution of the sperm aster after microinjection of isolated human sperm centrosomes into meiotically mature human oocytes. Hum Reprod. 1995; **10**, 2179–82.

[20]   Ugajin T, Terada Y, Hasgawa H, Nabeshima H, Suzuki K, Yaegashi N. The shape of the sperm midpiece in intracytoplasmic morphologically selected sperm injection relates sperm centrosomal function. J Assist Reprod Genet. 2010; **27**, 75–81.

[21]   Cassuto NG, Bouret D, Plouchart JM, Jellad S, Vanderzwalmen P, Balet R, et al. A new real-time morphology classification for human spermatozoa : a link for fertilization and improved embryo quality. Fertil Steril. 2009; **92**, 1616–25.

[22]   Leandri RD, Gachet A, Pfeffer J, Celebi C, Rives N, Carre–Pigeon F, et al. Is intracytoplasmic morphologically selected sperm injection (IMSI) beneficial in the first ART cycle? A multicentric randomized controlled trial. Andrology. 2013; **1**, 692–7.

[23]   Knez K, Zorn B, Tomazevic T, Vrtacnik–Bokal E, Virant–Klun I. The IMSI procedure improves poor embryo development in the same infertile couples with poor semen quality: a comparative prospective randomized study. Reprod Biol Endocrinol. 2011; **9**, 123.

[24]   Balaban B, Yakin K, Alatas C, Oktem O, Isiklar A, Urman B. Clinical outcome of intracytoplasmic injection of spermatozoa morphologically selected under high magnification: a prospective randomized study. Reprod Biomed Online. 2011; **22**, 472–6.

[25]   Setti AS, Braga DP, Figueira RC, Iaconelli A, Jr., Borges E. Intracytoplasmic morphologically selected sperm injection results in improved clinical outcomes in couples with previous ICSI failures or male factor infertility: a meta-analysis. Eur J Obstet Gynecol Reprod Biol. 2014; **183**, 96–103.

[26]   Shalom-Paz E, Anabusi S, Michaeli M, Karchovsky-Shoshan E, Rothfarb N, Shavit T, Ellenbogen A. Can intra cytoplasmatic morphologically selected sperm injection (IMSI) technique improve outcome in patients with repeated IVF-ICSI failure? A comparative study. Gynecol Endocrinol. 2015; **31**, 247–51.

[27]   Vanderzwalmen P, Hiemer A, Rubner P, Bach M, Neyer A, Astrid Stecher A, et al. Blastocyst development after sperm selection at high magnification is associated with size and number of nuclear vacuoles. Reprod Biomed Online. 2008; **17**, 617–27.

[28]   Knez K, Zorn B, Tomazevic T, Vrtacnik–Bokal E, Virant-Klun I. The IMSI procedure improves poor embryo development in the same infertile couples with poor semen quality: A comparative prospective randomized study Reprod Biol Endocrinol. 2011; **9**, 123–30.

[29]   Cassuto NG, Hazout A, Bouret D, Balet R, Larue L, Benifla JL, Viot G. Low birth defects by deselecting abnormal spermatozoa before ICSI. Reprod Biomed Online. 2014; **28**, 47–53.

[30]   Vanderzwalmen S, Jareno D, Vanderzwalmen P, Imber R, Murtinger M, Wirleitner B. Sperm selection for ICSI by morphology. Montag M. Morbeck D (Eds.) Principles of IVF Laboratory Practice: Optimizing Performance and Outcomes. Cambridge University Press 2017, 163–171.

[31]   Van der Zwalmen P, Bertin-Segal G, Geerts L, Debauche C, Schoysman R. Sperm morphology and IVF pregnancy rate: comparison between Percoll gradient centrifugation and swim-up procedures. Hum Reprod. 1991; **4**, 581–8.

[32]   Berkovitz A, Dekel Y, Goldstein R, Bsoul S, Machluf Y, Bercovich D. The significance of human spermatozoa vacuoles can be elucidated by a novel procedure of array comparative genomic hybridization. Hum Reprod. 2018; **33**, 563–71.

[33]   Peer S, Eltes F, Berkovitz A, Yehuda R, Itsykson P, Bartoov B. Is fine morphology of the human sperm nuclei affected by in vitro incubation at 37 C? Fertil Steril. 2007; **88**, 1589–94.

[34]   Neyer A, Vanderzwalmen P, Bach M, Stecher A, Spitzer D, Zech N. Sperm head vacuoles are not affected by in-vitro conditions, as analysed by a system of sperm-microcapture channels. Reprod Biomed Online. 2013; **26**, 368–77.

[35]   Denomme MM, McCallie BR, Parks JC, Schoolcraft WB, Katz–Jaffe MG. Alterations in the sperm histone-retained epigenome are associated with unexplained male factor infertility and poor blastocyst development in donor oocyte IVF cycles. Hum Reprod. 2017; **32**, 2443–55.

Chapter

6

Laser-Assisted ICSI

Roberta Maggiulli, Simona Alfano, Erminia Alviggi, Gemma Fabozzi, Danilo Cimadomo, Filippo Maria Ubaldi, and Laura Rienzi

Introduction

Since the achievement of the first pregnancy in 1992, intracytoplasmic sperm injection (ICSI) has been regarded as a prominent technological advancement that has revolutionized assisted reproductive technologies (ART), overturning the laboratory and clinical outcomes achieved until then with long-standing conventional in vitro fertilization (IVF) techniques.

This extremely successful technique is widely preferred to IVF as an insemination method because of its overall efficacy and reliability, primarily in the management of male factor infertility. Nevertheless, an increasing trend in the use of ICSI has been documented even when severe male factor is not the main indication, that is, in the management of couples with a history of failed fertilization, with a limited number of oocytes available or with borderline semen quality. Moreover, this trend has evolved in parallel to the increasing application of preimplantation genetic testing (PGT) and the involvement of cryopreserved or in vitro matured oocytes in ART [1]. The consistently high fertilization rates achieved opened the gate to a widespread application of ICSI to such an extent that according to the International Committee Monitoring Assisted Reproductive Technologies (ICMART) report, ICSI is used in around two-thirds of all ART treatment worldwide.

The Issue of Oocyte Degeneration

During conventional ICSI, a morphologically normal motile spermatozoon is selected and mechanically immobilized. Once the equatorial plane of the oocyte is focused, the zona pellucida is bypassed by the injection needle and a limited volume of oocyte cytoplasm is suctioned to induce breakage of the oolemma and activate the oocyte; the spermatozoon is then released within the oocyte cytoplasm and the injection needle is gently withdrawn [2]. Although conventional ICSI

is very effective in terms of fertilization rate, it has some technical drawbacks. Mechanical impairments to oocyte structures, such as the oolemma, cytoskeleton apparatus and meiotic spindle, may be involuntarily induced during penetration of the glass injection needle within the oocyte cytoplasm. Moreover, sudden (when lysis occurs immediately after withdrawal of the injection needle) or delayed (when no immediate sign of damage is visible but lysis is observed at the fertilization check) oocyte degeneration may be experienced during ICSI. Despite its popularity, ICSI still represents a highly demanding technique, with a defined learning curve to achieve sufficient expertise in performing the procedure at an acceptable standard and develop good proficiency to manage the heterogeneity of cases encountered. When skilled embryologists perform ICSI, the incidence of oocyte degeneration, estimated as the number of oocytes injured during ICSI and/or observed over the number of injected oocytes, is mainly deemed to be independent of the operator that performs the procedure. When Rosen and colleagues compared the ICSI outcomes of four experienced operators (6–10 years of experience) in 2006, no difference was reported with regard to oocyte survival [3]. Unexpected oocyte lysis is reportedly occurring between 0% and 30% of inseminated oocytes, even when ICSI is performed by an experienced embryologist, and extreme care is applied during the injection. Indeed, even when full technical competence is acquired, the incidence of oocyte degeneration should be monitored as a quality indicator of laboratory performances (key performance indicators, KPIs) [4]. According to the Vienna consensus on ART KPIs, suggested reference performance (competence) and target (benchmark) values for ICSI damage rate should be lower than 10% and 5%, respectively. The occurrence of an inconsistent and suboptimal ICSI technique with a degeneration rate that does not lie within the above-mentioned reference limits, may have a relevant clinical implication, especially for poor prognosis patients with a low number of oocytes retrieved, where the viability of every single oocyte must be preserved to maximize the efficacy of each treatment. The putative causes behind oocyte degeneration have been extensively reviewed by Rubino and colleagues [5] and are mainly ascribable to the patients' baseline characteristics and response to ovarian stimulation [3,6]. The hormonal environment induced by ovarian stimulation seems the presumptive cause of alteration of the composition of the outer layers of the oocytes, that is, the glycoprotein complex of the zona pellucida or the lipoproteic structure of the oolemma, and correlates with a higher incidence of degeneration after ICSI [6,7]. Moreover, the onset of unexpected technical pitfalls may induce deviance from optimal oocyte injection technique and subsequent irreversible oocyte damage: an excessive profound penetration of the injection needle into the oocyte may harm the distal region of the oolemma; similarly, the persistence of the spermatozoon on the spike of the injection pipette to release the gamete into the cytoplasm may require excessive detrimental oocyte manipulation to release the gamete into the cytoplasm. Lastly, any excessive pressure applied to the oocyte during injection may impair the cytoskeleton and therefore facilitate leakage of cytoplasm from the wound of the membrane with consequent gamete degeneration [8].

Fragile Oocytes

The oocyte membrane behavior and response to injection is a recognized predictor of oocyte survival after injection. In normal oocytes, the presence of the actin-tubulin cytoskeleton grants elasticity to the plasma membrane and confers to the oocyte the ability to survive the trauma induced by the injection. The pattern of a normal membrane response to injection consists of a funnel-shaped invagination of the oolemma followed by spontaneous breakage when the injection pipette is approximately located at the center of the oocytes. When the injection needle is withdrawn, the oocyte is then capable of sealing the breach and rearranging the organelles' ultrastructure to survive this invasive procedure. Otherwise, in fragile oocytes a membrane "sudden breakage" pattern is observed with an immediate tearing of the oolemma at the time of insertion of the injection pipette, occasionally accompanied by instantaneous leakage of the

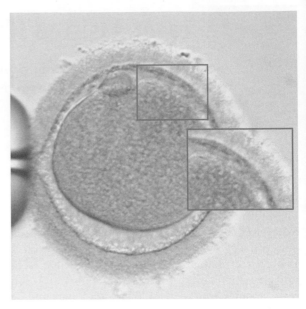

Figure 6.1 A fragile oocyte after ICSI. Cytoplasm leakage after ICSI is visible in the magnified box.

cytoplasm into the perivitelline space even before needle withdrawal [9] (Figure 6.1). Even when fragile oocytes survive the injection, their ability to achieve correct fertilization is remarkably reduced when compared to oocytes with other oolemma breakage patterns [9,10]. In this regard, a possible explanation for the reduced membrane resistance exhibited by fragile oocytes may be the absence of the protective effect of the funnel responsible for healing the membrane rupture thereby preventing cytoplasmic leakage. The discontinuity of the oolemma may affect the cortical component of the cytosol and subsequently the cytoskeleton, leading to disturbances in the microtubule apparatus which supports the chromatid segregation and extrusion of the polar body at the second meiotic division [6]. The above-mentioned hypothesis has been confirmed by further observations of a decreased incidence of cell degeneration after injection of oocytes displaying a persistent injection funnel compared to oocytes without such a persistent funnel. On the other hand, once fragile oocytes survive the injection procedure and correctly fertilize, their ability to develop as a blastocyst and support an ongoing pregnancy is comparable to normal oocytes [10]. The presence of a fragile oolemma with reduced elasticity is a common finding in murine oocytes [11], but occasionally reported also in a minority of human oocytes. In rare circumstances, however, most or even the totality of the oocytes injected may show an intrinsic fragility that results in deviations from the expected ICSI outcome because of increased oocyte lysis. When extensive oocyte degeneration occurs, the patients must face total fertilization failure and cycle cancellation. Obviously, the severity of these side effects is strictly dependent on each individual scenario and is less prominent in high-responder patients with a considerable number of oocytes available for insemination [12]. All these potential drawbacks of conventional ICSI encouraged embryologists to outline alternative methods to minimize oocyte trauma, leading to the development of a novel ICSI approach that involved a laser-drilled micro-opening of the zona pellucida before injection: the laser-assisted-ICSI (LA-ICSI).

LA-ICSI Procedure

In LA-ICSI protocol, all the steps preceding insemination, such as oocyte retrieval, sperm preparation and oocyte denudation, are performed according to standard protocols. As for conventional ICSI, each oocyte is immobilized by gentle aspiration on a holding pipette with the first polar body at the 6-o'clock position. This protocol requires a precise hole of 5–10 µm in diameter (Figure 6.2), which is made on the zona pellucida of the oocyte by a laser pulse, leaving intact its innermost layer. The hole produced expedites access of the injection needle containing the selected spermatozoon, which is then deposited into the cytoplasm. The employment of laser technology decreases the mechanical force required to penetrate the egg and

preserves the native morphology of the oocyte, even in the presence of morphological abnormalities such as increased zona pellucida thickness or excessive resistance to injection. In fact, LA-ICSI induces only a minimal deformation of the oocyte shape (Figure 6.3). However, besides the need for a costly laser, the presence of a hole in the zona pellucida throughout embryo preimplantation development might result in growth restriction, precocious hatching or monozygotic twinning [13]. To avoid these putative issues, Moser and colleagues conducted a prospective study on sibling oocytes from an unselected population of patients and tested a different approach for LA-ICSI: the zona pellucida was just thinned, and not totally drilled. Such an expedient allowed for lower degeneration and increased pregnancy rates after cleavage-stage embryo transfer [14]. To guarantee maximum safety during LA-ICSI and prevent the oolemma reaction, the inner layer is left intact (~0.5 µm) and the laser pulse applied is of short duration (2 ms), maintaining the maximum distance between the perivitelline space and the oolemma at the point of laser shot firing. The purpose of zona pellucida drilling is to thin its exterior layer avoiding the perforation of the inner layer. A tiny hole in the zona pellucida is created to allow the passage of the injection needle but the hole is not wide enough to cause embryo hatching.

Results of LA-ICSI

In the early 2000s, the clinical relevance of LA-ICSI was highlighted in two distinct papers [15,16] that reported successful clinical outcomes in patients who had previously suffered repeated ICSI failures because of oocyte degeneration. After these initial case reports, prospective studies were conducted showing consistently better results from LA-ICSI with respect to conventional ICSI in patients with a higher risk for fertilization failures, for example, with a history of increased incidence of oocyte degeneration (>20%) or remarkable sensitivity to the injection-induced damage [17–19]. The oocytes inseminated by LA-ICSI showed higher survival rates and two-pronucleated zygotes rates compared to sibling oocytes treated with conventional ICSI; similarly, also the embryo morphological quality on day 3 was better after LA-ICSI, suggesting minimized damage to subcellular oocyte components. More recently, in a RCT conducted in a general population of patients, Choi and colleagues performed a 70%

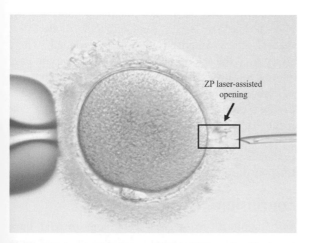

Figure 6.2 Laser-assisted zona pellucida (ZP) opening. The box highlights the hole on the ZP soon after exposure to the laser beam.

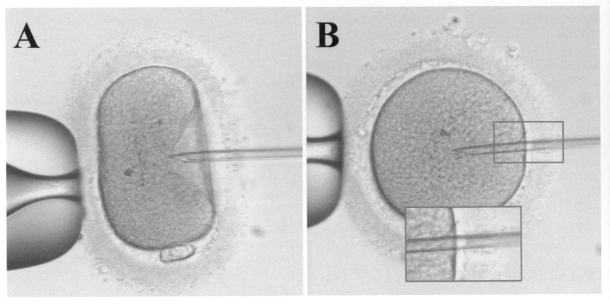

Figure 6.3 Oocyte characterized by a hard zona pellucida during (A) conventional ICSI and (B) laser-assisted ICSI.

zona thinning before ICSI and reported higher fertilization and pregnancy rates in patients both younger and older than 38 years [20]. A higher fertilization rate after LA-ICSI was also reported by Verza and colleagues in 2013 [21]. However, these data were not confirmed by Richter and colleagues' RCT on sibling oocytes published in 2006, in which LA-ICSI failed to provide a beneficial effect with respect to standard ICSI for any of the outcomes under investigation (i.e. fertilization, degeneration, embryo quality, compaction, blastocyst formation) [22]. In a more recent study published in 2016, Elhoussieny and colleagues randomized unselected patients to undergo either conventional-ICSI or LA-ICSI and did not report a benefit derived from the latter [23]. Figure 6.4 represents a summary of the conflicting results outlined by all these studies.

Laser Application and Safety Concerns

Several applications of laser-assisted technology in reproductive medicine have been proposed from the early 1990s promoting improvements and developments. However, when laser-assisted techniques were initially implemented, various concerns were raised about their safety. The oocytes hold most of the reproductive potential in humans, therefore it is pivotal to ensure the safety of techniques and avoid any putative damage. The main

concerns can be summarized as: (i) risk of inducing DNA damage, which may jeopardize oocyte competence to develop as a blastocyst and/or increase the incidence of single gene mutations; and (ii) length of laser exposure, which determines the diameter of the hole and increases local heating (the longer the exposure, the larger the diameter and higher the heating).

The mutagenicity-related issue mainly concerned the initial use of lasers with UV range wavelength. These were replaced by the last generation of infrared range emission-based lasers [24]. Specifically, the lasers in common use today are indium-gallium-arsenic-phosphorous (InGaAsP) semiconductor diode lasers that use infrared light at 1480 nm wavelength. These lasers avoid the risk of inducing DNA damage and have allowed for the widespread introduction of this tool into IVF laboratories. In fact, modern lasers are assembled as part of specialized microscope objectives of 40× or 20× magnification that can be installed on inverted microscopes with bright field, phase contrast and Hoffman modulation optics. This setup makes laser pulses easier to apply during ordinary manipulations [24].

Conclusion

Some applications of laser technology in ART have been successfully implemented, that is, embryo biopsy for preimplantation genetic testing, artificial

Comparison of clinical outcomes between C-ICSI and LA-ICSI according to different studies

C - conventional ICSI / LA - laser assisted ICSI

■ Oocyte degeneration rate   ■ Fertilization rate

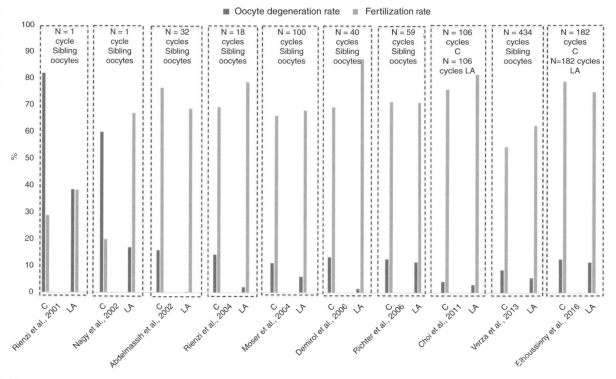

Figure 6.4 Summary of oocyte degeneration and fertilization rates achieved along the main studies that compared conventional-ICSI (C) to laser-assisted ICSI (LA). (A black and white version of this figure will appear in some formats. For the color version, please refer to the plate section.)

shrinkage, immobilization or selection of immotile spermatozoa, as well as LA-ICSI. Preliminary results from studies conducted in the early 2000s suggest that laser-assisted micro-drilling of the zona pellucida may be useful to make ICSI more successful when inseminating oocytes which are more prone to fertilization failure. Although this condition usually does not affect many couples, in case of full degeneration of all the injected oocytes, this leads to cycle cancellation. In these cases, LA-ICSI becomes a valuable option that deserves consideration.

The oolemma pattern and zona pellucida thickness are strongly related to oocyte survival and fertilization after ICSI. Both of these features depend on the hormonal milieu and the cause of infertility; therefore, adjusting ovarian stimulation and/or changing in vitro culture conditions might be beneficial, but LA-ICSI provides an immediately available solution [15,18]. Nevertheless, LA-ICSI has not been widely accepted by all clinics as some concern exists regarding its overall benefits. For

instance, in terms of oocyte survival, embryo quality or clinical results, in the unselected patient population [22]. Moreover, some authors have suggested that it is the strength and stretching capacity of the membrane under the zone pellucida and around the cells that are associated with a successful ICSI procedure, and that putative harm can be decreased through the use of excellent skills and high-quality injection needles [25].

Another effective way to prevent harm during ICSI, when oocytes characterized by fragile oolemma should be injected, is piezo-assisted ICSI [26]. With this method, a blunt injection needle operated by a piezo-electric device is used in a chosen population of patients characterized by enhanced oocyte fragility. Such a technique shows comparable benefits to LA-ICSI. However, LA-ICSI is still more convenient for all those laboratories already equipped with a microsurgical laser device, which might be exploited for IVF procedures other than ICSI (e.g. assisted hatching, artificial shrinkage, biopsy).

In conclusion, the efficacy of LA-ICSI compared to conventional ICSI in patients whose oocytes show a propensity for sudden oolemma breakage or a marked thickness of the zona pellucida, makes this method very useful to optimize the treatment by reducing oocyte damage and leading to better survival rates. This approach could provide patients with the highest level of care and optimize their chance of pregnancy.

References

[1] Rosenwaks Z, Pereira N. The pioneering of intracytoplasmic sperm injection: historical perspectives. Reproduction 2017;**154**:F71–7.

[2] Palermo G, Joris H, Devroey P, Van Steirteghem AC. Pregnancies after intracytoplasmic injection of single spermatozoon into an oocyte. Lancet 1992;**340**:17–18.

[3] Rosen MP, Shen S, Dobson AT, Fujimoto VY, McCulloch CE, Cedars MI. Oocyte degeneration after intracytoplasmic sperm injection: a multivariate analysis to assess its importance as a laboratory or clinical marker. Fertil Steril 2006;**85**:1736–43.

[4] ESHRE Special Interest Group of Embryology and Alpha Scientists in Reproductive Medicine. The Vienna consensus: report of an expert meeting on the development of ART laboratory performance indicators. Reprod Biomed Online 2017;**35**:494–510.

[5] Rubino P, Vigano P, Luddi A, Piomboni P. The ICSI procedure from past to future: a systematic review of the more controversial aspects. Hum Reprod Update 2016;**22**:194–227.

[6] Palermo GD, Alikani M, Bertoli M, Colombero LT, Moy F, Cohen J, *et al*. Oolemma characteristics in relation to survival and fertilization patterns of oocytes treated by intracytoplasmic sperm injection. Hum Reprod 1996;**11**:172–6.

[7] Ebner T, Yaman C, Moser M, Sommergruber M, Jesacher K, Tews G. A prospective study on oocyte survival rate after ICSI: influence of injection technique and morphological features. J Assist Reprod Genet 2001;**18**:623–8.

[8] Nagy ZP, Liu J, Joris H, Bocken G, Desmet B, Van Ranst H, *et al*. The influence of the site of sperm deposition and mode of oolemma breakage at intracytoplasmic sperm injection on fertilization and embryo development rates. Hum Reprod 1995;**10**:3171–7.

[9] Palermo GD, Cohen J, Alikani M, Adler A, Rosenwaks Z. Development and implementation of intracytoplasmic sperm injection (ICSI). Reprod Fertil Dev 1995;**7**:211–7; discussion 7–8.

[10] Mizobe Y, Oya N, Iwakiri R, Yoshida N, Sato Y, Onoue N, *et al*. Developmental ability of embryos produced from oocytes with fragile oolemma by intracytoplasmic sperm injection. J Assist Reprod Genet 2016;**33**:1685–90.

[11] Kimura Y, Yanagimachi R. Intracytoplasmic sperm injection in the mouse. Biol Reprod 1995;**52**:709–20.

[12] Liu J, Nagy Z, Joris H, Tournaye H, Smitz J, Camus M, *et al*. Analysis of 76 total fertilization failure cycles out of 2732 intracytoplasmic sperm injection cycles. Hum Reprod 1995;**10**:2630–6.

[13] Mantoudis E, Podsiadly BT, Gorgy A, Venkat G, Craft IL. A comparison between quarter, partial and total laser assisted hatching in selected infertility patients. Hum Reprod 2001;**16**:2182–6.

[14] Moser M, Ebner T, Sommergruber M, Gaisswinkler U, Jesacher K, Puchner M, *et al*. Laser-assisted zona pellucida thinning prior to routine ICSI. Hum Reprod 2004;**19**:573–8.

[15] Rienzi L, Greco E, Ubaldi F, Iacobelli M, Martinez F, Tesarik J. Laser-assisted intracytoplasmic sperm injection. Fertil Steril 2001;**76**:1045–7.

[16] Nagy ZP, Oliveira SA, Abdelmassih V, Abdelmassih R. Novel use of laser to assist ICSI for patients with fragile oocytes: a case report. Reprod Biomed Online 2002;**4**:27–31.

[17] Abdelmassih S, Cardoso J, Abdelmassih V, Dias JA, Abdelmassih R, Nagy ZP. Laser-assisted ICSI: a novel approach to obtain higher oocyte survival and embryo quality rates. Hum Reprod 2002;**17**:2694–9.

[18] Rienzi L, Ubaldi F, Martinez F, Minasi MG, Iacobelli M, Ferrero S, *et al*. Clinical application of laser-assisted ICSI: a pilot study. Eur J Obstet Gynecol Reprod Biol 2004;**115** Suppl 1:S77-9.

[19] Demirol A, Benkhalifa M, Sari T, Gurgan T. Use of laser-assisted intracytoplasmic sperm injection (ICSI) in patients with a history of poor ICSI outcome and limited metaphase II oocytes. Fertil Steril 2006;**86**:256–8.

[20] Choi KH, Lee JH, Yang YH, Yoon TK, Lee DR, Lee WS. Efficiency of laser-assisted intracytoplasmic sperm injection in a human assisted reproductive techniques program. Clin Exp Reprod Med 2011;**38**:148–52.

[21] Verza S, Schneider DT, Siqueira S, Esteves S. Laser-assisted intracytoplasmic sperm injection (LA-ICSI) is safe and less traumatic than conventional ICSI. Fertil Steril 2013;**100**:Supplement.

[22] Richter KS, Davis A, Carter J, Greenhouse SJ, Mottla GL, Tucker MJ. No advantage of laser-assisted over conventional intracytoplasmic

sperm injection: a randomized controlled trial [NCT00114725]. J Exp Clin Assist Reprod 2006;**3**:5.

[23] Elhoussieny A, El Mandooh M, Bahaa-Eldin A, Fathy H. Laser assisted zona thinning versus the conventional mechanical method for intracytoplasmic sperm injection in ICSI programs. *Int J Obstet Gynaecol Res* 2016;**3**:221–39.

[24] Davidson LM, Liu Y, Griffiths T, Jones C, Coward K. Laser technology in the ART laboratory: a narrative review. Reprod Biomed Online 2019;**38**:725–39.

[25] Tannus S, Son WY, Gilman A, Younes G, Shavit T, Dahan MH. The role of intracytoplasmic sperm injection in non-male factor infertility in advanced maternal age. Hum Reprod 2017;**32**:119–24.

[26] Furuhashi K, Saeki Y, Enatsu N, Iwasaki T, Ito K, Mizusawa Y, *et al.* Piezo-assisted ICSI improves fertilization and blastocyst development rates compared with conventional ICSI in women aged more than 35 years. Reprod Med Biol 2019;**18**:357–61.

Chapter

7

Piezo: The Add-On to Standardize ICSI Procedure

Tetsunori Mukaida, Kenichiro Hiraoka, Hideaki Watanabe, Kiyotaka Kawai, and Csaba Pribenszky

Background and History

Within 2 years of reports of the first success in humans, the number of ongoing pregnancies from ICSI was around 600 worldwide; however, oocyte survival and fertilization rates following sperm microinjection were (and still are) largely variable among institutions and embryologists [1–3]. Animal experiences were needed to further improve the technique, with mouse being the best candidate. However, the conventional spiked pipette used for ICSI cannot break the mouse oolemma because of its extraordinary flexibility, even when the pipette tip is pushed deep into the oocyte, reaching the cortex of the opposite side. As a consequence, use of the conventional ICSI technique rarely fertilizes mouse oocytes.

The direct piezoelectric effect was discovered by the Curie brothers, Pierre and Jacques in 1880. The word "piezoelectric" is derived from the Greek *piezein*, which means to squeeze, press, or push. The phenomena itself is the ability of certain materials to generate an electric charge in response to applied mechanical stress, or vice versa: the generation of stress (movement) when an electric field is applied. Kimura and Yanagimachi, at the University of Hawaii, School of Medicine, USA, aimed to improve the mouse ICSI technique by fixing a piezo module to the holder of the injection microcapillary. By applying controlled electricity to the module, mechanical pulses were generated and transferred to the holder. The vibrating, drilling movement was transmitted to the microcapillary and hence to the zona pellucida (ZP) and further on to the oolemma, making possible the piercing of both barriers. Thus, microinjection of mouse oocytes could be achieved with high survival and fertilization rates.

The idea of using piezo or other electro-mechanic effect to aid the microinjection procedures was not entirely new. In the early 1980s, it was reported that

piezoelectric drivers could be used for cell puncture [4]. Similarly, in the early 1990s, an electromechanically operated micropipette holder called the "Sonic sward" was developed to overcome the difficulties in penetrating the ZP during the procedure of SUZI [5]. The Sonic sward used an ultrasound pulse to "stab" the ZP. Fromm and co-workers used a commercial piezoelectric element made from a stacked column of monomorph ceramic discs that they fixed to a micromanipulator [4]. Kimura and Yanagimachi, whom we can credit with establishing the protocol for piezo-ICSI, used a brand developed for micropositioning micromanipulators, the PMM-01, by Prima Meat Packers (now called PrimeTech Ltd., Japan) [6]. This tool was further developed to be the first device on the market for piezo-ICSI. In their work, Kimura and Yanagimachi also described a way of immobilizing sperm using piezo, and they highlighted that application of a mercury droplet near the tip of the injection pipette increased the penetrative capability of the pipette through the ZP and oolemma and decreased the injuries made to the oocytes as a result of the procedure. In fact, today's method of piezo-ICSI is based on the principles and protocol described in their 1995 paper in *Biology of Reproduction* [6].

In 1996, again at the University of Hawaii, Huang and colleagues applied the piezo-ICSI technique to human oocytes for the first time, and reported that the fertilization rate of eggs injected and the rate of damaged oocytes and abnormal embryos, moreover the pregnancy rate, were comparable to conventional ICSI as reported in literature [7]. The achieved fertilization rate was 60.5%, which is indeed very low compared to results expected from a clinic currently. In 1999, Yanagida and colleagues reported significant improvement of both survival (81% vs. 89%) and fertilization (54% vs. 70%) rates when compared to conventional ICSI; however, the control group had suboptimal results [8]. Takeuchi and colleagues published a comparison of conventional and piezo-ICSI in 2001. In the study the control results were as expected: piezo-ICSI on human oocytes resulted in a fertilization rate of 90.3% compared to 83.1% with conventional ICSI, cleavage rates were comparable between the two groups (piezo-ICSI: 88.1%, conventional: 84.6%) [9]. Piezo-ICSI has since become standard in various fields of biotechnology procedures in which cell injection is required. The human ART field had to wait another 14 years for the next landmark publication: Hiraoka and Kitamura aimed to assess the clinical efficiency of piezo-ICSI and to improve the method of injection. They compared use of conventional ICSI to piezo-ICSI using normal micropipettes with flat tips, and did not report any differences in outcomes. However, significantly higher survival, fertilization, good-quality day-3 embryo rates and numerically better pregnancy, and live birth rates were obtained using piezo-ICSI if a micropipette of ultra-thin wall thickness was used [10]. Thus, Hiraoka and colleagues further standardized the piezo-ICSI technique by specifying the injecting micro-capillary for the setup. Of note, Nakayama and colleagues have pinpointed another application of the piezo-equipped microinjector, namely assisted hatching. In this application, about five times higher intensity and speed is applied compared to that used for piezo-ICSI. The injection needle vibrates vigorously; during the vibration, the orbit of movement of the needle tip is round. This circular movement carves a defined area into the ZP, which is conical in shape and about 30 μm in diameter. This procedure is used to thin the zona, thereafter, a hole of 20 μm in diameter is created in the thinned zona, using weaker vibrations [11].

Regardless of the limited number of publications and the lack of practical experiences, the piezo-ICSI technique has started to gain attention in human ART in Japan; an exponentially/steadily increasing number of clinics are using it since around 2013. In this chapter, we summarize experiences gained with piezo-ICSI so far and aim to make tangible what this technique could offer to IVF laboratories.

Mode of Action

In the piezo-ICSI application, a piezo element (actuator) is attached firmly to the microcapillary holder and a flat-tipped, thin-walled microcapillary is used instead of a spiked one. The flat tip of the micropipette is pressed gently to the ZP so that the circular edge of

the pipette tip makes continuous contact with the zona. The piezo-electric materials inside of the actuator convert electric energy into mechanical energy, thus the piezo-electric effect is generated (crystal deformation in response to an externally applied voltage). When voltage is applied, the piezo crystal creates a force as it tries to extend. The controller voltage is used to regulate the piezo force. A typical controlling unit allows the user to adjust three parameters of a given series of pulses: amplitude, frequency and duration. As these three parameters are adjusted, the user can tailor the series of pulses appropriately for penetrating the ZP and the membrane. The axial force series initiates oscillations at the tip of the holder, and ultimately on the injection pipette. As high voltages from the controller unit connected to the actuator cause only small changes in the width of the crystals, this can be manipulated with better-than-micrometer precision, making piezo crystals an important tool for positioning objects, in this case the microcapillary holder, with great accuracy. The extremely rapid signals propel the holder together with the microcapillary forward, producing ultra-fast sub-micron axial and also lateral momentum in a precise and rapid movement that allows for penetration of the opposing biological structures. In attempts to understand the governing physics, the considerable lateral tip oscillations of the injection pipette were also considered to be an important role in the piercing effect [12].

The application of "operating liquid" (heavy liquid – primarily/historically a mercury column inside the distal part of the micropipette) is advised for safe piercing of the oocyte. There is not yet a scientific consensus about the physical principles of the operating liquid, but it is likely that the added value in terms of safe piercing arise from its:

- modulating effect (reducing the amplitude) on the lateral vibrations of the microcapillary (ensuring a safe use on the oocytes)
- intensifying axial bursts
- creation of minimal negative pressure within the microcapillary when it touches the ZP.

It was reported that use of mercury inside the microcapillary significantly improved oocyte survival and fertilization rates and made procedures repeatable and robust [6].

Application of piezoelectric principles in the ICSI procedure provides the following benefits:

The finest resolution of movement: A piezoelectric actuator can produce extremely fine position changes down to the nanometer range. The smallest changes in operating voltage are converted into smooth movements. Motion is not influenced by friction.

Fastest response time: Piezo actuators offer the fastest response time available, in the microsecond range. Acceleration rates of more than 10 000 g can be obtained.

No electromagnetic field: Piezo actuators do not produce magnetic fields nor are they affected by magnetic fields.

Extreme durability: A piezo actuator has neither gears nor rotating shafts. Its movement is based on solid state dynamics. Endurance tests conducted on piezo actuators have shown no change in performance even after several billion cycles.

Clean room compatible: Piezo actuators are ceramic elements that do not need any lubricants and show no wear. They produce zero volatile organic compounds (VOCs).

Thus, the piezo-electric actuator offers the operator a highly repeatable motion with ultra-fine resolution [13].

The Operating Liquid

As mentioned, application of an "operating liquid" is advised for a safe and effective piercing procedure. The piezo-driven drilling effect is observed if there is media or oil only within the microcapillary; however, the efficacy is notably lower and there is a higher ratio of oocyte degeneration. The presence of a small amount of heavy liquid as an operating liquid inside the microcapillary helps the procedure of piezo-ICSI by minimizing and stabilizing lateral vibrations of the pipette tip, intensifying axial vibrations and generating a slight vacuum. It was shown that a small droplet of operating liquid (mercury) in the pipette creates higher shear forces at the membrane–pipette interface [14].

Mercury

The most evident and widely used heavy liquid as an operating liquid is mercury; however, its toxic effect was a big obstacle for safe use, and it is a definite no-go in human laboratories. Only few alternative fluid materials have been identified as possible candidates to replace mercury, which can provide sufficiently high density and low viscosity to moderate piezo effects, preventing injection-induced damage to the eggs. To date, the candidates found and used are fluorocarbons (perfluorocarbon liquids – PFCLs) and fluoroethers, namely Fluorinert and Novec.

Fluorinert and Novec (3M)

The fluorocarbons and fluoroethers used for piezo-ICSI of human (and animal) oocytes are from the Fluorinert and Novec families, produced by 3M (St. Paul, MN, USA). Fluorinert contains a mixture of fully fluorinated compounds together with a fraction of underfluorinated impurities. PFCLs, in general, are clear, colorless, odorless, non-flammable fluids having a viscosity similar to water. They are thermally and chemically stable, compatible with most sensitive materials, including metals or plastics, and are practically non-toxic through normal routes of industrial exposure. They have low surface tension and essentially no solvent action on non-fluorinated compounds. Water solubility is in the order of a few parts per million.

These liquids have been used in the electronics industry for over 40 years in a wide variety of applications, mainly in heat transfer, thermal management in various processes, equipment manufacturing applications and precision cleaning as lubricant deposition solvents for medical devices. When the product is used for applications in which the finished device is implanted into the human body, no residual Fluorinert solvent remains on the parts. Fluorinert has zero ozone depletion potential (ODP), but high global warming potential (GWP) and long atmospheric lifetime. As such, it should be carefully managed to minimize emissions, by employing good conservation practices, and by implementing recovery, recycling and/or proper disposal procedures.

A new liquid was introduced by 3M recommended for use as a replacement for perfluorocarbons: Novec 7300, a segregated hydrofluoroether, a non-flammable, thermally stable, non-ozone depleting liquid, with a more favorable GWP. It is also used as an alternative operating liquid for Fluorinert during piezo-ICSI.

As the producer of both Fluorinert and Novec, 3M discloses in its Safety Data Sheet that "3M Electronics Markets Materials Division (EMMD) will not knowingly sample, support, or sell its products for incorporation in medical and pharmaceutical products and applications in which the 3 M product will be temporarily or permanently implanted into humans or animals." The recommended uses, as stated, are as heat transfer agents, cooling agents, electrical insulators, solvents and laboratory chemicals, for industrial and professional use only. These are not intended for use as a medical device or drug.

An operating liquid is essential for the standard and effective piezo-ICSI procedure. The operating liquid, inside the microcapillary is in direct contact with the medium holding the sperm. Although the area of contact between the two liquids is very small (the area of the cross-section of the micropipette), accidental spill can also occur into the media holding the oocytes, sperm and presumptive zygotes. Consequently, the ideal operating liquid would be a pure, defined material with zero cytotoxicity. The unidentified constituents of Fluorinert and Novec and the undefined impurities coming essentially from their manufacturing processes, pose a risk for safe operation and an obstacle to human registration and widespread use of the technique.

Very recently, a new operating liquid has been developed that is completely free of toxic impurities and constituents. The studies show zero cytotoxicity and an improved efficacy in the piezo-ICSI procedure. For safe operations and also for regulatory purposes, the operating liquid has to be chemically inert, defined and pure, free of impurities. Fully fluorinated carbons (perfluorocarbon) contain only carbon and fluorine, with inert, favorable physical properties for piezo-ICSI. Among many, perfluoro-n-octane (PFNO) proved to be the most effective for piezo-ICSI (Pribenszky et al., unpublished results). However, under-fluorinated toxic compounds are essentially created during production even with PFNO. Impurities, perfluorocarbonic acids, C-H compounds, fluorinated alcohols and perfluorfuran altogether define the cytotoxicity and all are present in the currently used operating liquids, and, in lower quantities, even in PFNO. We

further processed and purified PFNO by a proprietary method and turned it into a pure, single-molecule medical product, increasing the opportunity for widespread use of piezo-ICSI in regulated human IVF.

The Micropipette

Piezo-ICSI application requires a special type of flat-tipped micropipette. Different types of these pipettes are available on the market from Origio (Humagen; Cooper Surgical), Eppendorf and Prime Tech:

Piezo Drill Tip Mouse ICSI capillary with blunt end tip, inner diameter (ID): 6 μm, angle: 25° (Eppendorf, Germany)

Piezo Drill Micropipettes ID: from 5 μm to 20 μm, angle 15–25° (Origio/Humagen/CooperSurgical, USA)

PINU06-20 FT, ID: 4.5 μm, angle 20° or 25° (Prime Tech, Japan).

As referred to in Table 7.2, there are critical attributes for a micropipette such as wall thickness and angle for successful piezo-ICSI in the human. Hiraoka and Kitamura [10,15] published details of the importance of the ultra-thin pipette wall (inner diameter: 5.1 μm, wall thickness: 0.45 μm) by comparing its efficacy to a standard sized micropipette used to perform piezo-ICSI (inner diameter: 5.25 μm, wall thickness: 0.85 μm). Oocyte survival after ICSI, fertilization rate, good-quality day-3 embryo rate, pregnancy, implantation and live birth rates of conventional ICSI, piezo-ICSI with standard micropipette and piezo-ICSI with ultra-thin micropipette were compared retrospectively in their study (Table 7.1). Results showed that an ultra-thin-walled flat-tipped micropipette was needed to confer low oocyte degeneration after

Table 7.1 Retrospective comparison of ICSI done in the conventional way (c-ICSI) or piezo-ICSI with normal flat-tipped or ultra-thin micropipettes

	c-ICSI	p-ICSI with normal pipette	p-ICSI with ultra-thin pipette
Number of oocytes injected	624	717	769
Oocytes survived after ICSI, %	90 [a]	95 [b]	99 [c]
Oocytes fertilized, %	68 [a]	75 [b]	89 [c]
Good-quality D3 embryos, %	37 [a]	43 [b]	55 [c]
Implantation rate, %	19 [a]	21 [a]	31 [b]

[a,b,c] different superscripts show significant difference between the groups at a given endpoint [10].

Table 7.2 Comparison of <u>materials</u> used in conventional ICSI and piezo-ICSI

	Conventional ICSI	Piezo-ICSI
Pipette type – angle	Generally between 20° and 40°, usually > 30°	< 25° Important as the lower the angle the better the transmission of the force.
Pipette type – tip	Spiked	Flat
Pipette type – wall thickness	Not specified, as the tip is spiked. Usually the thickness of the pipette wall is ~1 μm	Standard flat pipette has suboptimal results, ultra-thin is preferred
Injector type	Oil or air injector	Air is highly preferable because of significantly lower preparation time and less wasted material
Fluid used within the pipettes	PVP (5–10%) or media	PVP (5–7%) and/or media plus the operating liquid
Final adjustments of the pipettes	Check and modify alignment and angle	Check and modify alignment and angle. Then adjust the piezo pulses by observing the vibration of the tip and the meniscus within the pipette
Hardware	Standard setup	Additional hardware: two pedals for initiating pulses; a controller and an injector with piezo

ICSI Angle Options
0.5–0.7 mm
Angle
15°, 20°, 25°, 30°, 35°, 40°, 45°

thickness — 0.45μm
5.1 μm
6 μm

Mineral oil
Oil injector

ICSI, high fertilization and D3 good embryo quality. Implantation and live birth rates were also reported to be significantly higher for the ultra-thin group; however, these numbers were insufficient to draw strong conclusions.

The authors concluded that a pipette with an ultra-thin wall is needed for an effective piezo application. To date, the only product where wall thickness is specified and guaranteed is Prime Tech's ultra-thin micropipette.

Procedures

Conventional ICSI is performed by mechanical penetration of ZP followed by the membrane of the oocyte, using a spiked micropipette.

Procedures can differ greatly between practices. However, in general, polyvinylpyrrolidone (PVP) is used to ensure better control of the sperm because of the high viscosity of PVP. The most common approach to immobilize sperm is by mechanical breakage of the tail by pressing it against the bottom of a dish with a fine swift movement of the injection pipette. The immobilized sperm are then aspirated, usually tail first, into the injection pipette. Surplus PVP is expulsed from the micropipette away from the injection site when bringing the spermatozoon to the tip of the injection needle and before bringing the injection pipette close to the injection site of the oocyte. The injection pipette is then pushed through the ZP with a steady force applied manually by the operator. An important determinant of successful ICSI is reported to be breakage of the oocyte membrane by aspirating the membrane together with cytoplasm into the injection pipette [2], although not every research group has reached the same conclusion. In 2001, Dumoulin et al. showed that the type of membrane breakage does have a significant effect on fertilization rate: a lower fertilization rate was reported when there was no or immediate breakage of the membrane, while a higher fertilization rate was observed when the membrane broke following suction application. Furthermore, in cases where the breakage was obtained immediately, there were higher degeneration rates [16].

Not only does the manner of penetrating the ZP or the oolemma differ between users, but different oocytes seem to respond differently to the same stimulus and hence practice should be adjusted based on the uniqueness of the physicochemical characteristics of an oocyte as they are experienced empirically during the injection. In other words, it is uncertain how an oocyte will react to a harsher or smoother approach of injection technique, and hence flexibility during the procedure is key [17]. After the procedure, the micropipette is retreated from the oocyte.

Piezo-assisted injection includes a few steps, which are different from those of conventional ICSI. The preparation steps include the following actions:

1. Loading of the operating liquid into the injecting microcapillary:

About 10–15 μL of operating liquid is loaded into the injecting microcapillary. The most common and fastest technique is to grab a 1 mL syringe, fix a gel loading tip or microloader tip (Eppendorf) to the syringe, aspirate ~0.5 mL from the operating liquid, then backfill the injecting microcapillary by inserting the plastic loading tip into the large, back opening of the micropipette and inject an amount that occupies ~1–1.5 cm in the thick part of the glass microcapillary (Figure 7.1).

A further tip for backfilling the microcapillary is to take ~50 μL of operating liquid into the tip of a 100 μL pipette, then fix a microloader (Eppendorf) onto the 100 μL pipette tip, then use this setup to backload the injecting glass microcapillary. It is important to avoid air bubbles (Figure 7.2).

2. Fixing the injecting microcapillary into the micropipette holder

Follow the same protocol for fixing and adjustment as done during conventional ICSI. However, for piezo-ICSI the angle of the pipette is ~25°, so attention must be paid during the first setup to adjust the angle of the arm of the micromanipulator accordingly. It is advised to use an air injector.

3. Adjusting (verifying) the piezo function (checkpoint 1.)

Push the operating liquid, using the air injector, to the end of the glass microcapillary, and create a droplet at the tip. Initiate pulsations using the pedal to confirm the vibration of the pipette tip. Parameters can be readjusted under visual observation of the effect (Figure 7.3).

4. Aspirating the sperm holding medium

PVP or other sperm holding medium used according to

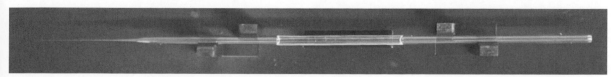

Figure 7.1 Operating liquid loaded into the injecting microcapillary. (A black and white version of this figure will appear in some formats. For the color version, please refer to the plate section.)

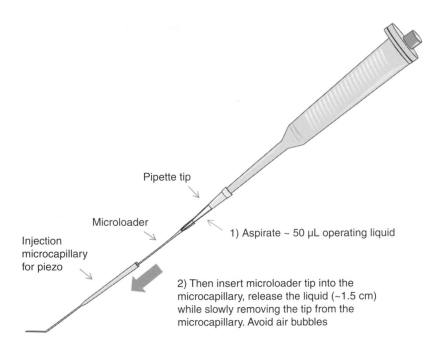

Figure 7.2 Backloading the injecting microcapillary with the operating liquid. (A black and white version of this figure will appear in some formats. For the color version, please refer to the plate section.)

Pipette tip

Microloader

Injection microcapillary for piezo

1) Aspirate ~ 50 μL operating liquid

2) Then insert microloader tip into the microcapillary, release the liquid (~1.5 cm) while slowly removing the tip from the microcapillary. Avoid air bubbles

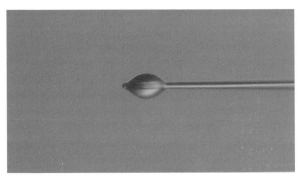

Figure 7.3 First checkpoint of the piezo function. (A black and white version of this figure will appear in some formats. For the color version, please refer to the plate section.)

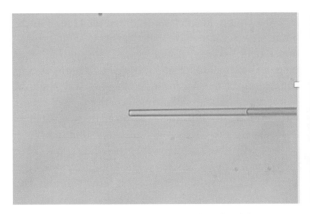

Figure 7.4 Phase border of the operating liquid and the sperm holding medium. (A black and white version of this figure will appear in some formats. For the color version, please refer to the plate section.)

the SOP of the clinic, should be aspirated in a way that it is in direct contact with the operating liquid (Figure 7.4).

5. Adjusting (verifying) the piezo function (checkpoint 2)

Initiate pulsations using the pedal to confirm the vibration of the interphase between the operating liquid and the sperm holding medium. Parameters can be readjusted under visual observation of the effect (Figure 7.4).

6. Sperm immobilization

A motile spermatozoon is aspirated, tail first, into the injection pipette, then two to three piezo-pulses are

applied while the sperm is let out of the micropipette with the tail of the sperm touching the edge of the tip of the micropipette (Figure 7.5).

7. Penetrating the zone pellucida

After sperm immobilization, the entire length of the spermatozoon is aspirated a couple of millimeters into the pipette. After bringing the micropipette tip to ZP of the oocyte at the 3 o'clock position, the pipette is excited by several piezo-pulses while being pushed

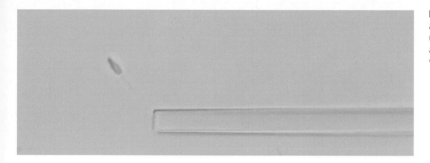

Figure 7.5 Immobilization of a spermatozoon by the piezo technique. (A black and white version of this figure will appear in some formats. For the color version, please refer to the plate section.)

through the zona using a gentle, steady pressure through the arm of the micromanipulator. When the tip of the pipette had passed through the zona, a cylindrical piece of the zona will remain within the pipette that should be expelled outside of the oocyte (in some practices it is expelled into the perivitelline space). After this, the spermatozoon is pushed forward until its head is at the tip of the pipette. The pipette is then advanced slowly and steadily through the ooplasm till it traverses ~80% of the distance of the oocyte itself (the oolemma can stretch that much without being broken). Upon application of a single piezo-pulse, the oolemma is punctured at the pipette tip, as indicated by its rapid relaxation. The spermatozoon is then gently released into the cytoplasm with the minimum amount of media, while the pipette is gently withdrawn from the oocyte. The fertilization process is thus complete (Figure 7.6).

Conditions That May Interfere with the Efficacy of Piezo-ICSI

Introducing piezo-ICSI into the workflow of the IVF laboratory yields promise for standardizing ICSI procedures and improving ICSI outcomes. However, consideration must be given to a few conditions that could interfere with the standardized setup and workflow (Table 7.3).

The flawless transfer of piezo vibrations from the piezo element to the injecting microcapillary is fundamentally important. Many factors can disturb this physical process by reducing intensity (drilling capacity), but these could be compensated for by changing the setup on the controlling unit. Special laboratory arrangements can exist that prevent the effective use of piezo, for example soft flooring can take away the strength of the pulse and prevent optimal performance of piezo-ICSI

(this may even be a cause for compete malfunction). A suboptimal setup could include wooden floors covered by plastic linoleum (as is often the case in Japan), especially if the manipulator table is placed far from the supporting walls and beams and the wooden floor is not laid directly on top of the concrete flooring. The harder the floor, the better the piezo effect. In the case of soft flooring, a solution could be to place a thick steel sheet under the legs of the micromanipulator table. More solid micromanipulators (XenoWorks or Takanome brands) may improve the situation but classic anti-vibration tables do not solve this issue. Electric anti-vibration tables such as the desktop active vibration isolation frame (Kurashiki Kako Co. Ltd., Japan), however, may eliminate the effect of suboptimal flooring. Thus, a combination of a hard floor plus an active anti-vibration frame and strong micromanipulator provides the safest operation and best support for piezo-ICSI.

The type of micromanipulator used for ICSI is also a variable. Major brands on the IVF market are Narishige (Japan), Takanome (a brand of Narishige), XenoWorks (Sutter Instrument, USA), TransferMan (Eppendorf, Germany) and Integra (ex-RI/Origio, Denmark). In general, Narishige and TransferMan work well; however, they do not have fixed positions for placing and fixing the pipette holders. Brands such as Takanome or XenoWorks are stronger, stiffer, easier to adjust in terms of angle and can also compensate partly for soft flooring. Takanome also provides a fixed and stable position for the pipette holders. All of these features support the proper functioning of piezo-ICSI.

Another variable is the oocyte itself. The elasticity and fragility of the oolemma can differ individually, and cases exist in which the oolemma is extra-fragile. In such case, piezo-ICSI does provide a solution as the blunt pipette tip and its steady, slow progress into the oocyte during the ICSI procedure avoids accidental rupture of the oolemma and disruption of cellular

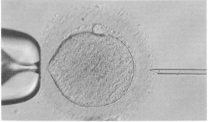
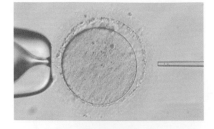

1) Piercing the zone pellucida

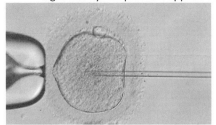
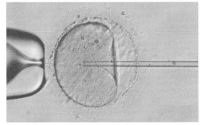

2) During c-ICSI a notable deformation of the oocyte is observed while there is significantly less pressure applied during piezo-ICSI

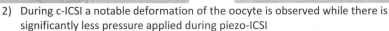

3) The micropipette is advanced to about 4/5 of the oocyte, stretching the membrane

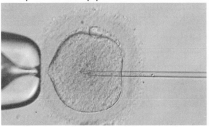
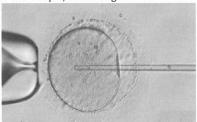

4) The oolemma and the cytoplasm is aspirated into the micropipette during c-ICSI whereas a single piezo pulse opens the membrane during piezo-ICSI (no aspiration is needed)

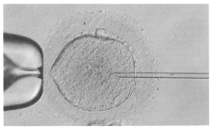
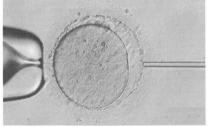

5) The micropipette is gently extracted after the sperm injection

Figure 7.6 Steps of conventional ICSI and piezo-ICSI. (A black and white version of this figure will appear in some formats. For the color version, please refer to the plate section.)

Table 7.3 Comparison of techniques used in conventional ICSI and piezo-ICSI

	Conventional ICSI	Piezo-ICSI
Preparation of the injector	Inserting the micropipette into the injector, aspiration of media	First backfilling the pipette with the operation liquid then all the steps as in c-ICSI
Manipulating with the injector	Different from place to place, user by user	Standard, steady, slow movements with the injector
Immobilization of the sperm	Mechanical breakage of the tail by pressing it against the bottom of the dish with a fine swift movement of the injection pipette	Sperm is aspirated into the pipette, then two piezo pulses are applied while the sperm tail touches the edge of the micropipette. (or the conventional technique)
Injecting the sperm into the oocyte	Movements and actions by the operator not standardized. Aspiration of the oolemma is advised for membrane breakage	Steady and slow progress forward through the zona (release the zona plug outside of the oocyte), slow progress into the cytoplasm, a single pulse then release of the sperm
Orientating the injection and the effect on the microtubules (spindle)	Orientating is important, the sharp tip and the aspiration of the cytoplasm may pose damage for the spindle or cytoskeleton	The slow progress with the blunt tip micropipette into the cytoplasm, the single piezo pulse to rupture the oolemma and the fact that no cytoplasm aspiration is necessary ensures safe procedures. Nevertheless positioning is important to avoid the spindle area

organelles. Special settings of the piezo-ICSI device can be applied for fragile oocytes.

Different conditions might be compensated for by adjustments of the controller (intensity/speed). The controlling unit is used to adjust the intensity of the axial vibration and the speed of the pulses. Different setups of the piezo element/micropipette holder/mount and type of liquids inside the micropipette can behave differently within the same settings. Intensity means the level of pulse strength applied. Speed means the number of pulses within a time-frame. Different setups can be fixed for piercing of the ZP or the oolemma. Settings for the ZP would usually be of higher intensity and a series of pulses, whereas for the oolemma a single pulse of milder intensity works better. There are recommended settings for different applications; however, the values can be finetuned based on the requirements of the local setup. Readjustment of the settings on the controlling unit can compensate for the variations caused by the different setups.

Summary of Clinical Experiences

Once the piezo-ICSI technique is set up within the lab routine, the ICSI technique itself can be standardized and consequently will provide more robust and increased success rates. According to general considerations, the benefits of piezo-ICSI include an increased fertilization rate, a decreased ratio of lyzed oocytes after ICSI, more embryos to cryopreserve or transfer and a shorter learning curve for the newcomer/novice embryologist to perform ICSI with good and standard efficacy.

A piezo-ICSI procedure requires a steady, slow progressive movement with the injecting microcapillary through the ZP, then into the oocyte while stretching the oolemma which will be pierced by a single piezo pulse. No changes of speed and momentum or cytoplasm aspiration are needed, only single dimensional one-way progression. This modification of the procedure makes it significantly simpler and easy to define

Table 7.4 Summarized data of nine Japanese clinics comparing the efficacy of piezo-ICSI and conventional ICSI

Study type	No. of studies	No. of oocytes		No. of 2 PN		Oocyte degeneration rate		Blastocyst rate	
		p-ICSI	c-ICSI	p-ICSI	c-ICSI	p-ICSI	c-ICSI	p-ICSI	c-ICSI
Retrospective + randomized	9	10043	7541	7674 (76%)	4976 (66%)	498 (5%)	674 (9%)	3171 (41%)	1551 (31%)
Sibling oocytes randomly allocated to groups	4	1273	1306	1047 (82%)	942 (72%)	57 (4%)	70 (5%)	572 (55%)	503 (53%)

Table 7.5 Retrospective analysis of rates of pregnancy (gestational sack confirmed), miscarriage and twinning of elective single embryo transfers at a single clinic. For fertilization, IVF or conventional ICS or piezo-ICSI was performed.

	Number of cycles	Av. age	n ET	Pregnancy rate/ET	Miscarriage rate	n births	Twinning Rate %
IVF	1253	36.4	1253	576 (46.0%)	134 (23.3%)	431	4 (0.32%)
Conventional-ICSI	1320	37.2	1320	512 (38.8%)	132 (25.8%)	382	7 (0.53%)
Piezo-ICSI	631	37.8	631	259 (41.0%)	59 22.8%)	210	3 (0.48%)

compared to conventional ICSI. Thus, the learning curve for a novice, newcomer embryologist becomes significantly shorter. In general, a novice embryologist would require ~100 tries on discarded material to develop an acceptable skill to perform piezo-ICSI with good results [18]. This requires, in general, two months of training at the clinic before an embryologist can be left alone to perform piezo-ICSI. For conventional ICSI, in general, a minimum of one year of training is required to achieve the same standard as that with two months of training for piezo-ICSI. Such a benefit may not be that tangible in the hands of well-trained, highly experienced embryologists; however, the differences between embryologists within a clinic in ICSI success rates will be significantly reduced because of the standardization of the piezo technique. This experience has been confirmed by interviews with staff at all of the clinics contacted by the authors, including the nine clinics referred to below that published clinical data.

Nine clinics provided data for an overall analysis of how piezo-ICSI performs in comparison to conventional ICSI [8, 19–25; Mukaida T, personal communication]. Five clinics analyzed laboratory success rates by comparing data retrospectively when piezo-ICSI or conventional ICSI was used for fertilization. Patient populations and other procedures might differ in these studies, so their evidence level is low. A further four studies compared piezo-ICSI with conventional ICSI by randomly allocating sibling oocytes to either piezo or to the conventional groups, thus providing a higher level of evidence. Data show that fertilization rate significantly improved with piezo-ICSI in all cases. In addition, in the retrospective analysis, there was lower oocyte degeneration after piezo-ICSI and higher blastocyst ratio (Table 7.4).

In a 2019 sibling oocyte study, Furuhashi et al. showed similar clinical results between piezo-ICSI and conventional ICSI when all ages were compared; however, for women >35 years of age, the fertilization (P = 0.008) and blastocyst development (P = 0.016) rates with piezo-ICSI on D5 and D6 were significantly higher than

with conventional-ICSI. These published data have been confirmed by several personal communications, stating that one of the special indications of piezo-ICSI would be fertilization of more fragile oocytes and oocytes from older age groups of women [25].

First clinical results with the medical PFNO operating liquid, from a parallel intervention trial, were published in 2021 [26]. The treatment group received oocytes injected with piezo-ICSI with medical PFNO, while the control group was fertilized by a conventional ICSI method. There was no difference in maternal/paternal age, AMH, BMI or average mature oocyte number. The authors found increased fertilization rate (80.6% vs. 65.9%, p<0.05), decreased oocyte degeneration rate (3.8% vs. 10.2%, p<0.05), and an average one extra embryo vitrified for piezo patients (3.8 vs. 2.7, p<0.05). Clinical pregnancy rate was comparable between the groups (55% vs. 50%).

Zona drilling by the piezo technique leaves a permanent opening in the ZP, which is cylinder-shaped and with a diameter of approximately 4–6 μm. To address the possible effect of this small opening on the twinning rate, we collected and compared retrospectively a clinic's past experience (2013–2018) of elective single embryo transfers using conventional IVF, conventional ICSI or piezo-ICSI for fertilization. Table 7.5 shows no differences in rates of pregnancy, miscarriage or twinning between the groups (Mukaida T, personal communication).

Conclusions

Piezo-ICSI has become part of the everyday clinical routine of many dozens of infertility labs in Japan in the last five years. Clinical experience, as well as data, has started to accumulate; in 2018 and 2019, an increasing number of clinics presented data at the annual congress of the Japanese Embryology Society.

The most important added value of piezo to the ICSI procedure is the simple, gentle and standard way in which the fertilization itself is performed. The procedure creates less stress for the oocyte and is easy to pick up and master by the embryologists. Thus, piezo might be the first step toward automatization of the ICSI procedure.

Primarily, the tangible benefit of introducing piezo-ICSI lies in the standardization and simplification of the ICSI procedure, as a result of which new embryologists would be able to perform ICSI in a considerably shorter time compared to the conventional technique. The success of the ICSI procedure becomes independent of the embryologist, providing the clinic with a more robust and predictable laboratory output.

Piezo-ICSI also has promised to be the method of choice in cases of more sensitive/fragile oocyte cases and in older age groups of patients. Evidence appears to show additional benefits for patients older than 35 years in terms of significantly decreased oocyte degeneration after ICSI and increased blastocysts.

Clinical experiences underline the spread of the technique in human IVF; however, the operating liquid currently used in the injecting microcapillary might be an obstacle for human registration.

References

[1] Palermo G, Joris H, Devroey P, Van Steirteghem AC. Pregnancies after intracytoplasmic injection of single spermatozoon into an oocyte. *Lancet* 1992; **340** : 17–18.

[2] Vanderzwalmen P, Bertin G, Lejeune B, Nijs M, Vandamme B, Schoysman R. Two essential steps for a successful intracytoplasmic sperm injection: injection of immobilized spermatozoa after rupture of the oolema. *Hum Reprod* 1996; **11** : 540–7.

[3] Van Steirteghem AC, Nagy P, Joris H, Verheyen G, Smitz J, Camus M, et al. The development of intracytoplasmic sperm injection. *Hum Reprod* 1996; **8** : 59–72.

[4] Fromm M, Weskamp P, Hegel U. Versatile piezoelectric driver for cell puncture. *Pflügers Arch* 1980; **384** : 69

[5] Fishel S, Dowell K, Lisi F, Rinaldi L. Subzonal insemination and breaching techniques for assisting conception in vitro. In: Fishel S. (Ed.) *Micromanipulation Techniques. 1994.* Bailliere's Clinical Obstetrics & Gynaecology Elsevier 65–84.

[6] Kimura Y, Yanagimachi R. Intracytoplasmic sperm injection in the mouse. *Biol Reprod* 1995; **52** : 709–20.

[7] Huang T, Kimura Y, Yanagimachi R. The use of piezo micromanipulation for intracytoplasmic sperm injection of human oocytes. *J Assist Reprod Genet* 1996; **13** : 320–8.

[8] Yanagida K, Katayose H, Yazawa H, Kimura Y, Konnai K, Sato A. The usefulness of a piezo-micromanipulator in intracytoplasmic sperm injection in humans. *Hum Reprod* 1999; **14** : 448–53.

[9] Takeuchi S, Minoura H, Shibahara T, Shen X, Futamura N, Toyoda N. Comparison of piezo-assisted micromanipulation with conventional micromanipulation for intracytoplasmic sperm injection into human oocytes. *Gynecol Obstet Investig* 2001; **52** : 158–62.

[10] Hiraoka K, Kitamura S. Clinical efficiency of Piezo-ICSI using micropipettes with a wall thickness of 0.625 μm. *J Assist Reprod Genet* 2015; **32** : 1827–33.

[11] Nakayama T, Fujiwara H, Tastumi K, Fujita K, Higuchi T, Mori T. A new assisted hatching technique using a piezo-micromanipulator. *Fertil Steril.* 1998; **69** : 784–8.

[12] Ediz K, Olgac N. Microdynamics of the piezo-driven pipettes in ICSI. *IEEE Trans Biomed Eng* 2004; **51** : 1262–8.

[13] Tan KK, Zhou HX, Dou HF, Ng SC. Piezo micromanipulation system for ICSI. *IFAC Proc Vols* 2001; **34** : 174–8.

[14] Karzar-Jeddi, Olgac N, Fan TH. Dynamic response of micropipettes during piezo-assisted intracytoplasmic sperm injection. *Phys Rev E Stat Nonlin Soft Matter Phys* 2011; **84** : 41908.

[15] Hiraoka K, Kitamura S. Erratum to: Clinical efficiency of Piezo-ICSI using micropipettes with a wall thickness of 0.625 μm. *J Assist Reprod Genet* 2016; **33** : 549.

[16] Dumoulin JM, Coonen E, Bras M, Bergers-Janssen JM, Ignoul-Vanvuchelen RC, van Wissen LC, et al. Embryo development and chromosomal anomalies after ICSI: effect of the injection procedure. *Hum Reprod* 2001; **16** : 306–12.

[17] Simopoulou M, Giannelou P, Bakas P, Gkoles L, Kalampokas T, Pantos K, Koutsilieris M. Making ICSI Safer and More Effective: A Review of the Human Oocyte and ICSI Practice *In Vivo* 2016; **30** : 387–400.

[18] Hiraoka K. Piezo-ICSI. Conference proceedings and hands-on workshop by the Pacific Society for Reproductive Medicine (PSRM) and the Association of the Thai Embryologists (ATE) 2018.

[19] Tsukamoto S, Hara N, Kubo A, Hoshino S, Tajima T. Comparison of culture outcomes between conventional-ICSI and piezo-ICSI. *Japanese Soc Fertil Implant* 2019; 157.

[20] Kawakami N, Hanatani M, Takahashi H, Inoue S, Taguchi K, Kawahara Y, et al. Comparison of culture

outcomes after introduction of piezo-ICSI at our clinic. *Japan Soc Fertil Implant* 2019; 158.

[21] Imajo A, Sakoi S, Iwaoka M, Takai Y, Matsuoka A, Kurata Y, et al. Comparison of clinical outcomes between conventional-ICSI and piezo-ICSI at our clinic. *Japan Soc Fertil Implant* 2018; 280.

[22] Koizumi A, Hirao A, Tokumoto A, Ohashi I, Yano K. Benefits of piezo-ICSI at our clinic. *J Assist Reprod* 2018; **21**: 66.

[23] Suzuki H, Takeda N, Abe A, Funayama M, Sato Y, Tanaka Y, et al. Does use of piezo-ICSI affect pregnancy rate? Clinical results of transfer of blastocysts derived from oocytes subjected to piezo-ICSI. *J Japanese Soc Reprod Med* 2017; **62**: 231.

[24] Kishi K, Shiotani M. Benefit of piezo-ICSI in patients aged ≥ 40 years. *J Assist Reprod* 2019; **22**: 59.

[25] Furuhashi K, Saeki Y, Enatsu N, Iwasaki T, Ito K, Mizusawa Y, et al. Piezo-assisted ICSI improves fertilization and blastocyst development rates compared with conventional ICSI in women aged more than 35 years. *Reprod Med Biol.* 2019; **18** : 357–61.

[26] Zander-Fox D, Lam K, Pacella-Ince L, Tully C, Hamilton H, Hiraoka K, McPherson O N, Tremellen K. PIEZO-ICSI increases fertilization rates compared with standard ICSI - A prospective cohort study. *Reprod BioMed Online.* 2021; 1ISSN 1472-6483.

Chapter

8

Artificial Oocyte Activation After ICSI

Thomas Ebner

Introduction

While conventional IVF has been successful in couples with tubal infertility or other female indications, it may fail in patients with compromised semen parameters. To overcome this limitation, certain micromanipulation techniques have been introduced. With any of these methods, for example, partial zona dissection (PZD) or subzonal insemination (SUZI), attempts were made to bring the male gamete closer to the oocyte so that fertilization could be achieved even in the presence of few sperm. In this context, the ultimate micromanipulation technique was introduced in 1992 by Palermo and co-workers when these authors placed a single spermatozoon within the ooplasm (ICSI), resulting not only in fertilization but also in healthy live birth [1].

There is general consent that in the case of ICSI the fertilization process is less physiological than with conventional IVF as several important steps are bypassed, such as penetration of the cumulus and binding to the zona pellucida to name but a few. Apart from concerns regarding this obvious shortcut, there is the additional risk to select and inject spermatozoa with deficits in genetic constellation, integrity of the centrosome, phospholipase C zeta (PLCζ) content, protamine ratio or DNA methylation. To avoid such an unwanted scenario, every effort should be taken to process and subsequently select sperm considered for use in the most physiological way [2]. Such "physiological ICSI" approaches aim for sperm with optimal morphology at higher magnification (IMSI), high head birefringence (polarization microscopy), completed maturation (hyaluronic acid binding) and/or DNA intactness.

However, even in the presence of a presumably normal spermatozoon oocyte, activation/fertilization cannot be guaranteed and, in fact, approximately 3% of all ICSI cycles result in complete fertilization failure. If this event is the consequence of a low number of mature eggs available for injection, repeated ICSI treatment in a subsequent cycle may prove useful. Some patients will still have to face repeated fertilization failure and remain without transfer in spite of normal sperm parameters and good ovarian response.

Investigation of Causes

Although less common causes, including premature sperm chromatin condensation, spindle or sperm aster defects and incorrect sperm injection, may play a role, lack of oocyte activation is considered to be the main cause of fertilization failure following conventional ICSI [3].

When a human egg is activated, the first detectable ooplasmic event is an increase in intracellular Ca^{2+} concentration. In ICSI this initial trigger is caused by an artificial calcium influx from the surrounding culture medium immediately after injection of the sperm. Subsequently, a typical oscillation-like Ca^{2+} pattern is generated, which is crucial for normal fertilization and further preimplantation development of the embryo [4]. These ooplasmic calcium oscillations are most likely provoked by the sperm-bound enzyme PLCζ. The capability to generate calcium peaks is developed within the oocyte during final maturation stages, which indicates that successful fertilization also depends on the inherent quality of the female gamete. Hence, both the sperm and the oocyte play an equal role in oocyte activation, fertilization and further embryo development to the blastocyst; the sperm by providing PLCζ and the oocyte by its responsiveness to this activating enzyme and associated downstream molecular pathways.

In the cohort of patients affected by fertilization problems, it is of utmost importance to distinguish between the two etiologies, that is whether any failure in fertilization is sperm or oocyte-borne. The identification of the respective cause of fertilization failure not only helps to tailor the optimal – preferably least invasive – fertilization technique, but also could be the basis of patient counseling where gamete donation is the only remaining option.

The most common methodology to distinguish between the deficiency of the oocyte-activating potential of the sperm and the inability of oocytes to respond to penetrated sperm is a heterologous ICSI model [5,6]. The so-called mouse oocyte activation test (MOAT) requires injection of sperm from affected patients into mature murine oocytes. The actual activation potential of such sperm is then estimated based on the rate of 2-cell formation. The MOAT results allow classification of patients with failed or low fertilization after ICSI into three groups: low (≤20% mouse egg activation, sperm factor very likely), intermediate (21–84%, oocyte and sperm may contribute to the problem) and high activation (≥85%, no sperm defect). To increase the predictive power, in particular, in the intermediate MOAT group, the same authors investigated mouse and human oocyte Ca^{2+} analysis (M-OCA and H-OCA, respectively) after injection of patient sperm. It was concluded that intermediate MOAT patients suffer from sperm-related activation deficiencies. H-OCA detected the presence of sperm activation deficiencies with greatest sensitivity [7].

Methods of AOA

Regardless of whether the spermatozoon or egg is the causative gamete with respect to the observed decline in activation and fertilization, any increase in ooplasmic calcium could rescue fertilization. However, in patients with such poor prognoses, physiological calcium requisition (e.g. in the form of oscillations) is not possible in oocytes, hence intracellular Ca^{2+} must be raised artificially (artificial oocyte activation, AOA). If deciding not to actively inject calcium (e.g. $CaCl_2$), culture medium and/or intracytoplasmic storage could act as a source of calcium.

Modified ICSI

The penetration of the zona pellucida and the oolemma during ICSI causes micromanipulation-driven calcium entry into the ovum. Tesarik and co-workers further increased this effect by modifying their ICSI technique [5]. In principle, the authors described a normal aspiration phase but, in contrast to conventional ICSI, the cytoplasm containing the sperm was not released in the center but in the oocyte periphery opposite to the injection site. Repeating this invasive procedure twice resulted in sufficient Ca^{2+} being recruited, mostly from intracellular storage, as a series of six cases (with either sperm or oocyte-borne fertilization failures) were successfully treated. However, a high oocyte degeneration rate (~25%) makes this technique less feasible.

Others have tried to combine the manipulation-related calcium flux with an ATP boost at the site of fertilization by dislocating metabolically active mitochondria (mICSI) from the periphery to the center of the oocyte [8]. In detail, the aspiration phase was performed at the 9-o'clock position near the cortex of the oocyte, but then the ooplasm containing sperm and active mitochondria was released centrally at the site where fertilization would occur. Overall, with mICSI a fertilization rate of 54% could be achieved in a group of 15 patients, who had never experienced fertilization before. One-third of these previously unsuccessful patients achieved clinical pregnancy with the mICSI technique [8].

Electrical Activation

Some embryologists take advantage of the fact that an electrical field can generate micropores in the oocyte membrane, which in turn leads to an influx of Ca^{2+} ions from the culture medium [9,10] to facilitate activation by means of Ca^{2+}-dependent processes.

In principle, use of direct or alternate current (or a combination) are both feasible options [9,10]. In the literature, it is recommended to apply piezoelectrical stimulation within 20–30 minutes after ICSI. Number and energy of required stimuli, however, seem to be variable. It should be highlighted that even with this approach total ICSI fertilization failure cannot be completely avoided (failure rate 2–5%). Apart from the equipment for piezoelectrical manipulation not being available in routine IVF labs, a slightly increased degeneration rate (6–12%) may hinder embryologists from using electrical activation techniques in routine IVF. Although more than 50 healthy children have been born so far [9,10], users recommend further investigation on the potential effect of electrical fields on the genetic composition of embryos before this technology can be applied in regular clinical use.

Chemical Activation

In terms of artificial oocyte activation after ICSI, chemical activation leads the way and is the most commonly used technique in IVF laboratories worldwide. There are various agents that can be used to artificially increase calcium concentration within the oocyte. These chemical approaches include unusual substances such as thimerosal, puromycin, 6-DMAP or phorbol esters, but these can be less effective, have use limited to some species, may cause spindle disruption or may be incapable of generating physiological Ca^{2+} oscillations (rather a single peak is achieved).

However, the story is different in the case of strontium chloride. It clearly provokes multiple Ca^{2+} transients in mouse oocytes and may do so in humans as well, although this is still subject to controversy [11]. The mechanism by which $SrCl_2$ induces Ca^{2+} oscillations is not fully understood, but seems to be related to depletion of internal calcium storage. Of note, AOA with strontium chloride may improve the rates of clinical and ongoing pregnancy as well as live birth compared with ICSI alone. This could be particularly valid for the subgroup of patients with previous cycles of low fertilization, that is <30%.

However, the most extensively studied activating agents in IVF are a group of mobile ion carriers, so-called ionophores, which chelate with divalent cations (charge of 2+) thus assisting them to cross membranes. Because of its physiological importance, calcium is the major player in this process.

As mentioned above, these complex compounds cause a single intracellular Ca^{2+} peak rather than a refined spatiotemporal series of oscillations. So why then do ionophores facilitate activation? This may be explained by mammalian studies that showed it is mainly the initial Ca^{2+} rise (or in case of ionophores the only peak) that drives further downstream events, in particular, calcium/calmodulin-dependent protein kinase II performance. Alternatively, there is evidence that this enzyme remains active even in the absence of calcium. Mammalian eggs can respond to a wide range of intracellular Ca^{2+} signals and, even more importantly, have a surprisingly high degree of tolerance for changes in ooplasmic calcium level.

In the literature, two such ionophores are considered relevant, ionomycin and calcimycin (also referred to as A23187). A review by Vanden Meerschaut and colleagues [12] elegantly illustrates one of the substantial problems with AOA – the lack of standardization of the procedure. It is not just a question of whether to use ionomycin or calcimycin, there are also major discrepancies in the dosage (5 μM to >10 μM), the mode (single versus double stimulus) and the timing of ionophore application (10 to 30 minutes). This inconsistency makes it difficult to draw meaningful conclusions from different IVF studies [3,6,13,14].

Recently, a ready-to-use A23187 (CultActive, Gynemed, Germany) was introduced [13], which could be considered a step forward toward the standardization of artificial activation. Using CultActive in diverse patient cohorts, scientists reported a total of 95 healthy children (one baby was not healthy) (Table 8.1). It is of interest that similar to $SrCl_2$ treatment, fertilization rates using calcimycin reach a plateau slightly above 50%. In this context, ionomycin might give better results, in particular, if combined with the direct injection of small volumes of $CaCl_2$ during ICSI [15].

Indications for AOA

At the beginning of the AOA era, mostly case reports were published [16], but when it became evident that ionophore application is a feasible and presumably safe option for many patients its utilization flourished. The classical indication for application of ionophores of whatever kind is complete activation failure (0% fertilization, no transfer) after ICSI in a previous cycle. Subsequently, a German group [17] realized that even if ICSI resulted in a low fertilization rate, the outcome could be increased if ICSI was combined with AOA in the following cycle. The threshold was found to be 30%; in other words, if less than a third of MII eggs are fertilized, a switch to AOA is recommended in the next treatment cycle. No such benefit was observed if the initial fertilization rate was 30–50% [17].

A significant proportion of patients who face no or low fertilization suffer from male infertility, hence "severe male factor sterility" is the third indication that would require reconsideration of AOA. Indeed, there is growing evidence that use of A23187 for patients with azoospermia, cryptozoospermia or Kartagener syndrome can yield high fertilization and pregnancy rates [14]. Although it is unclear whether ionophore treatment is justified in cases of isolated teratozoospermia, its utilization in globozoospermic patients is a prerequisite for successful fertilization and pregnancy. It should be highlighted that in this context calcimycin is less effective than ionomycin [15].

Safety of AOA

While the scientific community awaits more prospective studies with a larger number of patients to confirm the reassuring observations so far and to further substantiate the safety of AOA, a mounting body of evidence is being published indicating that neonatal and neurodevelopmental outcome (up to the age of 10) as well as language skills are within expected ranges [13,14,18]. Table 8.1 (table not intended to be exhaustive) lists published live births using different AOA protocols. A total of 324 children from 287 live births showed a major malformation rate of 1.2% and a minor malformation rate of 2.5%. It should be noted that 11/12 malformations came from one single study and it remains unclear whether this relatively high percentage is associated with ionomycin, the ICSI procedure or occurred by chance.

So far only one malformation, an anal atresia, has been reported after application of (ready-to-use) A23187 [13]. As this major complication is a late-onset malformation in gastrointestinal tract formation, a causal relation with ionophore treatment (applied before fusion of the gametes!) is very unlikely. And it should be noted that anal atresia in ART without artificial oocyte activation has also been reported.

In parallel with the efforts to collect data on children born after assisted oocyte activation, embryologists are aiming to increase their knowledge on the potential physiological effects of AOA. It is noteworthy that, in terms of gene expression, ICSI plus AOA ($SrCl_2$) was closer to IVF than ICSI alone. Even if used at a 10-fold concentration (e.g. 100μM), A23187 did not cause a widespread increase in chromosome segregation errors. Normal embryo quality and, particularly, comparable morphokinetic behavior (unpublished data) further assist acceptance of AOA in daily IVF work.

Although there is a steadily growing range of indications that would allow safe use of ionophores in IVF/ICSI, it should be stressed that AOA is not beneficial for all patients with a suspected oocyte- (or sperm-)related activation deficiency [3].

Future

There will be cases in whom the paternal and/or maternal Ca^{2+} machinery will not be the cause of fertilization problems or in whom the artificial Ca^{2+} transient will not be sufficient to pass the threshold required to initiate oocyte activation. In these patients, current AOA techniques will fail. In a first

Table 8.1 Neonatal health of published live births after artificial oocyte activation using different approaches

Method	Reference	Patients	Live births	Children	mMF	mjMF
Modified ICSI	Tesarik et al. [5]	6	5	6	0	0
	Ebner et al. [8]	60	20	20	0	0
Electrical activation	Yanagida et al. [21]	3	1	2	0	0
	Mansour et al. [9]	44	16	20	0	0
Chemical stimulation						
$SrCl_2$	Kyono et al. [11]	9	5	5	0	0
	Fawzy et al. [22]	115	46	46	0	0
	Kim et al. [23]	8	5	8	0	0
Ionomycin	Mateizel et al. [24]	237	39	47	8	3
	Nasr-Esfandari et al. [25]	54	25	25	0	0
	Heindryckx et al. [6]	30	17	21	0	0
Calcimycin (A23187)	Montag et al. [17]	89	25	25	0	0
	Kang et al. [26]	29	3	3	0	0
CultActive	Ebner and Montag [13]	100	28	35	0	1
	Ebner et al. [14]	66	25	32	0	0
	Ebner et al. [27]	57	25	25	0	0
	Ebner et al. [28]	1	1	2	0	0
	Darwish and Magdi [29]	4	1	2	0	0

mMF = minor malformation; mjMF = major malformation.

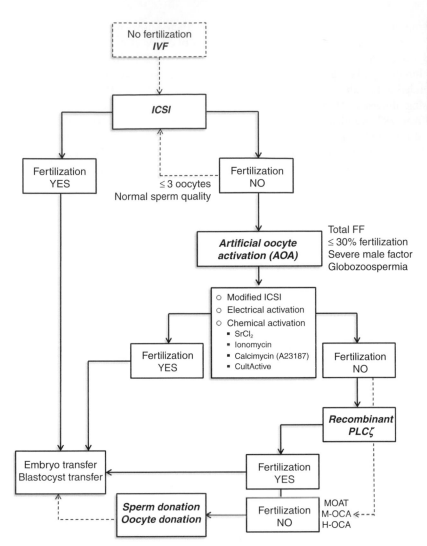

Figure 8.1 Treatment counseling algorithm based on fertilization outcome of the previous treatment cycle. Dashed lines mark alternative pathways. H-OCA = human oocyte calcium analysis; FF = fertilization failure; MOAT = mouse oocyte activation test; M-OCA = mouse oocyte calcium analysis; PLCζ = phospholipase C zeta; SRCl$_2$ = strontium chloride.

step, one could increase the number of stimuli to use the additive capacity of Ca^{2+} signals. If more invasive techniques are a feasible option after appropriate ethical and legal consideration, active injection of CaCl$_2$ (0.1 mol/L) preceding ionomycin treatment would be a feasible approach.

Alternatively, upcoming products, such as a ready-to-use ionomycin (Gynemed) could offer solutions. Preliminary data suggest that this compound can rescue cases in whom A231897 failed (unpublished data).

The ultimate and most physiological approach, however, would be application of (recombinant) PLCζ. This enzyme not only triggers Ca^{2+} oscillations, but also rescued failed oocyte activation in a prototype

of male infertility [19]. As murine oocytes [19] might differ in response to human recombinant PLCζ (compared with human eggs), finding the right dosage of the enzyme for clinical use remains a challenge.

As a valid ruling for all the AOA techniques mentioned, these should not be used without profound indication (Figure 8.1). Usually, AOA should not be used in the first stimulation cycle, except for globozoospermia or PLCζ mutations. In case of doubt that poor sperm quality might affect fertilization, a sibling oocyte model should be chosen. Although it has been stated that AOA is considered safe and ready for clinical application [20], the doctrine "primum non nocere" should always be kept in mind.

References

[1] Palermo G, Joris H, Devroey P, Van Steirteghem AC. Pregnancies after intracytoplasmic injection of single spermatozoon into an oocyte. *Lancet* 1992; **340**: 17–18.

[2] Parmegiani L, Cognigni GE, Bernardi S, Troilo E, Ciampaglia W, Filicori M. "Physiologic ICSI": hyaluronic acid (HA) favors selection of spermatozoa without DNA fragmentation and with normal nucleus, resulting in improvement of embryo quality. *Fertil Steril* 2010; **93**: 598–604.

[3] Vanden Meerschaut F, Nikiforaki D, De Gheselle S, Dullaerts V, Van den Abbeel E, Gerris J, Heindryckx B, De Sutter P. Assisted oocyte activation is not beneficial for all patients with a suspected oocyte-related activation deficiency. *Hum Reprod* 2012; **27**: 1977–1984.

[4] Kashir J, Heindryckx B, Jones C, De Sutter P, Parrington J, Coward K. Oocyte activation, phospholipase C zeta and human infertility. *Hum Reprod Update* 2010; **16**: 690–703.

[5] Tesarik J, Rienzi L, Ubaldi F, Mendozy C, Greco E. Use of a modified intracytoplasmic sperm injection technique to overcome sperm-borne and oocyte-borne oocyte activation failures. *Fertil Steril* 2000; **78**: 619–624.

[6] Heindryckx B, De Gheselle S, Gerris J, Dhont M, De Sutter P. Efficiency of assisted oocyte activation as a solution for failed intracytoplasmic sperm injection. *Reprod Biomed Online* 2008; **17**: 662–668.

[7] Ferrer-Buitrago M, Dhaenens L, Lu Y, Bonte D, Vanden Meerschaut F, De Sutter P, Leybaert L, Heindryckx B. Human oocyte calcium analysis predicts the response to assisted oocyte activation in patients experiencing fertilization failure after ICSI. *Hum Reprod* 2018; **33**: 416–425.

[8] Ebner T, Moser M, Sommergruber M, Jesacher K, Tews G. Complete oocyte activation failure after ICSI can be overcome by a modified injection technique. *Hum Reprod* 2004; **19**: 1837–1841.

[9] Mansour R, Fahmy I, Tawab NA, Kamal A, El-Demery Y, Aboulghar M, Serour G. Electrical activation of oocytes after intracytoplasmic sperm injection: a controlled randomized study *Fertil Steril* 2009; **91**: 133–139.

[10] Baltaci V, Ayvaz OU, Unsal E, Aktaş Y, Baltaci A, Turhan F, Ozcan S, Sönmezer M. The effectiveness of intracytoplasmic sperm injection combined with piezoelectric stimulation in infertile couples with total fertilization failure. *Fertil Steril* 2010; **94**: 900–904.

[11] Kyono K, Kumagai S, Nishinaka C, Nakajo Y, Uto H, Toya M, Sugawara J, Araki Y. Birth and follow-up of babies born following ICSI using SrCl2 oocyte activation. *Reprod Biomed Online* 2008; **17**: 53–8.

[12] Vanden Meerschaut F, Nikiforaki D, Heindryckx B, De Sutter P. Assisted oocyte activation following ICSI fertilization failure. *Reprod Biomed Online* 2014; **28**: 560–571.

[13] Ebner T, Montag M, Oocyte Activation Group. Live birth after artificial oocyte activation using a ready-to-use ionophore: a prospective multicentre study. *Reprod Biomed Online* 2015; **30**: 359–365.

[14] Ebner T, Köster M, Shebl O, Moser M, Van der Ven H, Tews G, Montag M. Application of a ready-to-use calcium ionophore increases rates of fertilization and pregnancy in severe male factor infertility. *Fertil Steril* 2012; **98**: 1432–1437.

[15] Nikiforaki D, Vanden Meerschaut F, de Roo C, Lu Y, Ferrer-Buitrago M, de Sutter P, Heindryckx B. Effect of two assisted oocyte activation protocols used to overcome fertilization failure on the activation potential and calcium releasing pattern. *Fertil Steril* 2016; **105**: 798–806.e2.

[16] Rybouchkin AV, Van der Straeten F, Quatacker J, De Sutter P, Dhont M. Fertilization and pregnancy after assisted oocyte activation and intracytoplasmic sperm injection in a case of round-headed sperm associated with deficient oocyte activation capacity. *Fertil Steril* 1997; **68**: 1144–1147.

[17] Montag M, Köster M, van der Ven K, Bohlen U, van der Ven H. The benefit of artificial oocyte activation is dependent on the fertilization rate in a previous treatment cycle. *Reprod Biomed Online* 2012; **24**: 521–526.

[18] Vanden Meerschaut F, D'Haeseleer E, Gysels H, Thienpont Y, Dewitte G, Heindryckx B, Oostra A, Roeyers H, Van Lierde K, De Sutter P. Neonatal and neurodevelopmental outcome of children aged 3–10 years born following assisted oocyte activation. *Reprod Biomed Online* 2014; **28**: 54–63.

[19] Nomikos M, Yu Y, Elgmati K, Theodoridou M, Campbell K, Vassilakopoulou V, Zikos C, Livaniou E, Amso N, Nounesis G, Swann K, Lai FA. Phospholipase Cζ rescues failed oocyte activation in a prototype of male factor infertility. *Fertil Steril* 2013; **99**: 76–85.

[20] Ebner T, Montag M. Artificial oocyte activation: evidence for clinical readiness. *Reprod Biomed Online* 2016; **32**: 271–273.

[21] Yanagida K, Katayose H, Yazawa H, Kimura Y, Sato A, Yanagimachi H, Yanagimachi R. Successful fertilization and pregnancy following ICSI and electrical oocyte activation. *Hum Reprod* 1999; **14**: 1307–1311.

[22] Fawzy M, Emad M, Mahran A, Sabry M, Fetih AN, Abdelghafar H, Rasheed S. Artificial oocyte activation with SrCl2 or calcimycin after ICSI improves clinical and embryological outcomes compared with ICSI alone: results of a randomized clinical trial. *Hum Reprod* 2018; 33: 1636–1644.

[23] Kim JW, Kim SD, Yang SH, Yoon SH, Jung JH, Lim JH. Successful pregnancy after SrCl2 oocyte activation in couples with repeated low fertilization rates following calcium ionophore treatment. *Syst Biol Reprod Med* 2014; 60: 177–182.

[24] Mateizel I, Verheyen G, Van de Velde H, Tournaye H, Belva F. Obstetric and neonatal outcome following ICSI with assisted oocyte activation by calcium ionophore treatment. *J Assist Reprod Genet* 2018; 35: 1005–1010.

[25] Nasr-Esfahani MH, Razavi S, Javdan Z, Tavalaee, M. Artificial oocyte activation in severe teratozoospermia undergoing intracytoplasmic sperm injection. *Fertil Steril* 2008; 90: 2231–2237.

[26] Kang HJ, Lee SH, Park YS, Lim CK, Ko DS, Yang KM, Park DW. Artificial oocyte activation in intracytoplasmic sperm injection cycles using testicular sperm in human in vitro fertilization. *Clin Exp Reprod Med* 2015; 42: 45–50.

[27] Ebner T, Oppelt P, Wöber M, Staples P, Mayer RB, Sonnleitner U, Bulfon-Vogl S, Gruber I, Haid AE, Shebl O. Treatment with Ca2+ ionophore improves embryo development and outcome in cases with previous developmental problems: a prospective multicenter study. *Hum Reprod* 2015; 30: 97–102.

[28] Ebner T, Maurer M, Oppelt P, Mayer RB, Duba HC, Costamoling W, Shebl O. Healthy twin live-birth after ionophore treatment in a case of theophylline-resistant Kartagener syndrome. *J Assist Reprod Genet* 2015; 32: 873–877.

[29] Darwish E, Magdi Y. A preliminary report of successful cleavage after calcium ionophore activation at ICSI in cases with previous arrest at the pronuclear stage. *Reprod Biomed Online* 2015; 31: 799–804.

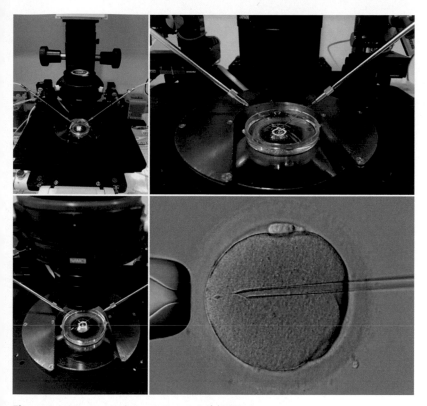

Figure 2.1 Micromanipulation station setup for ICSI.

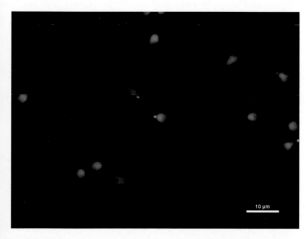

Figure 2.2 Pericentrin staining on spermatozoa assessing paternal centrosome.

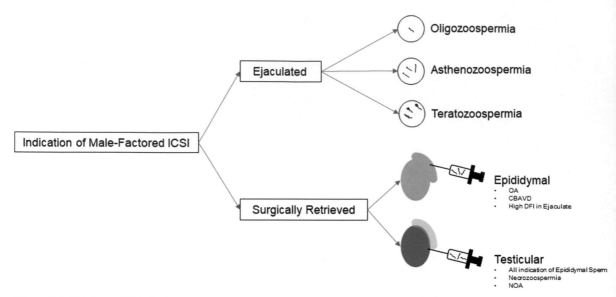

Figure 2.3 Male factor ICSI indications.

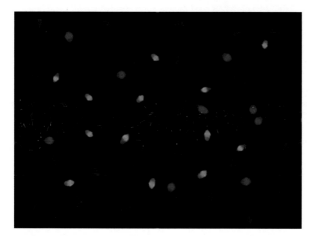

Figure 2.4 TUNEL assay depicting spermatozoa with fragmented DNA (green fluorescent signal).

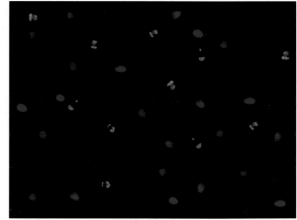

Figure 2.5 PLCζ, the putative soluble cytosolic factor, required for fertilization examined by immunofluorescence microscopy.

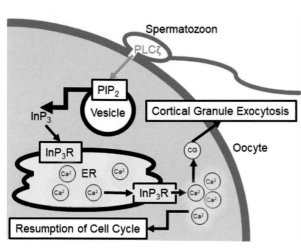

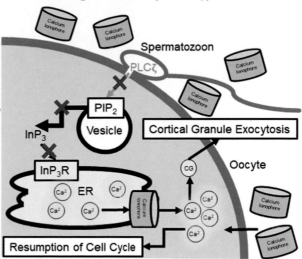

Figure 2.6 Mechanism of assisted oocyte activation.

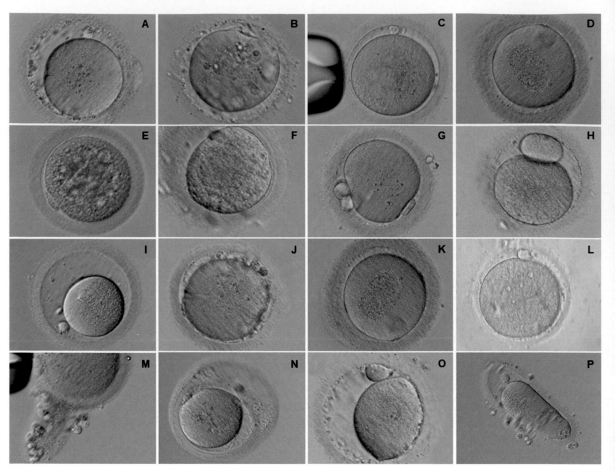

Figure 2.8 Different types of intraooplasmic dysmorphism: (A) inclusions, (B) refractile bodies, (C) smooth endoplasmic reticulum, (D) central granulation/dark center, (E) vacuoles, (F) granular ooplasm. Different types of extraooplasmic abnormalities: (G) fragmented PB, (H) large PB, (I) expanse of perivitelline space (PVS), (J) perivitelline debris. Different types of zona pellucida (ZP) deformities: (K) dark ZP, (L) thin ZP, (M) abnormal ZP, (N) bilayered ZP. Other types of oocyte dysmorphism: (O) irregular shape, (P) oval oocyte.

Fertilization Rates - Fresh vs. Frozen

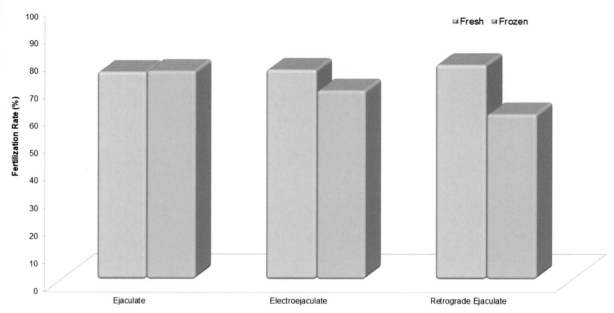

Figure 3.1 Comparison of ICSI fertilization rates with different sperm sources and whether fresh or frozen. Fertilization rates remain comparable throughout the different specimen origins and utilization conditions.

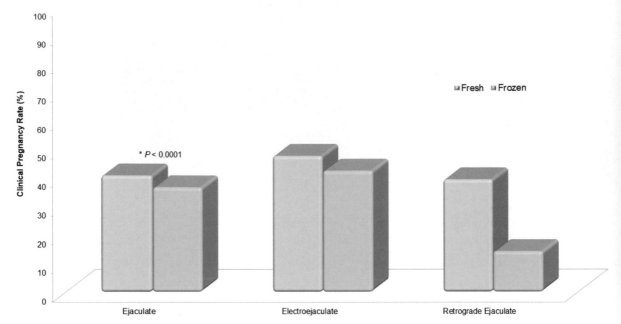

Figure 3.2 Comparison of ICSI fertilization rates with different sperm sources and whether fresh or frozen. Among the three groups, the clinical pregnancy rate appears higher when a fresh specimen is used, reaching significance ($P<0.0001$) in the ejaculated source. $*\chi^2$, 2x2, 1 df, effect of ejaculated sample status on clinical pregnancy rates, $P<0.0001$.

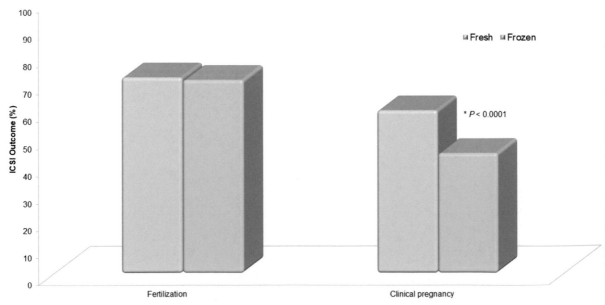

Figure 3.3 Comparison of ICSI fertilization and clinical pregnancy rates when utilizing fresh or frozen epididymal spermatozoa. While fertilization rates remain comparable, the utilization of a freshly retrieved epididymal specimen provides a higher clinical pregnancy rate. $*\chi^2$, 2x2, 1 df, effect of epididymal specimen status on clinical pregnancy rates, $P<0.0001$

ICSI Outcome with Testicular Spermatozoa

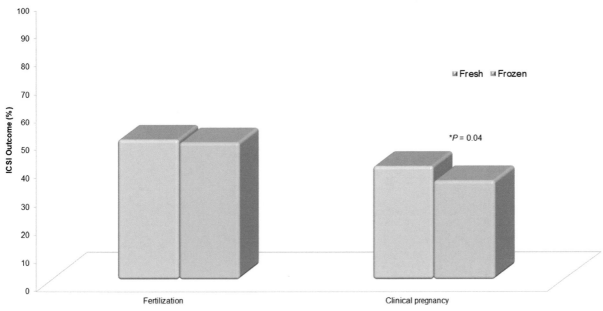

Figure 3.4 Comparison of ICSI fertilization and clinical pregnancy rates when utilizing fresh or frozen testicular spermatozoa. While fertilization rates remain comparable, the utilization of a freshly retrieved epididymal specimen provides a higher clinical pregnancy rate. *χ^2, 2x2, 1 *df*, effect of testicular specimen status on clinical pregnancy rates, *P*=0.04.

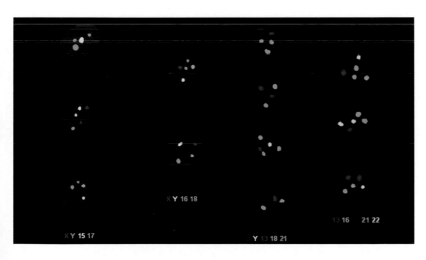

Figure 3.5 Fluorescent in situ hybridization assay depicting ploidy of spermatozoa.

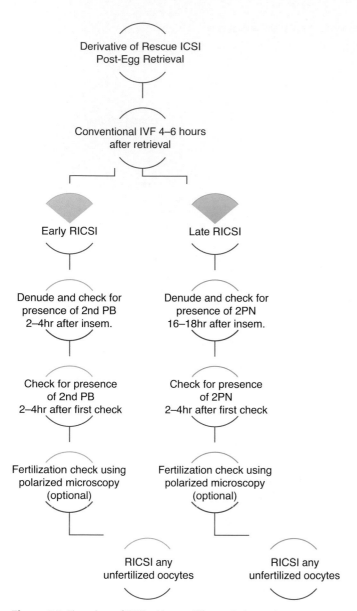

Figure 4.1 Flow chart of RICSI with two different timing options.

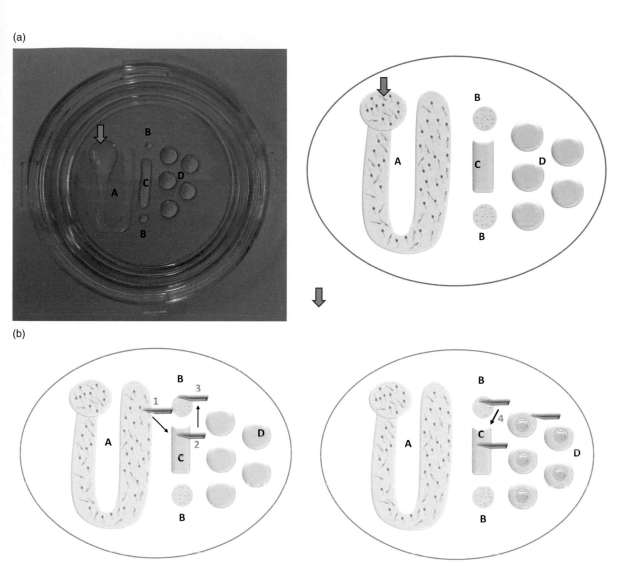

Figure 5.1 (a) Sperm selection under DIC optics followed by oocyte injection on a microscope equipped with HMC or bright field optics. (b) Left: sperm selection under DIC optics; right: oocyte injection with HMC or bright field optics. A: Swim out "snake" drop (HTF-HEPES-HSA); B: host-selected spermatozoa micro drops (HTF-HEPES-HSA); C: sperm immobilization drop (10% PVP); D: oocyte injection drops (HTF-HEPES-HSA); Arrow: position to deposit an aliquot of sperm suspension.

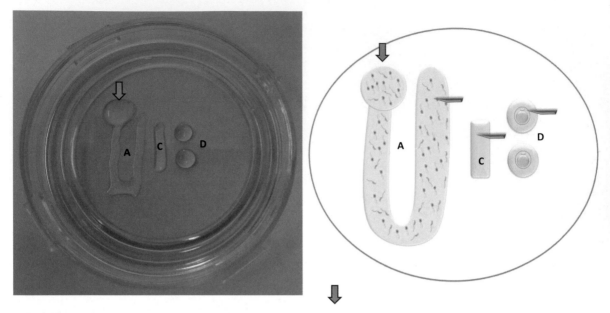

Figure 5.2 Sperm selection followed by oocyte injection on a microscope equipped with DIC optics. A: Swim out "snake" drop (HTF-HEPES-HSA); C: sperm immobilization drop (10% PVP); D: oocyte injection drops (HTF-HEPES-HSA); Arrow: position to deposit an aliquot of sperm suspension.

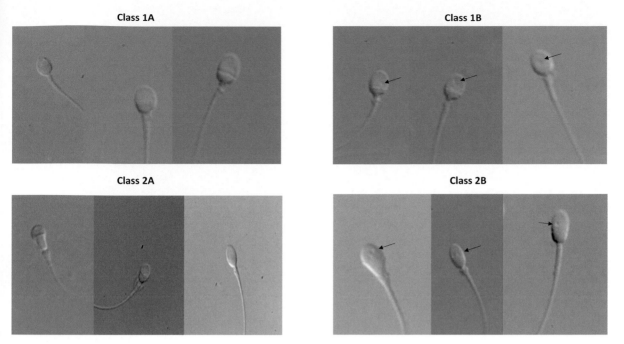

Figure 5.3 Class 1 and class 2 spermatozoa. Arrows indicate the presence of small, smooth VLS.

Class 3A   **Class 3B**

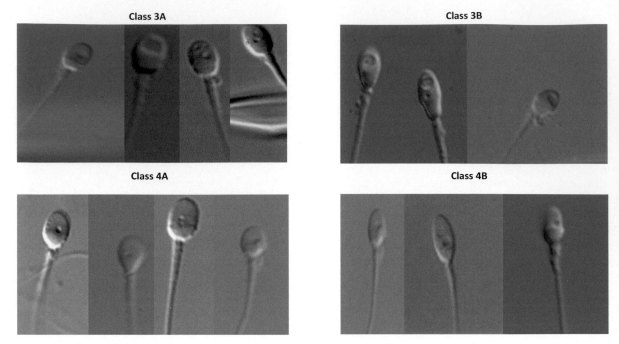

Class 4A   **Class 4B**

Figure 5.4 Class 3 and class 4 spermatozoa. Arrows indicate the presence of small, smooth VLS.

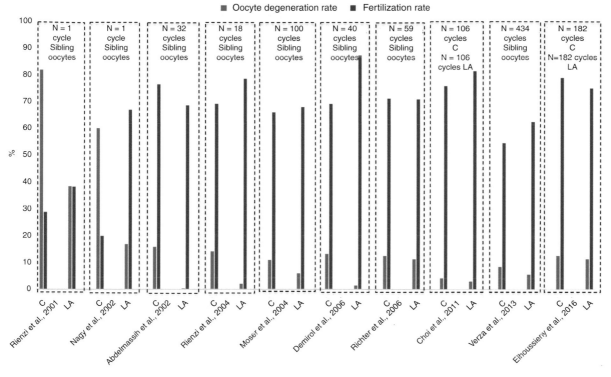

Figure 6.4 Summary of oocyte degeneration and fertilization rates achieved along the main studies that compared conventional-ICSI (C) to laser-assisted ICSI (LA).

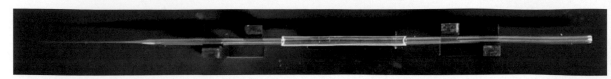

Figure 7.1 Operating liquid loaded into the injecting microcapillary.

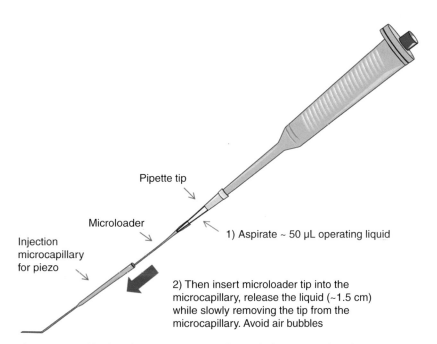

Pipette tip

Microloader

Injection
microcapillary
for piezo

1) Aspirate ~ 50 µL operating liquid

2) Then insert microloader tip into the
microcapillary, release the liquid (~1.5 cm)
while slowly removing the tip from the
microcapillary. Avoid air bubbles

Figure 7.2 Backloading the injecting microcapillary with the operating liquid.

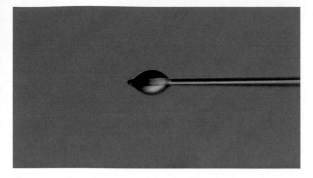

Figure 7.3 First checkpoint of the piezo function.

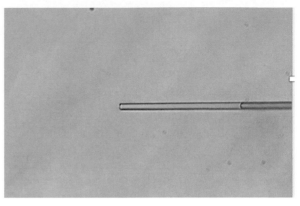

Figure 7.4 Phase border of the operating liquid and the sperm holding medium.

Figure 7.5 Immobilization of a spermatozoon by the piezo technique.

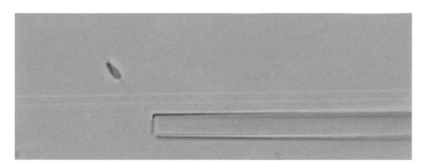

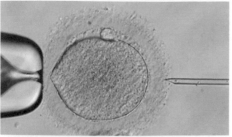 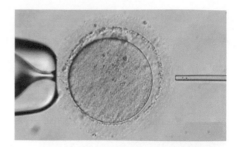

1) Piercing the zone pellucida

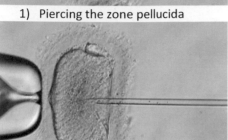 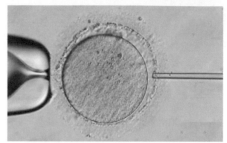

2) During c-ICSI a notable deformation of the oocyte is observed while there is significantly less pressure applied during piezo-ICSI

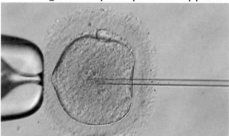 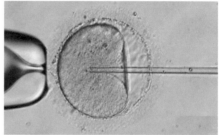

3) The micropipette is advanced to about 4/5 of the oocyte, stretching the membrane

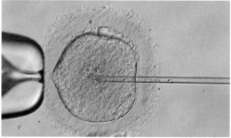 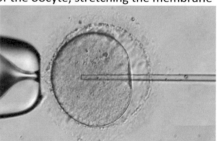

4) The oolemma and the cytoplasm is aspirated into the micropipette during c-ICSI whereas a single piezo pulse opens the membrane during piezo-ICSI (no aspiration is needed)

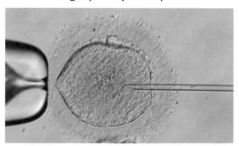 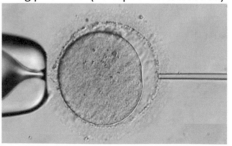

5) The micropipette is gently extracted after the sperm injection

Figure 7.6 Steps of conventional ICSI and piezo-ICSI.

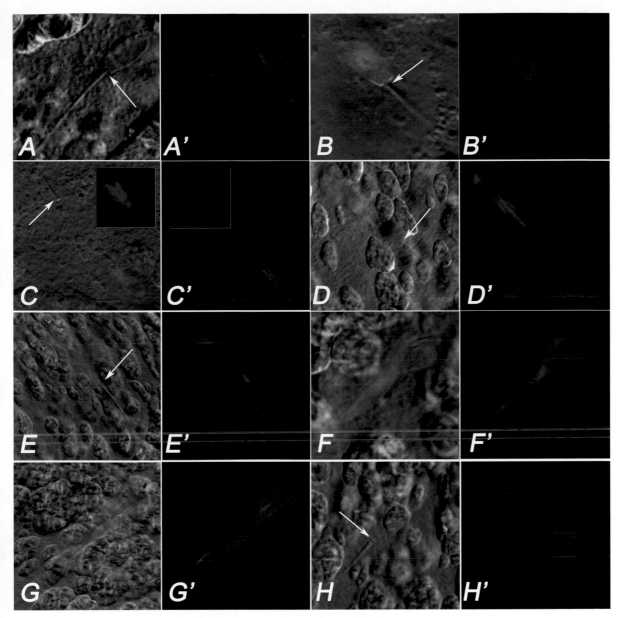

Figure 11.1 Release of putative SOAF component WBP2NL (red) after porcine ICSI. Before (A) and shortly after ICSI (B), the WBP2NL protein is confined to sperm head postacrosomal sheath, from which it is released into oocyte cytoplasm at the initial stage of sperm nucleus decondensation (C, D). As the sperm nucleus swells and elongates, WBP2NL also appears to invade the nuclear matrix in the postacrosomal area (E–G). Solubilization of WBP2NL is completed at the time of sperm tail (arrows in A, B, E and H) excision from the sperm head/nascent paternal pronucleus (H). Experimental details are described in Wu *et al.* [62]. Samples were DNA-stained with DAPI and fluorescent images superimposed onto parfocal differential interference contrast brightfield micrographs.

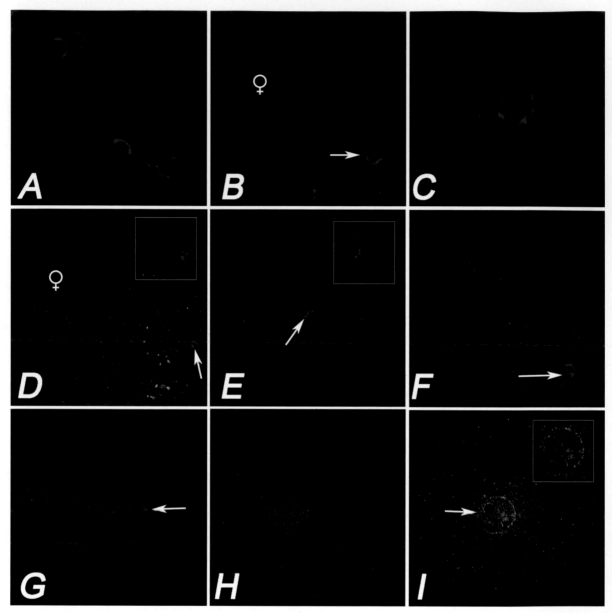

Figure 11.2 Fate of the subacrosomal perinuclear theca (PT) and inner acrosomal membrane (IAM) after porcine ICSI, traced by immunolabeling of sperm protein IAM32 (red). Before ICSI (A), the IAM32 protein is prominently detected on the inner acrosomal membrane of the acrosomal ridge and on the arch of the crescent-shaped equatorial segment. In many ICSI zygotes, the IAM-PT complex starts to dissociate from sperm nucleus even before the completion of oocyte meiosis (oocyte chromosomes are marked by ♀) while in other zygotes such a dissociation becomes detectable once the sperm nucleus begins to decondense (B). Clumped IAM-PT (arrows in E–G) often remains associated with paternal pronucleus at the time of pronuclear apposition (D, E), or drifts away from pronuclei in other zygotes (G), to eventually disappear (H). In some zygotes, the failure of IAM-PT removal blocks paternal pronucleus development without interfering with oocyte activation and formation of the maternal pronucleus and pronuclear apposition (I). Experimental details are described in Katayama *et al.* [56]. Samples were DNA-stained with DAPI and pronuclear nuclear envelope was labeled green (panel I).

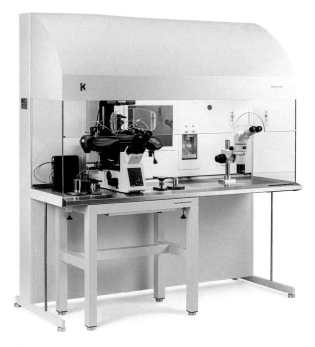

Figure 12.1 Workstation with integrated anti-vibration table.

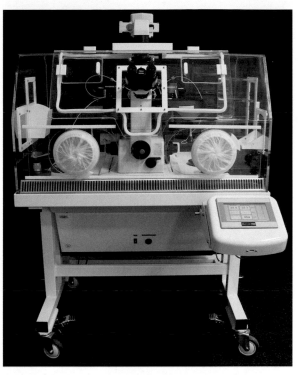

Figure 12.2 Biological cabinet with integrated anti-vibration pad.

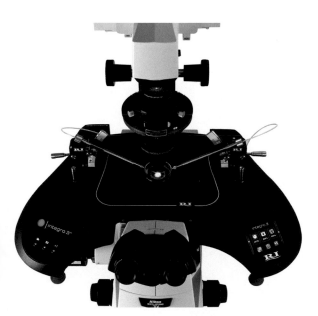

Figure 12.3 RI Integra 3™.

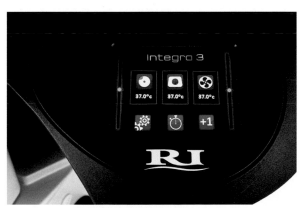

Figure 12.4 Touchscreen display of the RI Integra 3™.

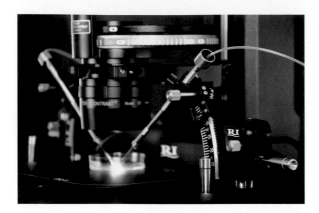

Figure 12.5 RI PL3 tool-holder and MPH micropipette holder.

(a)

(b)

(c)

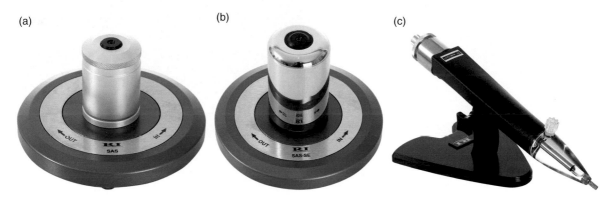

Figure 12.6 (a) RI SAS™,(b) SAS-SE™ and (c) SOS™ screw-actuated syringes.

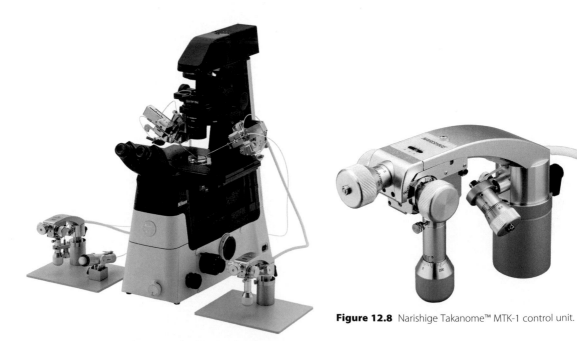

Figure 12.8 Narishige Takanome™ MTK-1 control unit.

Figure 12.7 Narishige Takanome™ MTK-1.

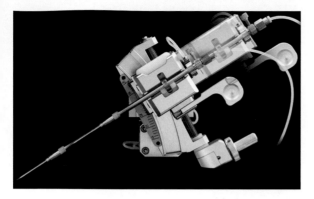

Figure 12.9 Narishige Takanome™ MTK-1 drive unit.

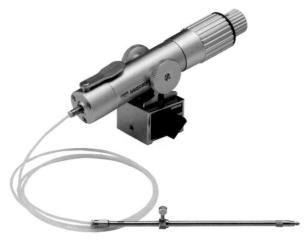

Figure 12.10 Narishige IM-11–2 pneumatic injector.

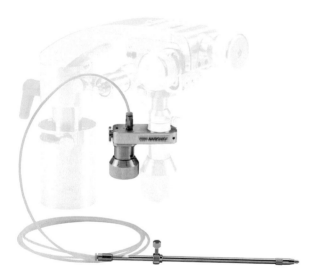

Figure 12.11 Narishige IM-HD1T pneumatic injector.

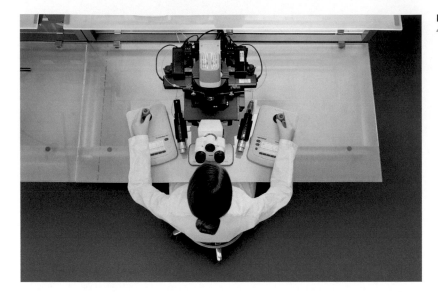

Figure 12.12 Eppendorf TransferMan®
4 m. © Eppendorf AG.

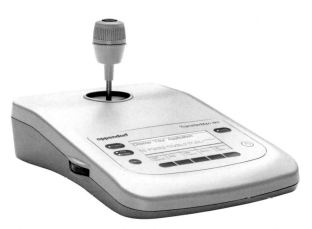

Figure 12.13 Eppendorf joystick control board © Eppendorf AG.

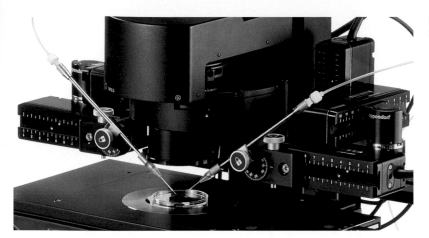

Figure 12.14 Eppendorf head-stage motor module © Eppendorf AG.

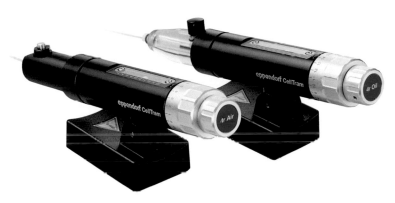

Figure 12.15 Eppendorf CellTram® 4 air and CellTram® 4 oil injectors © Eppendorf AG.

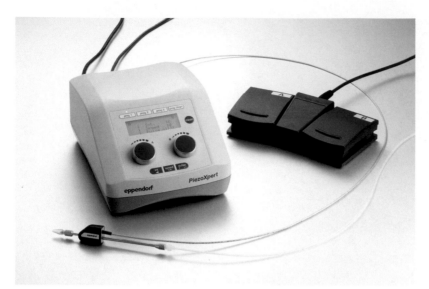

Figure 12.16 Eppendorf PiezoXpert®
© Eppendorf AG.

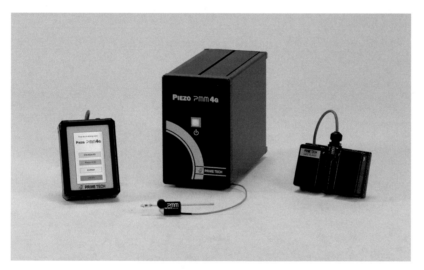

Figure 12.17 Prime Tech piezo PMM4G.

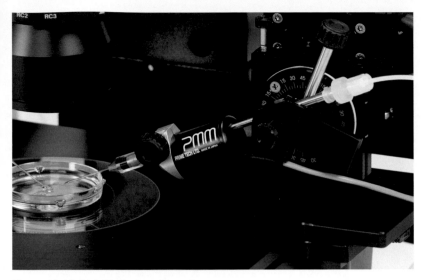

Figure 12.18 Prime Tech piezo drive unit.

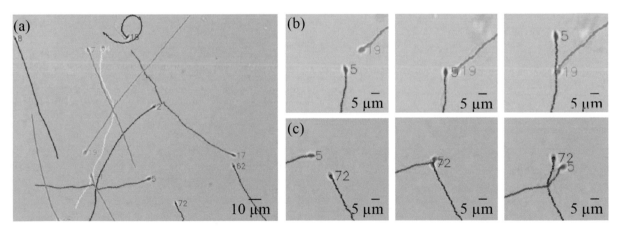

Figure 13.1 (a) Multiple sperm tracking using the JPDAF method. (b) The tracking of two sperm in close proximity. (c) The tracking of two sperm in intersection. Reproduced from [2].

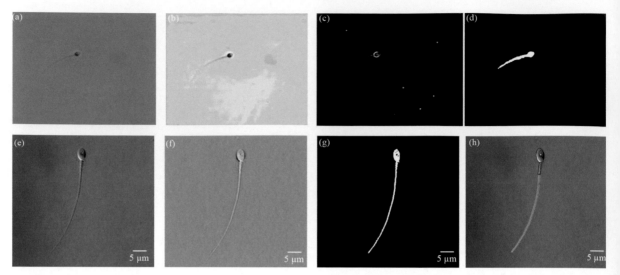

Figure 13.2 Live sperm morphology analysis. (a) Sperm image under 40× objective. (b) Denoising by wavelet transform. (c) Applying Sobel edge detection. (d) Sperm segmentation after median filter. Reproduced from [5]. (e) Sperm image under 100× objective and DIC imaging. (f) Image reconstruction to remove DIC side illumination effect. (g) Sperm segmentation by fuzzy c-means clustering. (h) Separation of head, midpiece, and tail, and the detection of vacuole. Reproduced from [2].

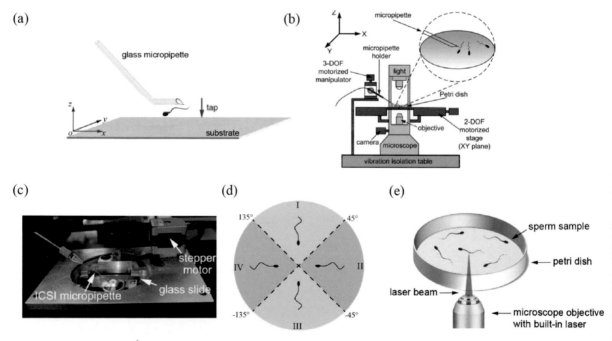

Figure 13.3 Robotic sperm immobilization. (a) Conventional manual immobilization uses a micropipette to tap the sperm tail against a substrate. Reproduced from [7]. (b) Schematic illustration of the robotic sperm immobilization system. Reproduced from [6]. (c) A rotational microscopy stage for actively adjusting sperm orientation to enable immobilization of sperm swimming in all directions. (d) Based on sperm head orientation, sperm swimming in all directions are classified into four quadrants for orientation adjustment. Reproduced from [7]. (e) Sperm immobilization using laser ablation. Reproduced from [8].

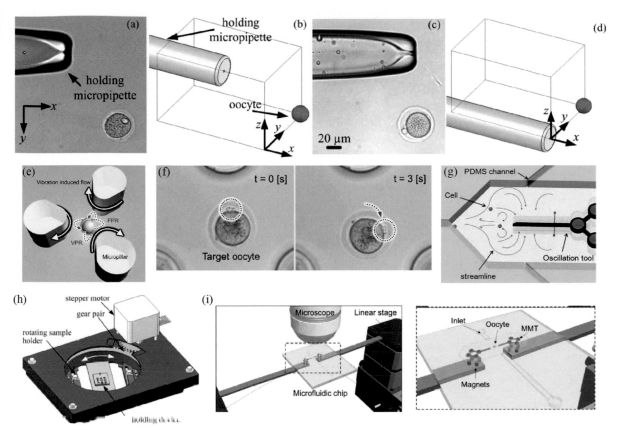

Figure 13.6 Oocyte orientation control using fluid flow and customized devices. (a, b) In-plane and (c, d) out-of-plane orientation control by the flow from the holding micropipette. Reproduced from [13]. (e, f) 3D oocyte rotation by the local whirling flow induced around the micropillars. Reproduced from [14]. (g) Oocyte rotation by local streamline generated by a magnetically driven oscillation tool. Reproduced from [15]. (h) Motorized rotational stage for 2D orientation control. Reproduced from [16]. (i) Magnetically driven microtools controlled to push an oocyte for 3D rotation of oocytes. FPR, focal plane rotation; VPR, vertical plane rotation; PDMS, polydimethylsiloxane; MMT, magnetically driven microtool. Reproduced from [17].

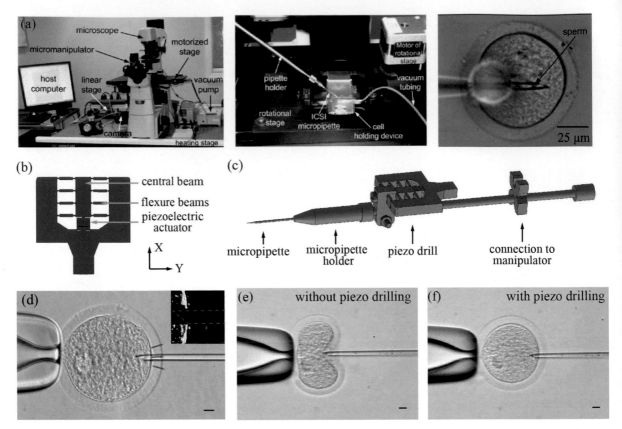

Figure 13.8 (a) Robotic sperm injection system. Reproduced from [19]. (b–f) Piezo drill developed to reduce oocyte deformation and prevent cytoplasm aspiration. (b) Flexure beams as lateral constraints to guide the micropipette motion along the axial direction, without the use of damping fluid such as mercury. (c) Eccentric configuration to be compatible with clinical setup. (d) Automated detection of membrane breakage to minimize the time delay between cell penetration and piezo stoppage. Motion history image of the membrane is shown in the inset. (e, f) Hamster oocyte penetration without and with piezo drilling. Reproduced from [23].

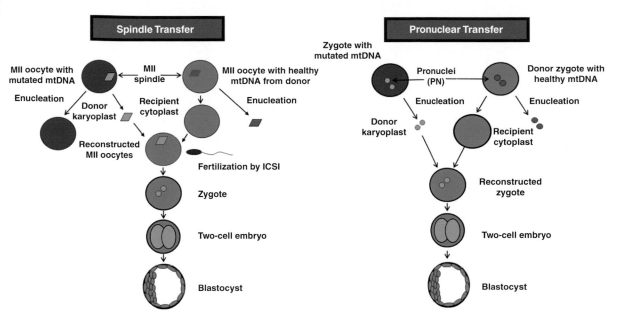

Figure 14.1 Diagrams outlining the procedures of spindle transfer (ST) and pronuclear transfer (PNT). The ST technique involves removing the metaphase II (MII) spindle-chromosome complex, and transferring it to an enucleated donor MII oocyte, followed by fertilization of the reconstructed oocyte. The method of PNT involves the removal of both pronuclei (PN) from a zygote and transferring them into an enucleated recipient zygote.

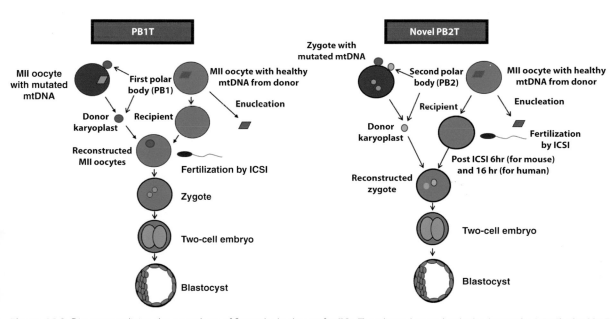

Figure 14.2 Diagrams outlining the procedures of first polar body transfer (PB1 T) and novel second polar body transfer (PB2 T). The PB1 T technique involves removal of PB1 from a MII oocyte, followed by transfer to an enucleated MII oocyte and fertilization of the reconstituted oocyte. The novel PB2 T approach, as described in the study by Tang *et al.* [17], circumvents the problem of distinguishing the female and male pronuclei, whereby the MII oocyte is first enucleated, followed by fertilization via ICSI. This oocyte then serves as the recipient for the transfer of the PB2 genome from a donor zygote.

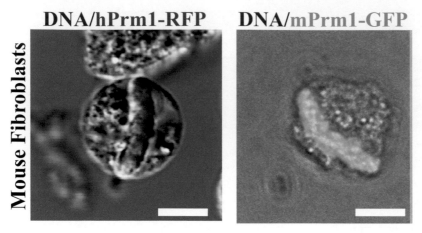

Figure 15.1 Nuclear remodeling of somatic cell nuclei expressing mouse and human Protamine 1 (Prm1).

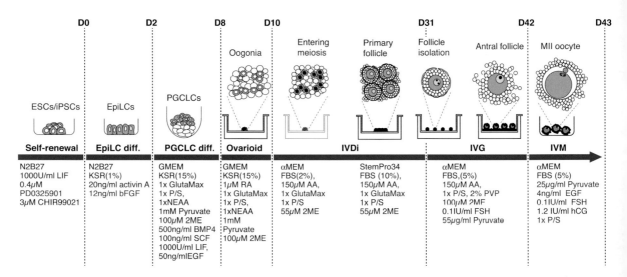

Figure 16.2 How to produce artificial eggs in mice. Shown are the condition of each culture term and days after differentiation from ESCs/iPSCs. IVDi, in vitro differentiation; IVG, in vitro growth; IVM, in vitro maturation.

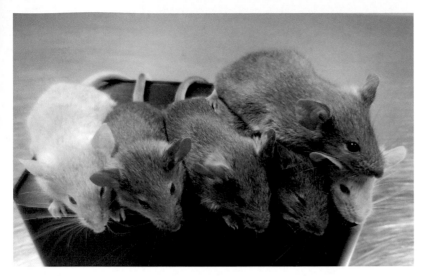

Figure 16.3 Mouse offspring from the tail. Shown are mice from artificial eggs derived from iPSCs that were established from adult tail-tip fibroblast.

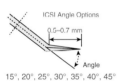

ICSI Angle Options

0.5–0.7 mm

Angle

15°, 20°, 25°, 30°, 35°, 40°, 45°

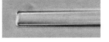

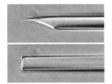

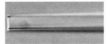

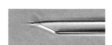

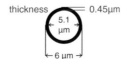

thickness ⎯ 0.45μm

5.1 μm

6 μm

Health of Children Born after Intracytoplasmic Sperm Injections (ICSI)

Shahad Sabti and Alastair G. Sutcliffe

Introduction

Intracytoplasmic sperm injection (ICSI) was first introduced in 1992, and its ability to permit almost any type of spermatozoa to fertilize an oocyte has made it a successful treatment for male factor infertility. Yet, despite this, concerns have been raised regarding its safety, largely as this methodology overrides the natural selection barrier which consequently means that fertilization can be achieved with poorer quality sperm leading to a higher risk of abnormalities in the offspring. Furthermore, the ICSI procedure may damage structures and processes in the oocyte and disturb the meiotic spindle. The role of the meiotic spindle is to equally separate the chromosomes in a parental cell into two daughter cells during the anaphase stage of meiosis, thus disruption to the spindle may lead to abnormal rearrangement of chromosomes, which can result in aneuploidy after fertilization. Additional risks involve the in vitro culture of zygotes produced with ICSI, which may disturb the methylation process that is part of epigenetic programming. This has the potential to lead to imprinting disorders such as Beckwith-Wiedmann syndrome and Angelman's syndrome. Studies looking at the safety of ICSI and the risks of these complications will be reviewed in this chapter.

Perinatal and Neonatal Outcomes

Studies have looked at perinatal and neonatal outcomes after ICSI (Table 9.1), with the majority concluding increased risks of preterm, very preterm, low birth weight, very low birth weight and small for gestational age infants. Initially, these risks were attributed to the higher rate of multiple pregnancies associated with ART. However, when this element was removed through the introduction of single embryo transfer (a process that substantially reduces the rate of multiple pregnancies), an increased risk was still observed in singleton pregnancies resulting from ICSI when compared to spontaneously conceived (SC). Pandey et al. conducted a systematic review looking at perinatal outcomes in singleton pregnancies conceived from IVF with ICSI. The review described a relative risk (RR) of 1.65 for low birth weight (<2500 g) and a RR of 1.54 for preterm delivery (<37weeks) [1]. As birth weight is affected by gestation, it could be argued that patterns of low birth weight seen may be secondary to prematurity. Yet, after adjusting for gestational age, birth weight was found to remain low, suggesting that this risk is particular to ICSI neonates. Comparing ICSI to IVF, Hourvitz et al. found that the mean birth weight of singletons conceived after ICSI was 3001 ± 703 g, similar to that of singletons conceived after IVF (3059 ± 643 g). Overall, the paper concluded that there was no significant difference in perinatal outcomes between pregnancies conceived after ICSI or indeed IVF [2]. However, ICSI-conceived neonates were more likely to be admitted to the neonatal intensive care unit (NICU) than IVF-conceived and SC neonates and spent more days in hospital [3]. This may be because of extra precautions taken by healthcare professions when treating ICSI-conceived neonates, although an increased risk of morbidity cannot be excluded. Furthermore, the increased number of complications is associated with a higher rate of perinatal mortality, for ICSI multiples, the RR was 6.6 [4], whereas for ICSI singletons, the RR was 1.27 [5].

All in all, pregnancies from IVF with ICSI were associated with an increased risk of perinatal complications when compared to spontaneous pregnancies. Although it remains unclear why this is the case, it is evident that these patients should be managed as high-risk pregnancies. It has been suggested that parental characteristics – which include subfertility factors, may play a role. Henriksen et al. compared the rates of preterm delivery in females conceiving within 6 months, between 7 and 12 months or after 12 months of attempts. The risk of preterm delivery

Table 9.1 Perinatal and neonatal outcomes after ICSI

Authors, year	Design	Sample size	Outcome measures	Conclusion
Pandey et al., 2012 [1]	Systematic review and meta-analysis	20 matched cohort studies 20 unmatched cohort studies	SGA Delivery <32 weeks Delivery <37 weeks Birth weight <2500g Birth weight <1500g APH PPROM Hypertensive disorders of pregnancy Gestational diabetes Induction of labor Cesarean section Congenital anomalies Perinatal mortality Neonatal admissions	Compared to SC pregnancies, IVF/ICSI singleton pregnancies were associated with a higher risk of obstetric and perinatal complications
Hourvitz et al., 2005 [2]	Retrospective cohort	219 ICSI pregnancies, 322 children 145 IVF pregnancies, 201 children	Parental characteristics Age Birthplace Origin Education Diseases Smoking Treatment (ICSI or IVF) Pregnancy complications Diabetes Hypertension Placenta previa Placental abruption Vaginal bleeding Poly/oligohydramnios Infectious diseases PROM Hospitalization Pregnancy outcome Duration Weight Apgar scores Multiple fetuses Method of delivery Neonatal problems and congenital malformations	No significant differences were found between pregnancies conceived after either ICSI or IVF, except for the lower birth weights of ICSI children No significant difference was found between ICSI and IVF, in terms of the risk of congenital malformations Compared to the general population, there was an increased risk of congenital malformation in ICSI and IVF pregnancies

Study	Design	Population	Parameters	
Nouri et al., 2013 [3]	Retrospective cohort	80 ICSI-conceived children 21 singletons 25 twins 3 triplets 450 IVF-conceived children 134 singletons 135 twins 14 triplets	Maternal parameters Age BMI Gravity Number of fetuses Pregnancy complications Pregnancy-induced hypertension Preeclampsia PROM Cervical insufficiency Premature uterine contractions Number of hospitalizations Fetal parameters Gestational age Birth weight Birth height pH of the umbilical artery APGAR after 1 minute and 10 minutes Congenital malformation Admission of the newborn to NICU Death of the infant	The course of pregnancies was more complicated after conventional IVF when compared to ICSI pregnancies Primary fetal outcome seemed to be better after IVF treatment when compared to ICSI treatment
McElrath and Wise, 1997 [8]	Retrospective cohort	9953 IVF conceived children	VLBW: birth weight <1500g	Fertility therapy is associated with VLBW, related only in part to an increased risk of multiple gestations

SGA, small for gestational age; APH, antepartum hemorrhage; PPROM, preterm premature rupture of membranes; PROM, premature rupture of membranes.

was 1.3 times higher in females conceiving between 7 and 12 months compared to those conceiving within 6 months. This risk further increased by 1.6 times in women conceiving after 12 months [6]. Regarding male infertility, the systematic review by Esteves et al. concluded that there was a higher rate of preterm delivery after ICSI in azoospermic fathers (17.9%) in comparison to non-azoospermic infertile fathers (9.7%) [7]. Interestingly, infertility alone is considered to be an independent risk factor for low birth weight and thus may be responsible for perinatal complications seen after ICSI [8].

Congenital Anomalies

Hansen et al. were the first to report the relationship between IVF with ICSI and congenital anomalies [9]. They described a two-fold increased risk of major birth defects in children conceived via IVF with ICSI. The major defects associated with ICSI can be divided into urogenital, cardiovascular, musculoskeletal and chromosomal.

Urogenital Anomalies

In the literature available, hypospadias (an opening of the urethra on the ventral aspect of the penis) seems to be the most common anomaly seen in male neonates born after ICSI (RR 3.0) [10]. However, it should be noted that hypospadias has often been linked with paternal infertility [11], and as such ICSI may not be directly related to this condition. A large proportion of male neonates born from ICSI were also found to have undescended testes [12], as well as low serum testosterone level at three months [13]. This could be suggestive of impaired Leydig function, which may be inherited from a subfertile father, as opposed to a result of ICSI. There were also high incidences of orofacial clefts [10], with similar rates observed in ICSI- and IVF-conceived neonates.

Cardiovascular and Musculoskeletal Anomalies

In terms of musculoskeletal anomalies, the RR of ICSI with IVF was 1.6, while the RR for cardiovascular defects was 1.4 [14]. Giorgione et al. carried out a meta-analysis focused on finding congenital heart defects in IVF with ICSI pregnancies. The study found that there was a 50% increased risk of congenital heart defects in IVF with ICSI pregnancies when compared

with SC and recommended echocardiography in all pregnancies from IVF with ICSI [15]. The reasoning behind the increased rate of cardiovascular anomalies remains unknown. Comparing ICSI to IVF, there was a 9.9% risk of birth defects after ICSI compared to a 7.2% risk after IVF.

Chromosomal Anomalies

The procedures of ART have been associated with imprinting disorders such as Beckwith-Wiedemann [16], and Angelman's syndrome [17]. Both syndromes are caused by an unmethylated maternal allele, so are unlikely to be related to paternal problems involving spermatic function. Instead, it seems more likely that ICSI disturbs the methylation of the maternal genome. As such, couples looking to use ICSI should be counseled regarding the risk of imprinting syndromes and genetic testing is advisable. Importantly, as the baseline risk of imprinting disorders is low, any small increase in risk still results in only rare occurrences of the disorder. Infertility may also play a role in causing these defects, Horsthemke and Ludwig found that a pregnancy interval of 24 months was associated with Angelman's syndrome [18]. Furthermore, infertile women and men undergoing ICSI usually have a higher rate of chromosomal abnormalities, further suggesting that infertility itself plays a role in causing major malformations in ICSI-conceived children [19,20].

Neurodevelopmental Outcomes

Neurodevelopmental outcomes include neuromotor, cognitive, speech/language and behavioral outcomes. Studies have been conducted on neurodevelopmental outcomes after ICSI with the majority concluding no significant difference when compared to SC.

Maternal Factors

Sutcliffe et al. compared 123 ICSI singletons with 123 SC singletons aged between 12 and 24 months [21]. Children were matched for social class, maternal educational level, sex and race. The study found that the mean mental age and mean Griffiths quotients were similar, with only a reduction in eye-hand coordination in the ICSI group. Likewise, Agarwal et al. (2005) compared 76 ICSI conceived children with 261 matched controls (SC neonates) [22]. They were matched for maternal age, sex, race and date of delivery. The study found that neurodevelopmental and functional outcomes were comparable in both groups. Remarkably, the ICSI group showed a higher-level performance than the control group, with a mean Bayley MDI score of 92 in the ICSI group and 90 in the naturally conceived group. Moreover, higher maternal educational status and family socio-economic status was found to correlate with higher performances. This was reflected by the international study conducted by Ponjaert-Kristoffersen et al. comparing 424 IVF-conceived, 511 ICSI-conceived and 488 naturally conceived 5-year-old children [23]. Although no significant differences were found in intelligence, IVF with ICSI offspring who were born to mothers at an older age had a lower full scale IQ (sum of scores in the performance scale and verbal scale) and verbal IQ score when compared to their SC counterparts. This suggests that factors such as maternal age have a greater effect on cognitive development, more so than the mode of conception. Paternal risk factors have also been tested, as with Bonduelle et al. but no associations were found with regards to infertility and psychomotor development [24].

It is difficult to assess the true impact of ICSI on neurodevelopment as not all studies are unified with regards to their findings. Sutcliffe et al. found no correlation between NICU admissions and development [21], unlike Hashem et al. who found that ICSI neonates admitted to NICU were more likely to have an abnormal DDST than those not hospitalized [25]. Hashem et al. also found a significant difference in height in the second and third years of life with SC children, whereas Place and Englert (2003) found no difference in height and weight between ICSI and SC children [26].

Cerebral Palsy

An association between ICSI and cerebral palsy has been reported. Pinborg et al. studied the incidence of cerebral palsy in IVF with ICSI children (>7 years old) and found a RR of 1.9 [27]. This could be attributed to a higher incidence of preterm and multiple births observed with ICSI, rather than the ICSI procedure itself. Pinborg et al. also proposed that the higher incidence may be the result of vanishing twins, with the surviving twin having cerebral palsy. In the study, 10% of singletons born from IVF with ICSI originated from twin pregnancies, with the surviving twin having a higher risk of low birth weight and prematurity.

Autism

Catford et al. found an increased risk of autistic spectrum disorder and intellectual impairment in ICSI-conceived children when compared to IVF-conceived children [28]. Although current studies assessing the risk of autistic spectrum disorder are inconsistent, this may be a result of the heterogenic etiology of autism.

Other Health Outcomes

Childhood Cancers

Few studies have reported the incidence of childhood cancers after IVF with ICSI treatment. A large meta-analysis carried out by Hargreave et al. looking at the relationship between childhood cancers and fertility treatment found an increased risk of all cancers, hematological cancers and CNS/neural cancers, in children born after fertility treatment [29]. As with the other outcomes mentioned above, it was unclear whether it was the fertility treatment or factors relating to fertility that led to the rise in risk. An Israeli study compared 9042 cases conceived by IVF with ICSI with 211,763 SC children for approximately 10 years [30]. The results showed an increased risk for retinoblastoma (RR 6.18) and renal tumors (RR 3.25) in the IVF with ICSI group when compared to the SC group. There were no differences in risk between ICSI- and IVF-conceived children. The etiology of childhood cancer is unknown, but it is thought that epigenetics may play a role.

Future Fertility of Offspring

In 18–22-year-old ICSI-conceived females, Belva et al. found no differences in levels of reproductive hormone including antimullerian hormone (AMH), follicle stimulating hormone (FSH) and luteinizing hormone (LH) when compared to SC females of the same age [31].

Similarly, FSH, LH, testosterone and inhibin B were also comparable between ICSI-conceived men and SC men. However, men conceived by ICSI were found to be low in sperm concentration, total sperm count and total motile sperm count when compared to their SC peers [32]. Furthermore, ICSI offspring were three times more likely to have a sperm concentration below the normal values defined by the World Health Organization (<15 million/mL of semen) and four times more likely to have total sperm counts below 39 million. Whether or not these altered semen parameters will impact these individual's future ability to have children is still unknown. This study was specific to those born from ICSI using ejaculated sperm because of impaired spermatogenesis, as such results cannot be applied to all offspring born after ICSI.

Cystic Fibrosis

The congenital absence of the vas deferens has been associated with cystic fibrosis, thus if ICSI is performed on an azoospermic father who has congenital bilateral absence or atrophy of the vas deferens, then the couple should be offered genetic counseling to discuss testing for cystic fibrosis.

Overall Outcome

Belva et al. followed up ICSI-conceived children at the age of 8 years, they found that ICSI-conceived children had similar outcomes in terms of physical examination including a neurological examination when compared to SC children with no increased rate of use of medical therapy, hospitalization or surgery [33]. Some common malformations seen with ICSI conceptions included inguinal hernias and strabism, but most were easily corrected with minor surgery. Similarly, Leunens et al. (2008) followed up ICSI-conceived children aged 10 years old and examined their cognitive, psychosocial and medical development [34]. The study determined that ICSI-conceived children showed comparable cognitive and motor development to SC children at least until the age of 10.

Some studies – such as the multicenter cohort study conducted by Bonduelle et al. – dispute these conclusions as these groups found increased rates of childhood illness, use of medical therapy, hospital admission and surgical operations in ICSI-conceived children [35]. Whilst the cause of hospitalization is unknown, it may be as a result of parental anxiety or concern, or secondary to conditions like cerebral palsy or cystic fibrosis.

Conclusion

ICSI treatment has been associated with an increased risk of prematurity, low birth weight and perinatal mortality, although the literature does not suggest these risks are specific to ICSI but more ART as a whole. Certain congenital and genetic anomalies have been associated with ICSI, particularly hypospadias, but this needs to be

researched further. Likewise, although the majority of studies have found no increased risk in neurodevelopmental abnormalities, this too needs to be researched. Overall it is still unclear whether the risks associated with ICSI are as a result of the procedure or of the inherent sperm abnormality. Regardless, couples seeking ICSI treatment should be advised about the possible increased risk in perinatal and neonatal complications including congenital and genetic anomalies and they should be made aware that long-term complications are still unknown.

References

[1] Pandey, S., Shetty, A., Hamilton, M., Bhattacharya, S. and Maheshwari, A. (2012). Obstetric and perinatal outcomes in singleton pregnancies resulting from IVF/ICSI: a systematic review and meta-analysis. Human Reproduction Update, 18(5),pp.485–503.

[2] Hourvitz, A., Pri-paz, S., Dor, J. and Seidman, D. (2005). Neonatal and obstetric outcome of pregnancies conceived by ICSI or IVF. Reproductive BioMedicine Online, 11(4),pp.469–475.

[3] Nouri, K., Ott, J., Stoegbauer, L., Pietrowski, D., Frantal, S. and Walch, K. (2013). Obstetric and perinatal outcomes in IVF versus ICSI-conceived pregnancies at a tertiary care center – a pilot study. Reproductive Biology and Endocrinology, 11(1),p.84.

[4] Luke, B. and Keith, L.G. (1992). The contribution of singletons, twins and triplets to low birth weight, infant mortality and handicap in the United States. Journal of Reproductive Medicine, 37,pp.661–666.

[5] Helmerhorst, F.M., Perquin, D.A., Donker, D. and Keirse, M.J.N.C. (2004). Perinatal outcome of singletons and twins after assisted conception: a systematic review of controlled studies. British Medical Journal, 328,pp.261–265.

[6] Henriksen, T.B., Baird, D.D., Olsen, J., Hedegaard, M., Secher, N.J. and Wilcox, A.J. (1997) Time to pregnancy and preterm delivery. Obstetrics and Gynecology, 89(4),pp.594–599.

[7] Esteves, S. and Agarwal, A. (2013). The azoospermic male: current knowledge and future perspectives. Clinics, 68(S1),pp.1–4.

[8] McElrath, T. and Wise, P.H. (1997). Fertility therapy and the risk of very low birth weight. Obstetrics and Gynecology, 90(4),pp.600–605.

[9] Hansen, M., Kurinczuk, J., Bower, C. and Webb, S. (2002). The risk of major birth defects after intracytoplasmic sperm injection and in vitro fertilization. New England Journal of Medicine, 346 (10),pp.725–730.

[10] Wennerholm, U., Bergh, C., Hamberger, L., Lundin, K., Nilsson, L., Wikland, M. and Källén, B. (2000). Incidence of congenital malformations in children born after ICSI. Human Reproduction, 15(4),pp.944–948.

[11] Sweet R.A., Schrott H.G., Kirland R., Culp,O.S. (1974). Study of the incidence of hypospadias in Rochester Minnesota 1940–1970 and a case control comparison of possible etiological factors. Mayo Clinic Proceedings, 49,pp.52–58.

[12] Ludwig, A., Katalinic, A., Thyen, U., Sutcliffe, A., Diedrich, K. and Ludwig, M. (2009). Physical health at 5.5 years of age of term-born singletons after intracytoplasmic sperm injection: results of a prospective, controlled, single-blinded study. Fertility and Sterility, 91(1),pp.115–124.

[13] Mau Kai, C., Main, K., Andersen, A., Loft, A., Skakkebæk, N. and Juul, A. (2007). Reduced serum testosterone levels in infant boys conceived by intracytoplasmic sperm injection. The Journal of Clinical Endocrinology & Metabolism, 92(7), pp.2598–2603.

[14] Lie, R., Lyngstadass, A., Ørstavik, K., Bakketeig, L., Jacobsen, G. and Tanbo, T. (2004). Birth defects in children conceived by ICSI compared with children conceived by other IVF-methods; a meta-analysis. International Journal of Epidemiology, 34(3), pp.696–701.

[15] Giorgione, V., Parazzini, F., Fesslova, V., Cipriani, S., Candiani, M., Inversetti, A., et al. (2018). Congenital heart defects in IVF/ICSI pregnancy: systematic review and meta-analysis. Ultrasound in Obstetrics & Gynecology, 51(1),pp.33–42.

[16] Maher, E.R., Brueton, L.A., Bowdin, S.C., Luharia, A., Cooper, W., Cole, T.R., Macdonald, F., Sampson, J.R., Barratt, C.L., Reik, W. and Hawkins, M.M. (2003). Beckwith-Wiedemann syndrome and assisted reproduction technology (ART). Journal of Medical Genetics, 40(1),pp.62–64.

[17] Ørstavik, K., Eiklid, K., van der Hagen, C., Spetalen, S., Kierulf, K., Skjeldal, O. and Buiting, K. (2003). Another case of imprinting defect in a girl with Angelman syndrome who was conceived by intracytoplasmic sperm injection. The American Journal of Human Genetics, 72(1),pp.218–219.

[18] Horsthemke, B. and Ludwig, M. (2005). Assisted reproduction: the epigenetic perspective. Human Reproduction Update, 11,pp.473–482.

[19] Schreurs A., Legius E., Meuleman C., Fryns J.P. and D'hooghe T.M. (2000). Increased frequency of chromosomal abnormalities in female partners of couples undergoing in vitro fertilization or intracytoplasmic sperm injection. Fertility & Sterility, 74,pp.94–96.

[20] Hansen M., Bower C., Milne E., de Klerk N. and Kurinczuk J.J. (2005). Assisted reproductive technologies and the risk of birth defects-a systematic review. Human Reproduction, 20,pp.328–333.

[21] Sutcliffe, A., Taylor, B., Saunders, K., Thornton, S., Leiberman, B. and Grudzinskas, J. (2001). Outcome in the second year of life after in-vitro fertilisation by intracytoplasmic sperm injection: a UK case-control study. The Lancet, 357(9274), pp.2080–2084.

[22] Agarwal, P., Loh, S., Lim, S., Sriram, B., Daniel, M., Yeo, S. and Heng, D. (2005). Two-year neurodevelopmental outcome in children conceived by intracytoplasmic sperm injection: prospective cohort study. BJOG: An International Journal of Obstetrics & Gynaecology, 112(10),pp.1376–1383.

[23] Ponjaert-Kristoffersen, I., Bonduelle, M., Barnes, J., Nekkebroeck, J., Loft, A., Wennerholm, U.-B., et al. (2005). International collaborative study of intracytoplasmic sperm injection-conceived, in vitro fertilization-conceived, and naturally conceived 5-year-old child outcomes: cognitive and motor assessments. Pediatrics, 115(3),pp.e283–e289.

[24] Bonduelle, M. Ponjaert, I., Van Steirteghem, A., Derde, M.-P., Devroey, P. and Liebaers, I. (2003). Developmental outcome at 2 years of age for children born after ICSI compared with children born after IVF. Human Reproduction, 18(2), pp.342–350.

[25] Hashem, M., Mahmoud, N., Aboulghar, H., Omar, A., El Shamaa, M. and Moustafa, R. (2010). Karyotyping and neurodevelopmental follow-up of intracytoplasmic sperm injection children up to 4 years of age. Middle East Fertility Society Journal, 15(1),pp.21–28.

[26] Place, I. and Englert, Y. (2003). A prospective longitudinal study of the physical, psychomotor, and intellectual development of singleton children up to 5 years who were conceived by intracytoplasmic sperm injection compared with children conceived spontaneously and by in vitro fertilization. Fertility and Sterility, 80(6),pp.1388–1397.

[27] Pinborg, A., Lidegaard, Ø., la Cour Freiesleben, N. and Andersen, A. (2005). Consequences of vanishing twins in IVF/ICSI pregnancies. Human Reproduction, 20(10),pp.2821–2829.

[28] Catford, S., McLachlan, R., O'Bryan, M. and Halliday, J. (2017). Long-term follow-up of intra-cytoplasmic sperm injection-conceived offspring compared with in vitro fertilization-conceived offspring: a systematic review of health outcomes beyond the neonatal period. Andrology, 5(4),pp.610–621.

[29]   Hargreave, M., Jensen, A., Toender, A., Andersen, K. and Kjaer, S. (2013). Fertility treatment and childhood cancer risk: a systematic meta-analysis. Fertility and Sterility, **100**(1),pp.150–161.

[30]   Lerner-Geva, L., Boyko, V., Ehrlich, S., Mashiach, S., Hourvitz, A., Haas, J., et al. (2016). Possible risk for cancer among children born following assisted reproductive technology in Israel. Pediatric Blood & Cancer, **64**(4), p.e26292.

[31]   Belva, F., Roelants, M., Vloeberghs, V., Schiettecatte, J., Evenepoel, J., Bonduelle, M. and de Vos, M. (2017). Serum reproductive hormone levels and ultrasound findings in female offspring after intracytoplasmic sperm injection: first results. Fertility and Sterility, **107** (4),pp.934–939.

[32]   Belva, F., Roelants, M., De Schepper, J., Van Steirteghem, A., Tournaye, H. and Bonduelle, M. (2016). Reproductive hormones of ICSI-conceived young adult men: the first results. Human Reproduction, **32**(2),pp.439–446.

[33]   Belva, F., Henriet, S., Liebaers, I., Van Steirteghem, A., Celestin-Westreich, S. and Bonduelle, M. (2006). Medical outcome of 8-year-old singleton ICSI children (born >=32 weeks' gestation) and a spontaneously conceived comparison group. Human Reproduction, **22**(2), pp.506–515.

[34]   Leunens, L., Celestin-Westreich, S., Bonduelle, M., Liebaers, I. and Ponjaert-Kristoffersen, I. (2007). Follow-up of cognitive and motor development of 10-year-old singleton children born after ICSI compared with spontaneously conceived children. Human Reproduction, **23**(1),pp.105–111.

[35]   Bonduelle, M., Wennerholm, U., Loft, A., Tarlatzis, B., Peters, C., Henriet, S., et al. (2005). A multi-centre cohort study of the physical health of 5-year-old children conceived after intracytoplasmic sperm injection, in vitro fertilization and natural conception. Human Reproduction, **20**(2), pp.413–419.

Chapter 10

Examining the Safety of ICSI Using Animal Models

Laura Hewitson

Introduction

In 1992, Palermo and colleagues reported the first clinical pregnancies conceived by intracytoplasmic sperm injection (ICSI) [1], which were followed soon after with the first live births [2]. Since then, an estimated 8 million births have resulted from assisted conceptions [3] with ICSI accounting for 70–80% of all the cycles performed world-wide [4]. Unlike IVF, which requires optimal sperm number and function for sperm–oocyte union, ICSI obviates these requirements and is routinely applied to alleviate severe male factor infertility resulting from both non-obstructive and obstructive azoospermia [5]. Notwithstanding these successes, the increasing evidence of the involvement of genetic factors in male infertility and the potential risk of transmission of genetic disorders to the offspring [6], suggests that a more judicious approach to the application of ICSI is warranted [7], especially as ICSI has been adopted by most fertility clinics over IVF even in the absence of male factor fertility [8].

While the success of clinical ICSI was reported well before animal models had been developed to study the potential health risks associated with this technique, one cannot ignore the overwhelming success it garnered. In fact, the discovery and development of ICSI followed an unusual path, with the clinical treatment pioneering the approach [9]. Even today, fundamental research in relevant animal models still lags behind. This chapter will examine the animal models of ICSI that have helped inform improvements to the technique *per se*; provided heterologous ICSI assays for testing human sperm function and oocyte activation; and addressed clinical concerns regarding long-term health of the offspring.

Development of Animal Models to Examine the Safety of ICSI

Except for a handful of papers experimenting with sperm microsurgical techniques in some animal species, the technique of ICSI was not well-developed in animal models until after live human births had been reported (reviewed by [10]). This included ICSI in the rabbit [11], mouse [12], rhesus macaque [13], rat [14], sheep [15], domestic cat and wild felids [16], pig [17], horse [18], and hamster [19], among others. The delay in the development of animal models for ICSI reflects the overwhelming success of clinical ICSI coupled with the many challenges of using animal gametes. For example, while the mouse seemed like the obvious choice as an animal model for ICSI, the use of mouse oocytes was hampered by low survival rates after ICSI without the aid of a piezo microinjector [12]. The piezo microinjector improved fertilization rates by enabling a wider injection pipette to be used to accommodate the hooked mouse sperm head in oocytes that are more susceptible to microsurgical techniques due to their smaller size (80 μm) [12]. By 1998, Yanagimachi and colleagues had perfected ICSI in mice by applying several technological advances [20] and since then, it has become the model of choice for most ICSI studies, especially those designed for producing offspring.

In cows and other ruminants, there are a different set of challenges for ICSI – primarily because the oocytes have a dark and opaque cytoplasm due to their high lipid content [21], which, unlike human oocytes, makes it difficult to visualize the meiotic spindle. An electrical or chemical activation stimulus is also required after ICSI in ruminants to ensure the resumption of meiosis [22]. Despite these differences, bovine oocytes have been used to develop heterologous ICSI models for assessing sperm function (discussed later in this chapter) but, as an animal model, they perhaps have greatest utility in biodiversity conservation and transgenic production [23]. Although animal models for ICSI provide some valuable tools, researchers still need to resolve some of the underlying technical challenges and practical limitations in using certain animal species.

Technical Aspects of ICSI

The ICSI procedure bypasses the complex series of events during sperm–oocyte union that would normally occur after spontaneous conception or fertilization by IVF (Table 10.1). Since a sperm is directly injected into the oocyte to initiate fertilization, a number of physical alterations can be observed including mechanical damage to the sperm from pretreatment prior to ICSI [24, 25]; introduction of the sperm acrosome [26, 27] and retention of sperm proteins typically lost during sperm–oocyte binding [28, 29]; injection of foreign materials, such as polyvinylpyrrolidone (PVP), into the oolemma [30]; disruption to the sperm plasma membrane [31, 32]; and the mechanical disruption of intracellular structures of the oocyte, such as the meiotic spindle [33, 34]. Additionally, mitotic spindle orientation and microtubule-cortex interactions during the first cleavage division differ between IVF- and ICSI-fertilized rhesus zygotes, suggesting that mechanical disruptions during fertilization impart cytoplasmic changes during first cleavage [35].

Shortly after the first clinical ICSI successes were reported, research began in earnest to examine aspects of the ICSI technique to evaluate its safety. A study using bovine zygotes sought to evaluate the use of PVP during ICSI [30] because of concerns over the toxicity of some commercially produced PVP solutions in mouse ICSI [36]. Using sham-ICSI (injection without a sperm), 2–3 pL of culture medium containing PVP or culture medium alone were injected into in vitro fertilized zygotes and then embryo development compared along with unmanipulated zygotes. Based on the development to the hatched blastocyst stage and blastocyst cell number, the authors concluded that the ICSI procedures currently used for human ICSI were not detrimental to embryonic development or embryo quality [30]. However, fertilization was not accomplished by ICSI and thus, the sperm itself was not exposed to PVP, which has been reported to cause submicroscopic damage to the sperm structure including changes in the shape and texture of chromatin [37], as well as developmental effects [38].

Cytoskeletal Dynamics of ICSI Fertilization

As a result of the low success rate of ICSI in mice and domestic species experienced in the 1990s, other animal models were sought to examine the safety of ICSI. Non-human primates share many similarities with the key aspects of human reproduction, such as gamete maturation, fertilization, embryonic development, embryo transfer and implantation. Thus, ICSI in rhesus macaques enjoyed many early successes [13, 39], including live births [29]. Efforts were expanded to include testicular sperm and elongated spermatids [40], as well as developing ICSI as a means to introduce foreign DNA into oocytes for transgenesis [41].

Fertilization of rhesus macaque oocytes by ICSI also provided some of the first images of the cytoskeletal events during fertilization [13] and identified unique structural changes occurring in the sperm [27, 29]. During IVF, the sperm binds to the zona pellucida, undergoes the acrosome reaction, and fuses with the oolemma. Conversely, ICSI bypasses the natural events of sperm binding and fusion. An analysis of rhesus monkey ICSI zygotes using transmission electron microscopy revealed that sperm decondensation is altered after ICSI compared to IVF [27]. The acrosome, which is typically lost at the oocyte membrane during sperm penetration, is injected along with the sperm during ICSI [26] and persists for several hours [28, 29]. Vesicle-associated membrane protein (VAMP), a constituent of the sperm acrosome, is detected as a constriction around the forming paternal pronucleus in rhesus monkey zygotes following ICSI [29]. The retention of VAMP following ICSI serves to separate the condensed and decondensing chromatin, persisting until paternal pronucleus formation is completed. In addition, the perinuclear theca, a structure found on the inner acrosomal membrane of the sperm and typically removed during fertilization at either the zona pellucida or the oocyte's plasma membrane, was found closely associated with the paternal pronucleus until at least 16 hours post-ICSI [29]. The persistence of the acrosome over the anterior part of the injected sperm may prevent the import of maternal nuclear proteins during sperm decondensation.

The significance of this asynchronous decondensation is not completely understood but it may lead to a diminished ability of the oocyte to express, or be exposed to, paternal genes or gene products, thus

Table 10.1 Differences in sperm–oocyte activities during fertilization by natural insemination versus ICSI

Activity	Natural fertilization	Fertilization by ICSI
Culture media	No (if naturally); Yes (if IVF)	Yes
Exposure to light	No (if naturally); Yes (dim, short illumination during IVF)	Yes (often extended exposure)
Temperature fluctuations	No	Yes
Capacitation of sperm	Yes (in vivo)	No (unless induced artificially)
Exposure to PVP	No	Yes (usually)
Selection of successful sperm	By oocyte (nature)	By embryologist
Use of immature or immotile sperm	No	Yes (if needed)
Sperm motility	Yes	Not required
Site of initial contact between sperm and oocyte cytoplasm	At oocyte cortex	At central cytoplasm
Acrosome reaction	Yes	No
Ionic triggers, including elevated Ca^{2+} concentration in sperm cytoplasm	During acrosome reaction	During oocyte activation
Sperm penetration through oocyte's outer vestments	Yes	No
Oocyte activation: ionic cascade	Initiated at oocyte surface	Initiated in oocyte cytoplasm
Deformation of oocyte membrane	No	Yes
Sperm entry site	Oocyte surface	Oocyte cytoplasm
Sperm membrane fate	Coalescence into oocyte's plasma membrane	Removal of small vesicles within oocyte cytoplasm
Sperm incorporation cone	Yes	No
Entry of sperm tail	Yes (always)	Yes/no (usually)
Perinuclear theca	Lost at cortex	Introduced with sperm
Decondensation of sperm nucleus	Uniform	Asynchronous with different choreography

leading to improper embryo formation [9]. Furthermore, in rhesus oocytes fertilized by ICSI, DNA synthesis, as detected by bromodioxyuridine (BrdU) incorporation, was delayed by several hours in both pronuclei while the paternal pronucleus was still undergoing decondensation in the apical region, and pronuclear migration was delayed, identifying a unique G1/S cell cycle checkpoint [29]. Conversely, after IVF, pronuclear migration was completed within 12 hours post-insemination and DNA synthesis was detected in both pronuclei [29].

Animal Models to Examine Potential Long-Term Health Effects of ICSI

Even with the global success of ICSI, a number of complications, including a higher risk of congenital anomalies, hypertensive disorders of pregnancy, disorders of the placenta, preterm birth, low birth weight, perinatal mortality, and small size for gestational age, have been reported [42–44]. There is also substantial evidence that infants born after ICSI have an increased risk of congenital malformations, chromosomal aberrations, and imprinting disorders when compared with peers born after spontaneous conception [43–45]. An excellent review by Belva and colleagues [46] summarized the currently available literature pertaining to the health of ICSI offspring and concluded with the following points: (i) endocrine gonadal function in pubertal ICSI boys is comparable with boys conceived by spontaneous conception (SC); (ii) reproductive hormone levels are comparable between ICSI young adults and control peers, but trend towards a higher risk of aberrant levels; (iii) sperm concentration, sperm count, and total motile count are lower in ICSI young adults compared with peers born after SC; and (iv) there is a greater risk of low sperm counts in ICSI young adults. The authors concluded that long-term follow-up of adults born after ICSI should be implemented in all centers treating couples with ICSI [46]. As more than 5 million ICSI babies have been born worldwide, this is an area of research that warrants diligent surveillance.

Animal models of ICSI with no underlying infertility issues can exhibit analogous complications, suggesting that these procedures may be causal as opposed to associated with infertility [42]. Furthermore, the long-term consequences extend well past fertilization and embryo development, potentially affecting genomic stability, health, and fertility of ICSI-conceived animals and their progeny [47, 48]. For example, in a mouse model of ICSI employing live-cell imaging by confocal microscopy, many embryos with apparent normal morphology viewed by conventional light microscopy had abnormal chromosome segregation (ACS) at the first mitotic division [49]. Around 50% of these ACS embryos developed into morphologically normal blastocysts resulting in implantation, although they did not develop to term. While this mouse ICSI model may provide insight to better understand the biological factors controlling the relationship between chromosomal abnormalities and subsequent in vitro embryonic development, it raises greater concerns. Perhaps less severely impaired, yet still abnormal, embryos produced by ICSI may be able to survive through pregnancy, resulting in potential long-term effects in the offspring that could extend into adult life [47, 48]. This is known as the Developmental Origins of Adult Health and Disease (DOHaD) [50], and has implications for assisted reproductive technologies (ART) [48]. For example, mice derived by ART can have alterations in glucose parameters [51] and cardiometabolic disease [52], and decreased testis weight, abnormal testicular tubule morphology, and increased testicular apoptosis [53]. Furthermore, if DNA-fragmented sperm is used for mouse ICSI, the offspring can develop aberrant growth, premature aging, abnormal behavior, and mesenchymal tumors [54].

Using Animal ICSI Models to Develop Human Sperm Function Tests

Fertilization, whether occurring naturally, by IVF, or by ICSI, requires accurate cytoplasmic events mediated by the sperm centrosome, the cell's microtubule organizing center (MTOC). The resultant sperm aster brings about the union of the paternal and maternal genomes at first mitosis [55]. This is true for nearly all species so far studied except rodents, which demonstrate maternally inherited centrosomes [56]. Defects in centrosomal functioning characterized by microtubule nucleation arrest, premature detachment of the sperm axoneme and aster from the paternal pronucleus, and sperm aster microtubule growth defects, have been identified in human oocytes fertilized by ICSI [34] and may result in infertility [57].

To assess sperm centrosomal function without using human oocytes, Terada and colleagues developed a novel assay based on heterologous ICSI, in which human sperm were injected into rabbit and bovine oocytes [58]. Several hours after ICSI, a sperm-derived microtubule aster was observed in both rabbit and bovine oocytes, indicating that heterologous ICSI may provide a unique opportunity to assay human sperm centrosomal function without the use of human oocytes [59]. Similar experiments injecting human sperm into mouse and hamster oocytes have been performed but since fertilization in rodents relies on maternally derived centrosomes, they are not an appropriate heterologous ICSI for assessing human sperm function [60].

While developing the assay for assessing human sperm centrosome function, the authors noted that human sperm injected into rabbit oocytes also displayed aberrant nuclear decondensation [61], as has been reported in rhesus ICSI oocytes [29]. As the X chromosomes in the sperm head are located in the apical region [62, 63], and decondensation of human sperm nuclei after ICSI occurs asynchronously, delayed processing of the sex chromosomes is likely. It is possible that a delay in entry into S-phase may result in mitotic errors during first cleavage [29, 61] and have implications regarding the increase in sex chromosome anomalies that has been reported in ICSI-derived babies [64].

Oocyte activation and sperm nuclei remodeling has also been examined in a heterologous ICSI model using mouse oocytes injected with three types of human sperm: intact, immobilized, and sperm treated with Triton X-100. Following human sperm injection, the fastest and most efficient oocyte activation and sperm head decondensation occurred when sperm were treated with Triton X-100 [65]. Intact human spermatozoa were the least effective at activating oocytes. Thus, the rate of mouse oocyte activation following human sperm injection is greatly influenced by the state of the sperm plasma membrane during injection [65]. In a heterologous ICSI model using human sperm injected into hamster oocytes, asynchronous decondensation of sperm nuclei was also reported when acrosome intact sperm were utilized [66]. Nuclear decondensation occurred more rapidly and was less asynchronous when human sperm pre-treated with Triton X-100 were injected into hamster oocytes. Heterologous assays using human sperm provide an effective ICSI model for studying sperm chromosomal processing during pronuclear development [66, 67].

Utility of a Mouse Model for 'Rescue' ICSI

In some ICSI treatment cycles, all of the available oocytes from a given collection fail to fertilize [68, 69]. The main cause of ICSI failure in such cases is typically the lack of oocyte activation because of a deficiency or relative lack of Ca^{2+} oscillations, which are necessary for oocyte activation [70]. Several artificial oocyte activation (AOA) methods using calcium ionophores have been used to overcome complete fertilization failure after ICSI but have met with mixed success [71]. Phospholipase C zeta (PLCζ) is one of the primary factors involved in oocyte activation during fertilization [72]. Abnormal localization patterns and reduced or deficient PLCζ protein in human sperm fail to induce calcium oscillations [73] resulting in complete fertilization failure after ICSI [74]. These studies suggest that the injection of PLCζ protein into oocytes that fail to fertilize, could be used as a potential therapy to overcome such cases of infertility [73]. In mouse oocytes that express dysfunctional PLCζ, recombinant human PLCζ was used to rescue failed activation after ICSI, and this intervention culminated in efficient blastocyst formation [75]. PLCζ has also been used to activate mouse oocytes in a model of male factor infertility [76].

Several case reports have examined the use of AOA after fertilization failure resulting from ICSI in patients with abnormal sperm. For example, sperm from a globozoospermic patient that was deficient in PLCζ resulted in high rates of fertilization and pregnancy after ICSI was followed by AOA [77]. In another case report, fertilization failure as a result of sperm PLCζ deficiency was overcome using ICSI followed by AOA leading to normal embryo development [78]. Finally, in a prospective clinical trial to evaluate ICSI success using sperm with a PLCζ deficiency, with and without AOA [79],

the fertilization rate was significantly lower in the group without AOA compared to the control group, but cleavage rate and embryo quality were similar across groups. There has only been one small study evaluating neonatal, developmental, and behavioral assessments of children born following ICSI with AOA, and although it revealed no serious adverse effects [80], AOA does not accurately mimic the physiological fertilization process and may have harmful effects on oocytes and embryos [72, 81, 82]. Finally, as PLCζ is not species-specific, the injection of human sperm into mouse oocytes can cause Ca^{2+} oscillations as well as oocyte activation [68]. The use of heterologous ICSI provides a non-invasive method for evaluating cases of oocyte activation failure after human ICSI [68, 83].

Summary

The development of animal models to assess the safety of ICSI was somewhat preempted by the overwhelming success of clinical ICSI, and its subsequent global application. Early attempts at ICSI in most animals were also hampered by technical challenges. With improvements in oocyte activation techniques, sperm pre-treatment protocols, and imaging methodologies, ICSI has now been accomplished in a large number of species. This has led to animal models for studying cytoskeletal changes after ICSI including altered sperm decondensation and DNA synthesis, as well as the development of heterologous models to study human sperm function and oocyte activation. The relatively short pregnancy and juvenile periods in the mouse have enabled studies of prenatal and postnatal outcomes, especially as the mouse appropriately phenocopies the complications observed in humans after ART. With more recent studies demonstrating that ART-conceived children may be at increased risk for postnatal effects, animal ICSI models also have great utility for addressing potential adverse outcomes in adult offspring.

References

[1] Palermo, G., et al., *Pregnancies after intracytoplasmic injection of single spermatozoon into an oocyte.* Lancet, 1992. **340**(8810): pp. 17–8.

[2] Van Steirteghem, A.C., et al., *Higher success rate by intracytoplasmic sperm injection than by subzonal insemination. Report of a second series of 300 consecutive treatment cycles.* Hum Reprod, 1993. **8**(7): pp. 1055–60.

[3] Fauser, B.C.J.M. *Towards the global coverage of a unified registry of IVF outcomes. Reprod Biomed Online*, 2019. 38: pp. 133–7.

[4] Nyboe Andersen, A., E. Carlsen, and A. Loft, *Trends in the use of intracytoplasmatic sperm injection marked variability between countries.* Hum Reprod Update, 2008. 14(6): pp. 593–604.

[5] Vernaeve, V., et al., *Pregnancy outcome and neonatal data of children born after ICSI using testicular sperm in obstructive and non-obstructive azoospermia.* Hum Reprod, 2003. 18(10): pp. 2093–7.

[6] Palermo, G.D., Q.V. Neri, and Z. Rosenwaks, *To ICSI or not to ICSI.* Semin Reprod Med, 2015. 33(2): pp. 92–102.

[7] Merchant, R., G. Gandhi, and G.N. Allahbadia, *In vitro fertilization/intracytoplasmic sperm injection for male infertility.* Indian J Urol, 2011. 27(1): pp. 121–32.

[8] O'Neill, C.L., et al., *Development of ICSI.* Reproduction, 2018. 156(1): pp. F51–F58.

[9] Schatten, G., et al., *Cell and molecular biological challenges of ICSI: ART before science?* J Law Med Ethics, 1998. 26(1): pp. 29–37.

[10] Salamone, D.F., N.G. Canel, and M.B. Rodriguez, *Intracytoplasmic sperm injection in domestic and wild mammals.* Reproduction, 2017. 154(6): pp. F111–F124.

[11] Hosoi, Y. and A. Iritani, *Rabbit microfertilization.* Mol Reprod Dev, 1993. 36(2): pp. 282–4.

[12] Kimura, Y. and R. Yanagimachi, *Intracytoplasmic sperm injection in the mouse.* Biol Reprod, 1995. 52(4): pp. 709–20.

[13] Hewitson, L.C., et al., *Microtubule and chromatin configurations during rhesus intracytoplasmic sperm injection: successes and failures.* Biol Reprod, 1996. 55(2): pp. 271–80.

[14] Dozortsev, D., et al., *Intracytoplasmic sperm injection in the rat.* Zygote, 1998. 6(2): pp. 143–7.

[15] Gomez, M.C., et al., *Sheep oocyte activation after intracytoplasmic sperm injection (ICSI).* Reprod Fertil Dev, 1998. 10(2): pp. 197–205.

[16] Pope, C.E., et al., *Development of embryos produced by intracytoplasmic sperm injection of cat oocytes.* Anim Reprod Sci, 1998. 53(1–4): pp. 221–36.

[17] Kolbe, T. and W. Holtz, *Intracytoplasmic injection (ICSI) of in vivo or in vitro matured oocytes with fresh ejaculated or frozen-thawed epididymal spermatozoa and additional calcium-ionophore activation in the pig.* Theriogenology, 1999. 52(4): pp. 671–82.

[18] Cochran, R., et al., *Production of live foals from sperm-injected oocytes harvested from pregnant mares.* J Reprod Fertil Suppl, 2000(56): pp. 503–12.

[19] Yamauchi, Y., R. Yanagimachi, and T. Horiuchi, *Full-term development of golden hamster oocytes following intracytoplasmic sperm head injection.* Biol Reprod, 2002. 67(2): pp. 534–9.

[20] Yanagimachi, R., *Intracytoplasmic sperm injection experiments using the mouse as a model.* Hum Reprod, 1998. 13 Suppl 1: pp. 87–98.

[21] Singh Parmer, M., et al., *Intracytoplasmic sperm injection (ICSI) and its applications in veterinary sciences: An overview.* Sci Int, 2013. 1(8): pp. 266–270.

[22] Oikawa, T., et al., *Evaluation of activation treatments for blastocyst production and birth of viable calves following bovine intracytoplasmic sperm injection.* Anim Reprod Sci, 2005. 86(3–4): pp. 187–94.

[23] Garcia-Rosello, E., et al., *Intracytoplasmic sperm injection in livestock species: an update.* Reprod Domest Anim, 2009. 44(1): pp. 143–51.

[24] Li, M.W., et al., *Long-term storage of mouse spermatozoa after evaporative drying.* Reproduction, 2007. 133(5): pp. 919–29.

[25] Li, M.W., et al., *Damage to chromosomes and DNA of rhesus monkey sperm following cryopreservation.* J Androl, 2007. 28(4): pp. 493–501.

[26] Ramalho-Santos, J., et al., *ICSI choreography: fate of sperm structures after monospermic rhesus ICSI and first cell cycle implications.* Hum Reprod, 2000. 15(12): pp. 2610–20.

[27] Sutovsky, P., et al., *Intracytoplasmic sperm injection for Rhesus monkey fertilization results in unusual chromatin, cytoskeletal, and membrane events, but eventually leads to pronuclear development and sperm aster assembly.* Hum Reprod, 1996. 11(8): pp. 1703–12.

[28] Ramalho-Santos, J., et al., *SNAREs in mammalian sperm: possible implications for fertilization.* Dev Biol, 2000. 223(1): pp. 54–69.

[29] Hewitson, L., et al., *Unique checkpoints during the first cell cycle of fertilization after intracytoplasmic sperm injection in rhesus monkeys.* Nat Med, 1999. 5(4): pp. 431–3.

[30] Motoishi, M., et al., *Examination of the safety of intracytoplasmic injection procedures by using bovine zygotes.* Hum Reprod, 1996. 11(3): pp. 618–20.

[31] Yanagimachi, R., *Intracytoplasmic injection of spermatozoa and spermatogenic cells: its biology and applications in humans and animals.* Reprod Biomed Online, 2005. 10(2): pp. 247–88.

[32] Mansour, R., *Intracytoplasmic sperm injection: a state of the art technique.* Hum Reprod Update, 1998. 4(1): pp. 43–56.

[33] Rubino, P., et al., *The ICSI procedure from past to future: a systematic review of the more controversial*

aspects. Hum Reprod Update, 2016. **22**(2): pp. 194–227.

[34] Asch, R., et al., *The stages at which human fertilization arrests: microtubule and chromosome configurations in inseminated oocytes which failed to complete fertilization and development in humans.* Hum Reprod, 1995. **10**(7): pp. 1897–906.

[35] Simerly, C.R., et al., *Fertilization and cleavage axes differ in primates conceived by conventional (IVF) versus intracytoplasmic sperm injection (ICSI).* Sci Rep, 2019. **9**(1): p. 15282.

[36] Bras M, et al., *The use of a mouse zygote quality control system for training purposes and toxicity determination in an ICSI programme.* Hum Reprod, 1994. **9**: pp. 23–24.

[37] Strehler, E., et al., *Detrimental effects of polyvinylpyrrolidone on the ultrastructure of spermatozoa (Notulae seminologicae 13).* Hum Reprod, 1998. **13**(1): pp. 120–3.

[38] Kato, Y. and Y. Nagao, *Effect of PVP on sperm capacitation status and embryonic development in cattle.* Theriogenology, 2009. **72**(5): pp. 624–35.

[39] Hewitson, L., et al., *Fertilization and embryo development to blastocysts after intracytoplasmic sperm injection in the rhesus monkey.* Hum Reprod, 1998. **13**(12): pp. 3449–55.

[40] Hewitson, L., et al., *Rhesus offspring produced by intracytoplasmic injection of testicular sperm and elongated spermatids.* Fertil Steril, 2002. **77**(4): pp. 794–801.

[41] Chan, A.W., et al., *Foreign DNA transmission by ICSI: injection of spermatozoa bound with exogenous DNA results in embryonic GFP expression and live rhesus monkey births.* Mol Hum Reprod, 2000. **6**(1): pp. 26–33.

[42] Feuer, S.K., L. Camarano, and P.F. Rinaudo, *ART and health: clinical outcomes and insights on molecular mechanisms from rodent studies.* Mol Hum Reprod, 2013. **19**(4): pp. 189–204.

[43] Fauser, B.C., et al., *Health outcomes of children born after IVF/ICSI: a review of current expert opinion and literature.* Reprod Biomed Online, 2014. **28**(2): pp. 162–82.

[44] Hansen, M., et al., *Assisted reproductive technologies and the risk of birth defects–a systematic review.* Hum Reprod, 2005. **20**(2): pp. 328–38.

[45] Manipalviratn, S., A. DeCherney, and J. Segars, *Imprinting disorders and assisted reproductive technology.* Fertil Steril, 2009. **91**(2): pp. 305–15.

[46] Belva, F., M. Bonduelle, and H. Tournaye, *Endocrine and reproductive profile of boys and young adults conceived after ICSI.* Curr Opin Obstet Gynecol, 2019. **31**(3): pp. 163–169.

[47] Sanchez-Calabuig, M.J., et al., *Potential health risks associated to ICSI: insights from animal models and strategies for a safe procedure.* Front Public Health, 2014. **2**: p. 241.

[48] Vrooman, L.A. and M.S. Bartolomei, *Can assisted reproductive technologies cause adult-onset disease? Evidence from human and mouse.* Reprod Toxicol, 2017. **68**: pp. 72–84.

[49] Yamagata, K., R. Suetsugu, and T. Wakayama, *Assessment of chromosomal integrity using a novel live-cell imaging technique in mouse embryos produced by intracytoplasmic sperm injection.* Hum Reprod, 2009. **24**(10): pp. 2490–9.

[50] Barker, D.J., *The developmental origins of adult disease.* J Am Coll Nutr, 2004. **23**(6 Suppl): pp. 588S–595S.

[51] Scott, K.A., et al., *Glucose parameters are altered in mouse offspring produced by assisted reproductive technologies and somatic cell nuclear transfer.* Biol Reprod, 2010. **83**(2): pp. 220–7.

[52] Rexhaj, E., et al., *Mice generated by in vitro fertilization exhibit vascular dysfunction and shortened life span.* J Clin Invest, 2013. **123**(12): pp. 5052–60.

[53] Yu, Y., et al., *Microinjection manipulation resulted in the increased apoptosis of spermatocytes in testes from intracytoplasmic sperm injection (ICSI) derived mice.* PLoS One, 2011. **6**(7): p. e22172.

[54] Fernandez-Gonzalez, R., et al., *Long-term effects of mouse intracytoplasmic sperm injection with DNA-fragmented sperm on health and behavior of adult offspring.* Biol Reprod, 2008. **78**(4): pp. 761–72.

[55] Schatten, G., *The centrosome and its mode of inheritance: the reduction of the centrosome during gametogenesis and its restoration during fertilization.* Dev Biol, 1994. **165**(2): pp. 299–335.

[56] Schatten, G., C. Simerly, and H. Schatten, *Microtubule configurations during fertilization, mitosis, and early development in the mouse and the requirement for egg microtubule-mediated motility during mammalian fertilization.* Proc Natl Acad Sci U S A, 1985. **82**(12): pp. 4152–6.

[57] Simerly CR, et al., *Male infertility as a result of disorders in the paternally inherited human centrosome.* South African J Sci 1997. **92**: pp. 548–557.

[58] Terada, Y., et al., *Human sperm aster formation after intracytoplasmic sperm injection with rabbit and bovine eggs.* Fertil Steril, 2002. **77**(6): pp. 1283–4.

[59] Terada, Y., *Human sperm centrosomal function during fertilization, a novel assessment for male sterility.* Hum Cell, 2004. **17**(4): pp. 181–6.

[60] Terada, Y., et al., *Use of Mammalian eggs for assessment of human sperm function: molecular and cellular analyses of fertilization by intracytoplasmic sperm injection.* Am J Reprod Immunol, 2004. **51**(4): pp. 290–3.

[61] Terada, Y., et al., *Atypical decondensation of the sperm nucleus, delayed replication of the male genome, and sex chromosome positioning following intracytoplasmic human sperm injection (ICSI) into golden hamster eggs: does ICSI itself introduce chromosomal anomalies?* Fertil Steril, 2000. **74**(3): pp. 454–60.

[62] Luetjens, C.M., C. Payne, and G. Schatten, *Non-random chromosome positioning in human sperm and sex chromosome anomalies following intracytoplasmic sperm injection.* Lancet, 1999. **353**(9160): p. 1240.

[63] Zalenskaya, I.A. and A.O. Zalensky, *Non-random positioning of chromosomes in human sperm nuclei.* Chromosome Res, 2004. **12**(2): pp. 163–73.

[64] Feichtinger, W., A. Obruca, and M. Brunner, *Sex chromosomal abnormalities and intracytoplasmic sperm injection.* Lancet, 1995. **346**(8989): p. 1566.

[65] Kasai, T., K. Hoshi, and R. Yanagimachi, *Effect of sperm immobilisation and demembranation on the oocyte activation rate in the mouse.* Zygote, 1999. **7**(3): pp. 187–93.

[66] Jones, E.L., O. Mudrak, and A.O. Zalensky, *Kinetics of human male pronuclear development in a heterologous ICSI model.* J Assist Reprod Genet, 2010. **27**(6): pp. 277–83.

[67] Heindryckx, B., et al., *Treatment option for sperm- or oocyte-related fertilization failure: assisted oocyte activation following diagnostic heterologous ICSI.* Hum Reprod, 2005. **20**(8): pp. 2237–41.

[68] Vanden Meerschaut, F., et al., *Diagnostic and prognostic value of calcium oscillatory pattern analysis for patients with ICSI fertilization failure.* Hum Reprod, 2013. **28**(1): pp. 87–98.

[69] Vanden Meerschaut, F., et al., *Assisted oocyte activation following ICSI fertilization failure.* Reprod Biomed Online, 2014. **28**(5): p. 560–71.

[70] Swann, K. and F.A. Lai, *PLCzeta and the initiation of Ca(2+) oscillations in fertilizing mammalian eggs.* Cell Calcium, 2013. **53**(1): pp. 55–62.

[71] Vanden Meerschaut, F., et al., *Assisted oocyte activation is not beneficial for all patients with a suspected oocyte-related activation deficiency.* Hum Reprod, 2012. **27**(7): pp. 1977–84.

[72] Amdani, S.N., et al., *Sperm factors and oocyte activation: current controversies and considerations.* Biol Reprod, 2015. **93**(2): p. 50.

[73] Nomikos, M., et al., *Phospholipase Czeta rescues failed oocyte activation in a prototype of male factor infertility.* Fertil Steril, 2013. **99**(1): pp. 76–85.

[74] Yoon, S.Y., et al., *Human sperm devoid of PLC, zeta 1 fail to induce Ca(2+) release and are unable to initiate the first step of embryo development.* J Clin Invest, 2008. **118**(11): pp. 3671–81.

[75] Nomikos, M., K. Swann, and F.A. Lai, *Starting a new life: sperm PLC-zeta mobilizes the Ca2+ signal that induces egg activation and embryo development: an essential phospholipase C with implications for male infertility.* Bioessays, 2012. **34**(2): pp. 126–34.

[76] Sanusi, R., et al., *Rescue of failed oocyte activation after ICSI in a mouse model of male factor infertility by recombinant phospholipase Czeta.* Mol Hum Reprod, 2015. **21**(10): pp. 783–91.

[77] Taylor, S.L., et al., *Complete globozoospermia associated with PLCzeta deficiency treated with calcium ionophore and ICSI results in pregnancy.* Reprod Biomed Online, 2010. **20**(4): pp. 559–64.

[78] Chithiwala, Z.H., et al., *Phospholipase C-zeta deficiency as a cause for repetitive oocyte fertilization failure during ovarian stimulation for in vitro fertilization with ICSI: a case report.* J Assist Reprod Genet, 2015. **32**(9): pp. 1415–9.

[79] Nazarian, H., et al., *Effect of artificial oocyte activation on intra-cytoplasmic sperm injection outcomes in patients with lower percentage of sperm containing phospholipase Czeta: a randomized clinical trial.* J Reprod Infertil, 2019. **20**(1): pp. 3–9.

[80] Vanden Meerschaut, F., et al., *Neonatal and neurodevelopmental outcome of children aged 3–10 years born following assisted oocyte activation.* Reprod Biomed Online, 2014. **28**(1): pp. 54–63.

[81] Nasr-Esfahani, M.H., M.R. Deemeh, and M. Tavalaee, *Artificial oocyte activation and intracytoplasmic sperm injection.* Fertil Steril, 2010. **94**(2): pp. 520–6.

[82] van Blerkom, J., J. Cohen, and M. Johnson, *A plea for caution and more research in the 'experimental' use of ionophores in ICSI.* Reprod Biomed Online, 2015. **30**(4): pp. 323–4.

[83] Nomikos, M., et al., *Human PLCzeta exhibits superior fertilization potency over mouse PLCzeta in triggering the Ca(2+) oscillations required for mammalian oocyte activation.* Mol Hum Reprod, 2014. **20**(6): pp. 489–98.

Cellular and Molecular Events after ICSI in Clinically Relevant Animal Models

Lauren E. Hamilton, Richard Oko, and Peter Sutovsky

Introduction

In *Brave New World* (published 1932), Aldous Huxley prophesied that the future Earth would be populated by test tube babies, of which our planet now happily carries more than 5 million. Such an explosion was brought about by the revolutionary IVF work of Sir Robert Edwards and Patrick Steptoe [1], and greatly accelerated by the development of intracytoplasmic sperm injection (ICSI) [2], which for the first time enabled asthenozoospermic men to become fathers through assisted reproductive therapy (ART). While ICSI zygotes share most early developmental events with those conceived naturally by spermatozoa penetrating oocyte vestments on their own, there are notable deviations from natural developmental patterns in that ICSI protocols bypass important early interactions between the male and female gametes. These include sperm capacitation, acrosomal exocytosis, and gamete membrane adhesion and fusion. As a result, a more or less intact spermatozoon is deposited in the ooplasm, with sperm head structures potentially interfering with oocyte activation and paternal pronucleus development, and intact sperm tail structures hindering the formation of sperm-contributed zygotic centrosome and pronuclear apposition. A deep understanding of the differences between ICSI and natural fertilization is important for optimization and safeguarding of ICSI procedures, but difficult to gain solely from the study of failed-fertilized human ICSI oocytes. Developmental choreography of ICSI has thus been investigated in relevant rodent, large animal and non-human primate models, to which the present chapter is dedicated.

Oocyte Activation

The main molecular signal of oocyte activation is a triggered depletion of calcium stores from the endoplasmic reticulum (ER). In amphibians, this results in a relatively short-lived, large intracellular calcium release, whereas in mammals a series of episodic calcium oscillations occur [3]. The exact molecular mechanisms surrounding the initiation of the calcium release have yet to be resolved, but the most accepted hypothesis is that of sperm-induced oocyte activation, first introduced in 1990 by two independent groups of investigators [4,5]. It proposes that following sperm-oocyte plasma membrane fusion, the spermatozoon releases the sperm-borne oocyte activating factors (SOAF) into the oocyte cytoplasm and triggers the initiation of the mature oocyte to embryo transition.

For a molecule to be considered as a candidate SOAF it must possess specific developmental and functional characteristics. The localization of the SOAF as a component of the perinuclear theca (PT) was determined through work lead by Yanagimachi, using the mouse as a model [6]. Microinjections of isolated sperm heads that were devested of all membranous components and retained only the perinuclear theca (PT) and nucleus were shown to maintain the ability to successfully activate MII arrested oocytes and promote normal embryonic development [6]. Spermatozoa from male N-butyldeooxynojirimycin (NB-DNJ) mice that lacked an acrosome, equatorial segment and subacrosomal layer region of the PT (SAL-PT), but successfully formed the post-acrosomal sheath region of the PT (PAS-PT) [7,8], were also able to elicit full oocyte activation during IVF studies, thus narrowing the SOAF localization to the PAS-PT [9]. These findings were supported through bovine IVF studies that showed PAS-PT solubilization alone was sufficient to initiate oocyte activation and embryo development [10].

Functionally, SOAF candidates must also be able to elicit the aforementioned intracellular calcium release that triggers various downstream events such as the initiation of the polyspermy block, the maternal resumption of meiosis and pronuclear formation. The current candidate SOAF molecules are PLCZ1 and

WBP2NL. PLCZ1 is the smallest documented phospholipase C (PLC) isoform and is made from a novel testis-expressed sequence, but is also present within the epididymis [11]. Developmentally, PLCZ1 is first seen within the round spermatid stage of sperm development and has been reported to reside within various compartments of mature spermatozoa, such as the acrosome, equatorial segment region, the PAS-PT and the sperm tail [12]. Conversely, WBP2NL is a testis-specific ortholog of WBP2 that, developmentally, is first seen during the elongation phase of spermiogenesis and resides solely in the PAS-PT of mature spermatozoa [8]. While only WBP2NL release has been unambiguously demonstrated to solubilize from the sperm head after IVF and ICSI in animal models (Figure 11.1), both candidates have been shown to elicit calcium oscillations when either the recombinant protein or cRNA was microinjected into human or mouse MII arrested oocytes, and both have been subjected to knockout mouse models [13,14]. In the WBP2NL knockout mouse model, male mice remained fertile and the absence of WBP2NL was not shown to have a significant effect on oocyte activation [15]. In contrast, the PLCZ1 knockout males showed subfertility but during natural mating, the null males were still able to successfully sire some pups. Interestingly, PLCZ1 null spermatozoa showed elevated levels of WBP2NL, suggesting that perhaps there was a compensatory mechanism at play [16]. Identification of the SOAF molecule(s) has tremendous clinical implications because a large percentage of ICSI failures are attributed to an oocyte activation deficiency [12]. In assisted reproduction, artificial activation methods can be used to ensure successful activation, but caution and rigorous testing should be performed before they are used in humans to ensure that there are no longstanding effects.

Oocyte activation initiates biochemical signaling cascades within the newly fertilized oocyte and triggers its development into an embryo. The activation results in stimulation of anti-polyspermy defense mechanisms, maternal resumption of meiosis and zygotic entry into mitosis. The dynamics of calcium have been shown to be central to oocyte activation, and a good indicator of oocyte quality and developmental outcomes [17]. The initial rise of calcium within the cytoplasm has been shown to trigger cortical granule exocytosis (CGE), releasing the vesicular contents of the cortical granules into the perivitelline space [18,19]. The CGE results in formation of a proteinaceous layer that surrounds the newly fertilized ovum and acts as a polyspermy defense

[19]. Additionally, CGE release also elicits changes to the architecture of the zona pellucida (ZP), resulting in a less porous matrix that lacks ZP sperm receptors, a transformation known as the zona or cortical reaction [19], attributable to proteolytic cleavage of ZP2/ZPB protein by CGE protease ovastacin [20]. Of note, anti-polyspermy activation appears to be incomplete in mouse ICSI oocytes [21], a deviation that could be attributed to differences in SOAF release kinetics or the absence of early gamete adhesion events that may contribute to the induction of the cortical reaction. Further considerations with regards to ICSI are the recently discovered anti-polyspermy supporting, sperm-oocyte fusion-triggered mechanisms such as shedding of the sperm receptor JUNO from the oolemma [22] and the oocyte zinc spark, which will be discussed next [23].

The rise in intracellular calcium initiates the maternal resumption of meiosis through the downstream activation of enzymes such as the calcium-calmodulin kinase (CCK) and the anaphase promoting complex (APC) [24]. Interestingly, in mammalian fertilization, the continuation of the calcium oscillations results in repetitive activation of CCK molecules. This continuous reactivation of CCK activity is proposed to be responsible for the steady increase in cyclin B degradation that is maintained by APC [25]. Moreover, the loss of cyclin B, a regulatory factor for the maturation promoting factor (MPF), a key molecule responsible for the maintenance of meiosis II in the oocyte, allows for the oocyte to developmentally transition out of meiosis II [26]. The completion of meiosis results in extrusion of the secondary polar body and coordinates the maternal and paternal cell cycles as the two pronuclei develop and proceed into S phase. The role of calcium in the instigation of meiotic resumption has been extensively studied but may not be the only factor required. Recent work on zinc dynamics during oocyte activation have demonstrated that the large decrease in intracellular zinc minutes after fertilization results in modulation of cell cycle proteins such as EMI2, which also lead to the maternal resumption of meiosis [17]. The large depletion of intracellular zinc following fertilization was coined the "zinc spark" and has been shown to depend on and occur in coordination with intracellular calcium transients [17]. Along with their influence on meiotic resumption, zinc dynamics were also shown to promote the polyspermy block and to be good indicators of blastocyst quality [27].

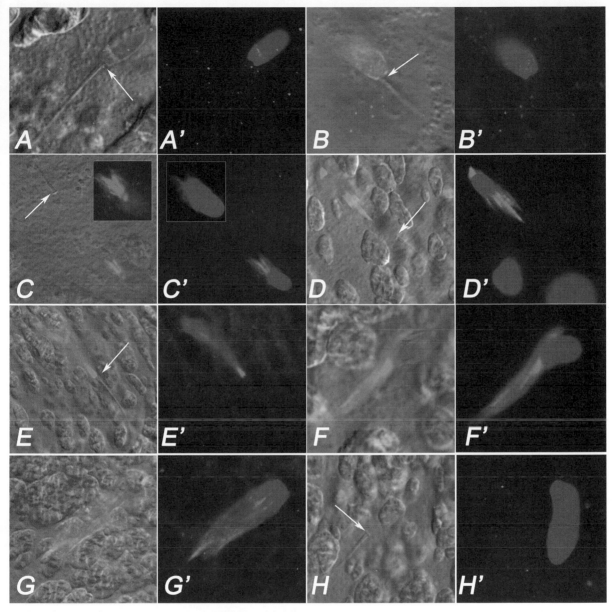

Figure 11.1 Release of putative SOAF component WBP2NL (red) after porcine ICSI. Before (A) and shortly after ICSI (B), the WBP2NL protein is confined to sperm head postacrosomal sheath, from which it is released into oocyte cytoplasm at the initial stage of sperm nucleus decondensation (C, D). As the sperm nucleus swells and elongates, WBP2NL also appears to invade the nuclear matrix in the postacrosomal area (E–G). Solubilization of WBP2NL is completed at the time of sperm tail (arrows in A, B, E and H) excision from the sperm head/nascent paternal pronucleus (H). Experimental details are described in Wu *et al.* [62]. Samples were DNA-stained with DAPI and fluorescent images superimposed onto parfocal differential interference contrast brightfield micrographs. (A black and white version of this figure will appear in some formats. For the color version, please refer to the plate section.)

In assisted reproduction, and ICSI in particular, the molecular mechanisms of oocyte activation should be largely unchanged. However, the exact timing of oocyte activation may be altered because of the absence of sperm–oocyte plasma membrane fusion and its influence on the efficiency and mechanism of SOAF release. Additionally, the use of artificial activators (e.g. calcium ionophore, recombinant SOAF proteins) may be required for spermatozoa that have a low fertilizing competency. While artificial activators are effective in achieving the required changes in intracellular calcium and zinc concentrations, their influence on other aspects of the zygotic molecular network cannot be fully realized without the knowledge and analysis of precise activation pathways.

The Nuclear Transition

Fertilization kickstarts the nuclear transition of both gametes from being genetically quiescent structures into pronuclei capable of DNA synthesis. This transformation must synchronously encompass chromatin reorganization of both the sperm and oocyte, and changes to microtubular and other cytoskeletal structures. Incorporation of the spermatozoon into the oocyte cytosol exposes it to an environment that has been enriched with large pools of endogenous molecules produced during oocyte maturation. It is during oocyte maturation that the stores of reduced glutathione (GSH) rapidly increase, reaching their highest concentration right before fertilization occurs [28]. Equipped with a sulfhydryl group, GSH provides a large reservoir of reducing power to the cell that is required not only for maintenance of the maternal meiotic spindle but also to transform sperm structures into zygotic components [29]. Both the sperm nucleus and sperm tail require reduction of disulfide bonds to unlock the paternal genetic and microtubular contributions to the zygote [29]. The sperm's nuclear decondensation process has also been shown to require the GSH-centered catalytic activity of both sperm-borne and oocyte-borne enzymes to initiate and maintain its timely disassembly [30]. Furthermore, it has also been shown that the reduction of disulfide bonds, which facilitates the breakdown of sperm tail structures such as the mitochondria sheath and the striated columns of the connecting piece, is required before the paternally inherited centrioles can begin to form into zygotic centrosomes.

In mammalian zygotes, four centrioles are speculated to arrange into two centrosomes and eventually form spindles at either pole. However, to date, four centrioles have never been observed in a developing zygote [31]. While the centrioles have been shown to be paternally derived in most non-murid mammals, only the proximal centriole was proposed to be incorporated into the egg. Until recently, the distal centriole was thought to be eliminated during the centriolar reduction that occurs in spermiogenesis. However, recent reports suggest that the distal centriole is not

fully reduced, but rather compositionally altered into an atypical centriole that migrates to the base of the sperm axoneme [31]. The newly discovered atypical centriole has been shown to be functionally active, retaining the ability to recruit pericentriolar material from the cytoplasm, form a daughter centriole and localize to the spindle pole during embryonic development [31]. These findings suggest that the altered distal centriole may have a role during fertilization and that two structurally and compositionally different centrioles are paternally inherited in the fertilization of most non-murid mammals.

Almost immediately after fertilization, the sperm centrioles interact with maternally derived γ-tubulin and centrosomal proteins to form the sperm aster, a radially symmetrical microtubule array that extends from the sperm centrosome [31]. The sperm aster is nucleated by the sperm-derived centriole near the developing paternal pronucleus and the microtubules grow out into the surrounding cytoplasm [32]. As the sperm aster grows, it also facilitates movement of the paternal pronucleus towards the center of the egg [32]. The elongating microtubules of the sperm aster eventually interact with the female pronucleus, as both pronuclei become centered within the cytoplasm [32]. Early in development, the centrosome also duplicates and the daughter centrosomes separate to form the poles of the first mitotic spindle. In the prophase of the first mitosis, these microtubule arrays develop into bipolar structures [32]. The microtubules are subsequently disassembled during metaphase and begin to form a fusiform anastral mitotic spindle [32]. In anaphase and telophase, asters are assembled at each pole that expand to create new centrosomes for the newly forming blastomeres of the embryo [32]. As the cell splits, the cleavage axis is largely determined by the position of the sperm aster, and has been found to correlate with the initial site of sperm entry [32]. Sperm centrosomal competence is crucial for pronuclear apposition and accurate chromosome partitioning during first embryo cleavage after ICSI [33], as researched in detail in non-human primate zygotes [34,35]. Furthermore, sperm aster formation has been developed as a diagnostic and potentially predictive tool in interspecific ICSI introducing patients' spermatozoa into bovine or rabbit oocytes [36,37] or in cell free systems combining patients' spermatozoa with amphibian egg extracts [38].

Sperm nuclear decondensation is intimately linked to the reorganization of the newly forming embryonic microtubular network, and must have a timely progression for development to be successful. Past studies in the bovine in vitro fertilization (IVF) system demonstrated how high concentrations of GSH are required for initiation of sperm nuclear decondensation [29]. The study further demonstrated that quenching GSH levels before fertilization also impacted sperm aster development, but that both phenotypes could be rescued through addition of a reducing agent [29]. Furthermore, the addition of GSH precursor amino acid cysteine to oocyte and embryo culture media increased the efficiency of ICSI in the porcine model, measured by blastocyst development rates and live births [39]. Recently, these findings were expanded upon, through ICSI studies in the mouse model that implicated glutathione-s-transferases of the omega class (GSTO), from both the sperm and oocyte in the sperm nuclear decondensation process [30]. Inhibition of the enzymatic active site of sperm-borne GSTO2 enzymes before ICSI injection resulted in a developmental delay of the male nuclear transition that ultimately impacted blastocyst survival rates [30]. Furthermore, the study also notes that inhibition of oocyte-borne GSTO enzymes within the cytosol of unfertilized MII arrested oocytes before sperm injection had a detrimental effect on development and resulted in high developmental arrest at the first cleavage [30]. Therefore, the male nuclear transition in mammals is proposed to rely on the reducing power of GSH found within the ooplasm, and the catalytic activity of enzymes from both the spermatozoa and the oocyte.

The unique nuclear architecture of the sperm head and how its chromatin associates with protamines, histones and the nuclear matrices before and after fertilization has a large impact on how it reorganizes in the developing egg [40]. The spermatozoon presents its DNA in a structural context that is required for the embryo to access the paternal genome in a proper sequence of developmental events [40]. Throughout spermatogenesis, the sperm nuclear architecture is dramatically transformed from open and organized by both somatic and testis-specific histones, to highly condensed and structured by protamines. During the early stages of spermiogenesis/spermatid elongation, histones are replaced first by transition proteins and then protamines, creating the extremely condense mature nuclear structure. This highly compacted nuclear conformation is fortified with zinc bridges and disulfide bonds providing protection from DNA damage during sperm transit [41].

However, once the sperm head is incorporated into the ooplasm, it must be able to rapidly decondense. Hammoud et al., and others, demonstrated that the spermatozoon nucleus is not homogenously organized and retains a small number of histones at specific genes associated with early embryonic development [42]. Moreover, Van der Heijden et al. demonstrated that histones with specific modifications in the sperm cell are also present in the paternal pronucleus [43]. This suggests that when sperm protamines are replaced by maternally derived histones, two to four hours post fertilization, sperm-derived histones are retained. These findings suggest that the male pronuclear architecture may be paternally inherited by the newly fertilized egg. The paternal contribution to nuclear structure is also further supported by the discovery of somatic histones within the post-acrosomal sheath region of the perinuclear theca [44]. Proteomic analysis of the histones housed within the perinuclear theca showed no significant post-transcriptional modifications that would suggest they had ever been within the nucleus [44]. Additionally, developmental studies demonstrated that they were newly formed during round spermatid stage, suggesting they may have a role post-fertilization [44]. The structure of the sperm nuclear matrices has also been shown to be essential for DNA replication [40]. ICSI studies have highlighted the importance of the nuclear matrix, demonstrating that when sperm with damaged nuclear matrices are injected into MII arrested oocytes, they do not support embryonic development [40]. Therefore, the nuclear matrix may act as a DNA integrity checkpoint following fertilization and artificial reproductive technologies should work to ensure it is not damaged during sperm processing [40].

The formation of the paternal pronucleus after ICSI is conditional upon timely and complete removal of sperm perinuclear theca structures, first the SOAF-bearing post-acrosomal sheath, followed by the sub-acrosomal PT layer anchoring the residual inner acrosomal membrane. These structures are removed in an orderly manner at sperm-oolemma fusion and sperm head incorporation in the oocyte cortex during natural fertilization and after IVF. As will be discussed below, ICSI with intact spermatozoa is prone to partial retention of these rigid perinuclear structures, promoting aberrant paternal chromosome positioning if not complete arrest of pronuclear development [10,45].

Post-Fertilization Sperm Mitophagy

Mitochondria are functionally known as the power-houses of the cell, generating energy through oxidative phosphorylation. They are essential organelles that also participate in cellular homoeostasis, steroidogenesis and the regulation of apoptosis [46]. They contain their own unique genome, equipped with 37 genes that intimately interact with the nuclear genome of the cell and are thought to have evolved through bacterial symbiosis. In the context of mammalian reproduction, mitochondria are found both within the cytosol of the oocyte and tightly surrounding the midpiece of the sperm tail, forming the helical structure known as the mitochondrial sheath (MS) [46]. However, mitochondrial inheritance has been shown to be exclusively maternally derived, with sperm-borne mitochondria undergoing degradation during post-fertilization development.

Researchers have been fascinated by mitochondrial inheritance from as early as the 1940s [47], and today, the paradigm of maternal mitochondrial inheritance is popularly referred to as "the Mitochondrial Eve Paradigm." Sperm mitochondrial DNA (mtDNA) has been shown to have a high rate of mutation at the onset of the journey to fertilize [48]. Large amounts of mitochondrion-produced ATP are required to ensure spermatozoa have adequate motility and speed, but this comes at the expense of being exposed to a high level of free radicals and oxidative stress [49]. This may therefore make the overall quality of the sperm mitochondria lower than that of their oocyte counterparts. Elimination of paternal mitochondria after fertilization may thus prevent mitochondrial heteroplasmy (co-existence of paternal and maternal mitochondrial genomes in an individual) and reduce the likelihood of deleterious mtDNA mutations being transmitted from father's gametes to progeny. Recent studies have focused on the mechanisms of sperm mitochondrial degradation or sperm mitophagy and have shown that in mammals, this process is driven by the ubiquitin proteasome system (UPS) in combination with autophagic pathways [50].

The current working hypothesis of sperm mitophagy proposes that sperm mitochondrial proteins are initially ubiquitinated during the secondary spermatocyte stage of spermatogenesis [50]. Once the spermatozoon is incorporated at fertilization, ubiquitin-tagged proteins interact with the oocyte-derived protein dislocase VCP, which removes these proteins from the mitochondrial sheath structure and delivers them to the 26S proteasome system [50]. The VCP activity destabilizes

the structure of the mitochondrial sheath and may also prime the sperm mitochondria for interactions with the ooplasmic enzyme SQSTM1 [50]. SQSTM1 has been shown to interact with the sperm mitochondrial sheath early in post-fertilization development and is proposed to play a central role during sperm mitophagy [50]. Furthermore, interactions between SQSTM1 and GABARAP are suggested to promote the sequestering of the sperm mitochondrial cargo to autophagosomes within the ooplasm [50]. This action may also be aided by interactions with LC3 [50]. The autophagosomes would eventually bind with the lysosome and full degradation would occur. Additionally, sperm mitophagy may also involve the action of endonucleases that directly target mtDNA and mitochondrial proteins, decreasing the replication and persistence of paternal mtDNA [46]. Although species specificity is believed to play a role in sperm mitophagy, the involvement of the UPS and autophagy do persist in most models [46,50]. Performing future studies in higher-level mammals such as pigs, which have more developmental similarities to humans may also allow for a better understanding of how sperm mitophagy dysregulation may result in some of the mitochondrial diseases observed in human populations [51]. Studying interactions between the oocyte and foreign mitochondria and how they are tagged for degradation may also help in ART techniques that use donor mitochondria to rejuvenate oocytes. With regard to human ICSI safeguarding, there are, to our knowledge, no reported cases of paternally derived heteroplasmy. However, ART babies are not routinely screened for mtDNA mutations, and the recently confirmed association of heteroplasmy with multigenerational mitochondrial disease [52] along with research on biparental mtDNA inheritance associated with ICSI in lower vertebrates [53], raise the specter of adult-onset mitochondrial dysfunction starting to increase in the ART-conceived population as they grow older. Animal models of sperm mitophagy are discussed in detail by Zuidema and Sutovsky [51].

The Influence of Assisted Reproductive Techniques on the Molecular Foundations of Fertilization

The development of ICSI has provided a new spark of hope for infertile couples diagnosed with male-factor and/or unexplained infertility. ICSI expedites sperm–egg interactions and bypasses many sperm maturation and priming events that happen during natural fertilization. While ICSI exponentially increases fertilization rates, it may lead to changes in sperm composition and progression of fertilization in certain species because of a lack of capacitation and acrosomal exocytosis and the bypassing of sperm–oocyte interactions and natural sperm selection barriers.

ICSI has been implemented in many species, each with their own obstacles and challenges. The differences in sperm structure and composition between species change how sperm structures are processed and the tools used to insert them into the oocyte cytosol. In most mouse ICSI protocols, spermatozoa are obtained from the cauda epididymis, bypassing any interactions with components of the seminal plasma or prostatic fluid that may be required for sperm priming at the time when spermatozoa are deposited in the female reproductive tract. They are artificially capacitated, to varied extents, and as a result of their unique lack of a sperm centriole within the sperm tail, are separated at the head tail junction, before solely the head of the spermatozoon is injected into the oocyte. This process negates the impact of seminal plasma and prostatic components and may bypass important structural priming events that are pertinent in post-fertilization development. To enhance rodent ICSI, a piezo-driven ICSI technique was developed in Yanagimachi's laboratory to reduce oocyte damage, facilitate sperm head-tail excision and acrosome disruption, and to promote SOAF release from the perinuclear theca [54], which can also be applied to human ICSI [55]. Piezo micromanipulation also enables and dramatically improves fertilization and development rates in ungulate ICSI [56,57].

Throughout mammalian sperm development, Zn^{2+} ions are recruited to the sperm nucleus and incorporated into the compacting nuclear structure of the sperm head through the formation of zinc bridges [41]. This compacted architecture of the sperm chromatin is proposed to offer protection from DNA damage during transit but must then be rapidly decondensed to allow for male pronuclear formation during zygotic development [41]. In natural fertilization, spermatozoa are ejaculated in the acidic and zinc-rich environment of the prostatic fluid, which would gradually become diluted as the spermatozoa progress further into the female reproductive tract [41]. The dilution of environmental zinc available to the spermatozoa as well as the zinc efflux associated with sperm capacitation within female oviduct [58], lead to zinc removal from the chromatin and progressively contributes to a loosening

of the chromatin structure, allowing for a rapid nuclear decondensation once the sperm head is incorporated into the ooplasm [41]. However, during in vitro manipulation, there is a scarce consideration of how ion concentrations ultimately control sperm structural remodeling, which could hinder the progression of early embryonic development, particularly after ICSI. Additionally, as spermatozoa in vitro are no longer limited by their successful completion of the acrosomal exocytosis, spermatozoa that are used for ICSI may not be fully primed before microinjection.

Studies by De Lamirande et al. revealed that in addition to changes in zinc, sperm chromatin was progressively remodeled during sperm capacitation and the acrosomal exocytosis, through changes in chromatin conformation and histone orientation that lead to a greater ability to decondense [59]. These findings further emphasize the importance of sperm priming. Their oversight may contribute to the complications observed in some models, such as bovine ICSI, that are known to have post-fertilization problems associated with nuclear decondensation. In addition to the structural differences imparted by a lack of complete capacitation and acrosome exocytosis, the elimination of gametic fusion may also contribute to a slower degradation of sperm cytoskeletal structures. Sutovsky et al. showed that the microvilli that cover the surface of the oocyte interact with components of the PT during IVF and lead to a quicker dissociation of the PT from the sperm nucleus upon sperm head incorporation in the bovine model [60]. This quick dissociation of the PT from the sperm head was not seen in oocytes that were microinjected, which may lead to a delayed nuclear decondensation [60]. These remodeling events in combination with the removal of the acrosomal contents are all intrinsic ways the sperm readies itself for the molecular events of fertilization, and bypassing any one of them could have consequences on the development of the newly forming zygote. A particular concern has been raised about the post-ICSI fate of the subacrosomal PT which remains associated with sperm nucleus and can cause a delay or complete arrest of paternal pronucleus development, as studied in ICSI zygotes of Rhesus monkey [34,35,45] and domestic pig (Figure 11.2), with piezo-ICSI relieving this potential hurdle in the latter model [39,56]. Uneven decondensation of chromatin in the subacrosomal compartment, preferentially housing the sex chromosome, has been implicated as a mechanism responsible for a slight increase in sex chromosome abnormalities seen in ICSI children [61].

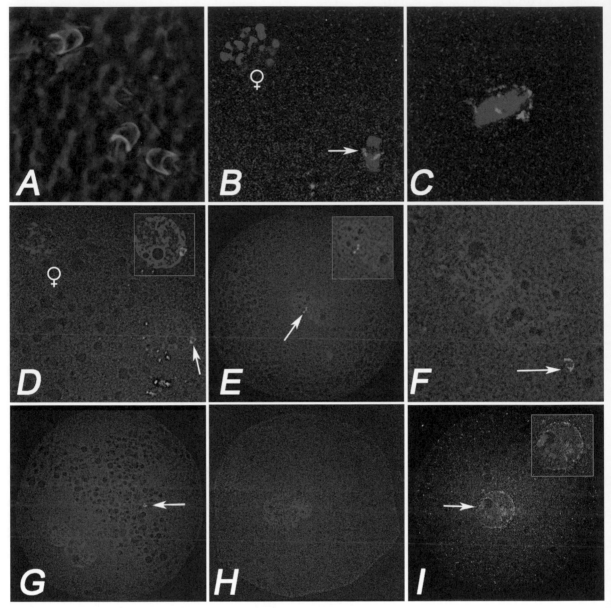

Figure 11.2 Fate of the subacrosomal perinuclear theca (PT) and inner acrosomal membrane (IAM) after porcine ICSI, traced by immunolabeling of sperm protein IAM32 (red). Before ICSI (A), the IAM32 protein is prominently detected on the inner acrosomal membrane of the acrosomal ridge and on the arch of the crescent-shaped equatorial segment. In many ICSI zygotes, the IAM-PT complex starts to dissociate from sperm nucleus even before the completion of oocyte meiosis (oocyte chromosomes are marked by ♀) while in other zygotes such a dissociation becomes detectable once the sperm nucleus begins to decondense (B). Clumped IAM-PT (arrows in E–G) often remains associated with paternal pronucleus at the time of pronuclear apposition (D, E), or drifts away from pronuclei in other zygotes (G), to eventually disappear (H). In some zygotes, the failure of IAM-PT removal blocks paternal pronucleus development without interfering with oocyte activation and formation of the maternal pronucleus and pronuclear apposition (I). Experimental details are described in Katayama *et al.* [56]. Samples were DNA-stained with DAPI and pronuclear nuclear envelope was labeled green (panel I). (A black and white version of this figure will appear in some formats. For the color version, please refer to the plate section.)

Epigenetically, the exposure to the different medias and processing techniques may also have hidden impacts on the embryos and how they develop, not only throughout embryonic development but also during pregnancy and postnatally. While the overall impact of artificial reproductive techniques such as

ICSI, that involve a higher degree of human interference have not yet been fully understood in the human population, updating medias and procedures to better mimic those found in vivo may help limit their overall influence. Improvements in sperm selection techniques that take DNA damage and chromatin structure into consideration may help increase the overall fitness of fertilizing sperm. Allowing sperm to fully undergo capacitation and the acrosome exocytosis may provide for a better and more natural priming for post-fertilization events and thus demembranating spermatozoa to start their disassembly before insertion may allow for more accurately timed development.

Conclusion

The molecular foundations of post-fertilization processes are greatly influenced by the fitness of the fertilizing spermatozoa and the surrounding environmental conditions. Ensuring that spermatozoa undergo adequate priming prior to micromanipulation can greatly increase the overall success of fertilization and developmental progression in human ART. While the overall sequence of the post-fertilization developmental processes is largely unchanged by the utilization of ICSI, human interference in the very intimate process of fertilization can cause changes in synchrony, developmental timing and epigenetics. These changes may not always present themselves in overt ways during pre- or post-implantation development but may have unforeseen consequences postnatally and even in adult life. In animal model studies, such alterations and means of mitigating them can be dependent on experimental approaches and the species that are used. Ethical guidelines surrounding the use of human embryos may also limit how much knowledge we can gather on the exact dynamics of human post-fertilization development. The more knowledge that we can gather about assisted mammalian fertilization from relevant animal models will ultimately help in creating and safeguarding the best artificial reproductive technology protocols that hopefully cause the least disruption to the natural process while continuing to garner high fertilization efficiency.

Acknowledgements

We thank our past and present collaborators on ICSI research who contributed to our studies cited in this chapter. Currently, LH and RO are supported by the Canadian Institute of Health Research (84440) and the Natural Science and Engineering Research Council of Canada (RGPIN/05305) to RO. PS is supported by Agriculture and Food Research Initiative Competitive Grant no. 2020-67015-31017 and 2021-67015-33404 from the USDA National Institute of Food and Agriculture, NIH-USDA Dual Purpose with Dual Benefit Program grant number NIH 1R01HD084353 and seed funding from the Food for the 21st Century Program of the University of Missouri.

References

[1] Johnson, M. H. Robert Edwards: the path to IVF. *Reprod. Biomed. Online* **23**, 245–262 (2011).

[2] Palermo, G., Joris, H., Devroey, P. & Van Steirteghem, A. C. Pregnancies after intracytoplasmic injection of single spermatozoon into an oocyte. *Lancet* **340**, 17–18 (1992).

[3] Parrington, J., Swann, K., Shevchenko, V. I., Sesay, A. K. & Lai, F. A. Calcium oscillations in mammalian eggs triggered by a soluble sperm protein. *Nature* **379**, 364 (1996).

[4] Stice, S. L. & Robl, J. M. Activation of mammalian oocytes by a factor obtained from rabbit sperm. *Mol. Reprod. Dev.* **25**, 272–280 (1990).

[5] Swann, K. A cytosolic sperm factor stimulates repetitive calcium increases and mimics fertilization in hamster eggs. *Development* **110**, 1295–1302 (1990).

[6] Kimura, Y. *et al.* Analysis of mouse oocyte activation suggests the involvement of sperm perinuclear material. *Biol. Reprod.* 58, 1407–1415 (1998).

[7] Oko, R., Donald, A., Xu, W. & van der Spoel, A. C. Fusion failure of dense-cored proacrosomal vesicles in an inducible mouse model of male infertility. *Cell Tissue Res.* **346**, 119 (2011).

[8] Wu, A. T. H. *et al.* The postacrosomal assembly of sperm head protein, PAWP, is independent of acrosome formation and dependent on microtubular manchette transport. *Dev. Biol.* **312**, 471–483 (2007).

[9] Suganuma, R. *et al.* Alkylated imino sugars, reversible male infertility-inducing agents, do not affect the genetic integrity of male mouse germ cells during short-term treatment despite induction of sperm deformities. *Biol. Reprod.* **72**, 805–813 (2005).

[10] Sutovsky, P., Manandhar, G., Wu, A. & Oko, R. Interactions of sperm perinuclear theca with the oocyte: Implications for oocyte activation, anti-polyspermy defense, and assisted reproduction. *Microsc. Res. Tech.* **61**, 362–378 (2003).

[11] Aarabi, M. *et al.* The testicular and epididymal expression profile of PLCζ in mouse and human

does not support its role as a sperm-borne oocyte activating factor. *PLoS One* 7, e33496 (2012).

[12] Amdani, S. N., Yeste, M., Jones, C. & Coward, K. Sperm factors and oocyte activation: current controversies and considerations. *Biol. Reprod.* **93**, 50–51 (2015).

[13] Aarabi, M. *et al.* Sperm-derived WW domain-binding protein, PAWP, elicits calcium oscillations and oocyte activation in humans and mice. *FASEB J.* **28**, 4434–4440 (2014).

[14] Saunders, C. M. *et al.* PLCζ: a sperm-specific trigger of Ca2+ oscillations in eggs and embryo development. *Development* **129**, 3533–3544 (2002).

[15] Satouh, Y., Nozawa, K. & Ikawa, M. Sperm postacrosomal WW domain-binding protein is not required for mouse egg activation. *Biol. Reprod.* **93**, 91–94 (2015).

[16] Hachem, A. *et al.* PLCζ is the physiological trigger of the Ca2+ oscillations that induce embryogenesis in mammals but offspring can be conceived in its absence. *Development* **144**, 2914–2924 (2017).

[17] Duncan, F. E. *et al.* The zinc spark is an inorganic signature of human egg activation. *Sci. Rep.* **6**, 1–8 (2016).

[18] Austin, C. R. Cortical granules in hamster eggs. *Exp. Cell Res.* **10**, 533–540 (1956).

[19] Liu, M. The biology and dynamics of mammalian cortical granules. *Reprod. Biol. Endocrinol.* **9**, 149 (2011).

[20] Burkart, A. D., Xiong, B., Baibakov, B., Jiménez-Movilla, M. & Dean, J. Ovastacin, a cortical granule protease, cleaves ZP2 in the zona pellucida to prevent polyspermy. *J. Cell Biol.* **197**, 37–44 (2012).

[21] Wortzman-Show, G. B., Kurokawa, M., Fissore, R. A. & Evans, J. P. Calcium and sperm components in the establishment of the membrane block to polyspermy: studies of ICSI and activation with sperm factor. *Mol. Hum. Reprod.* **13**, 557–565 (2007).

[22] Bianchi, E., Doe, B., Goulding, D. & Wright, G. J. Juno is the egg Izumo receptor and is essential for mammalian fertilization. *Nature* **508**, 483–487 (2014).

[23] Que, E. L. *et al.* Zinc sparks induce physiochemical changes in the egg zona pellucida that prevent polyspermy. *Integr. Biol.* **9**, 135–144 (2017).

[24] Yamamoto, T. M., Iwabuchi, M., Ohsumi, K. & Kishimoto, T. APC/C–Cdc20-mediated degradation of cyclin B participates in CSF arrest in unfertilized Xenopus eggs. *Dev. Biol.* **279**, 345–355 (2005).

[25] Dupont, G. Link between fertilization-induced Ca2+ oscillations and relief from metaphase II arrest in mammalian eggs: a model based on calmodulin-dependent kinase II activation. *Biophys. Chem.* **72**, 153–167 (1998).

[26] Gautier, J. *et al.* Cyclin is a component of maturation-promoting factor from Xenopus. *Cell* **60**, 487–494 (1990).

[27] Zhang, N., Duncan, F. E., Que, E. L., O'Halloran, T. V. & Woodruff, T. K. The fertilization-induced zinc spark is a novel biomarker of mouse embryo quality and early development. *Sci. Rep.* **6**, 1–9 (2016).

[28] Luberda, Z. The role of glutathione in mammalian gametes. *Reprod Biol* **5**, 5–17 (2005).

[29] Sutovsky, P. & Schatten, G. Depletion of glutathione during bovine oocyte maturation reversibly blocks the decondensation of the male pronucleus and pronuclear apposition during fertilization. *Biol. Reprod.* **56**, 1503–1512 (1997).

[30] Hamilton, L. E. *et al.* Sperm-borne glutathione-s-transferase omega 2 accelerates the nuclear decondensation of spermatozoa during fertilization in mice. *Biol. Reprod.* **101**, 368–376 (2019).

[31] Fishman, E. L. *et al.* A novel atypical sperm centriole is functional during human fertilization. *Nat. Commun.* **9**, (2018).

[32] Navara, C. S., Simerly, C., Zoran, S. & Schatten, G. The sperm centrosome during fertilization in mammals: implications for fertility and reproduction. *Reprod. Fertil. Dev.* **7**, 747–754 (1995).

[33] Palermo, G. D., Colombero, L. T. & Rosenwaks, Z. The human sperm centrosome is responsible for normal syngamy and early embryonic development. *Rev. Reprod.* **2**, 19–27 (1997).

[34] Hewitson, L. C. *et al.* Microtubule and chromatin configurations during rhesus intracytoplasmic sperm injection: successes and failures. *Biol. Reprod.* **55**, 271–280 (1996).

[35] Sutovsky, P. *et al.* Fertilization and early embryology: Intracytoplasmic sperm injection for Rhesus monkey fertilization results in unusual chromatin, cytoskeletal, and membrane events, but eventually leads to pronuclear development and sperm aster assembly. *Hum. Reprod.* **11**, 1703–1712 (1996).

[36] Nakamura, S. *et al.* Human sperm aster formation and pronuclear decondensation in bovine eggs following intracytoplasmic sperm injection using a piezo-driven pipette: a novel assay for human sperm centrosomal function. *Biol. Reprod.* **65**, 1359–1363 (2001).

[37] Terada, Y. *et al.* Human sperm aster formation after intracytoplasmic sperm injection with rabbit and bovine eggs. *Fertil. Steril.* **77**, 1283–1284 (2002).

[38] Simerly, C. *et al.* Biparental inheritance of γ-tubulin during human fertilization: molecular reconstitution of functional zygotic centrosomes in inseminated human oocytes and in cell-free extracts nucleated by human sperm. *Mol. Biol. Cell* **10**, 2955–2969 (1999).

[39] Katayama, M. *et al.* Improved fertilization and embryo development resulting in birth of live piglets after intracytoplasmic sperm injection and in vitro culture in a cysteine-supplemented medium. *Theriogenology* **67**, 835–847 (2007).

[40] Ward, W. S. Function of sperm chromatin structural elements in fertilization and development. *MHR Basic Sci. Reprod. Med.* **16**, 30–36 (2009).

[41] Björndahl, L. & Kvist, U. Human sperm chromatin stabilization: a proposed model including zinc bridges. *Mol. Hum. Reprod.* **16**, 23–29 (2009).

[42] Hammoud, S. S. *et al.* Distinctive chromatin in human sperm packages genes for embryo development. *Nature* **460**, 473 (2009).

[43] van der Heijden, G. W. *et al.* Sperm-derived histones contribute to zygotic chromatin in humans. *BMC Dev. Biol.* **8**, 34 (2008).

[44] Tovich, P. R. & Oko, R. J. Somatic histones are components of the perinuclear theca in bovine spermatozoa. *J. Biol. Chem.* **278**, 32431–32438 (2003).

[45] Ramalho-Santos, J. *et al.* ICSI choreography: fate of sperm structures after monospermic rhesus ICSI and first cell cycle implications. *Hum. Reprod.* **15**, 2610–2620 (2000).

[46] Sutovsky, P. & Song, W. H. Post-fertilisation sperm mitophagy: The tale of Mitochondrial Eve and Steve. *Reprod. Fertil. Dev.* **30**, 56–63 (2018).

[47] Gresson, R. A. R. Presence of the sperm middle-piece in the fertilized egg of the mouse (Mus musculus). *Nature* **145**, 425 (1940).

[48] St. John, J. C., Jokhi, R. P. & Barratt, C. L. R. The impact of mitochondrial genetics on male infertility. *Int. J. Androl.* **28**, 65–73 (2005).

[49] Kramer, P. & Bressan, P. Mitochondria inspire a lifestyle. In Sutovsky, P. (ed.) *Cellular and Molecular Basis of Mitochondrial Inheritance.* Springer International Publishing, 105–126 (2019).

[50] Song, W. H., Yi, Y. J., Sutovsky, M., Meyers, S. & Sutovsky, P. Autophagy and ubiquitin-proteasome system contribute to sperm mitophagy after mammalian fertilization. *Proc. Natl. Acad. Sci. U. S. A.* **113**, E5261–E5270 (2016).

[51] Zuidema, D. & Sutovsky, P. The domestic pig as a model for the study of mitochondrial inheritance. *Cell Tissue Res.* **380**, 263–271 (2020).

[52] Luo, S. *et al.* Biparental inheritance of mitochondrial DNA in humans. *Proc. Natl. Acad. Sci.* **115**, 13039–13044 (2018).

[53] Peng, L. *et al.* Persistence and transcription of paternal mtDNA dependent on the delivery strategy rather than mitochondria source in fish embryos. *Cell. Physiol. Biochem.* **47**, 1898–1908 (2018).

[54] Kuretake, S., Kimura, Y., Hoshi, K. & Yanagimachi, R. Fertilization and development of mouse oocytes injected with isolated sperm heads. *Biol. Reprod.* **55**, 789–795 (1996).

[55] Huang, T., Kimura, Y. & Yanagimachi, R. The use of piezo micromanipulation for intracytoplasmic sperm injection of human oocytes. *J. Assist. Reprod. Genet.* **13**, 320–328 (1996).

[56] Katayama, M. *et al.* Increased disruption of sperm plasma membrane at sperm immobilization promotes dissociation of perinuclear theca from sperm chromatin after intracytoplasmic sperm injection in pigs. *Reproduction* **130**, 907–916 (2005).

[57] Katayose, H. *et al.* Efficient injection of bull spermatozoa into oocytes using a piezo-driven pipette. *Theriogenology* **52**, 1215–1224 (1999).

[58] Kerns, K., Zigo, M., Drobnis, E. Z., Sutovsky, M. & Sutovsky, P. Zinc ion flux during mammalian sperm capacitation. *Nat. Commun.* **9**, 2061 (2018).

[59] De Lamirande, E., San Gabriel, M. C. & Zini, A. Human sperm chromatin undergoes physiological remodeling during in vitro capacitation and acrosome reaction. *J. Androl.* **33**, 1025–1035 (2012).

[60] Sutovsky, P., Oko, R., Hewitson, L. & Schatten, G. The removal of the sperm perinuclear theca and its association with the bovine oocyte surface during fertilization. *Dev. Biol.* **188**, 75–84 (1997).

[61] Luetjens, C. M., Payne, C. & Schatten, G. Non-random chromosome positioning in human sperm and sex chromosome anomalies following intracytoplasmic sperm injection. *Lancet* **353**, 1240 (1999).

[62] Wu, A. T. H. *et al.* PAWP, a sperm-specific WW domain-binding protein, promotes meiotic resumption and pronuclear development during fertilization. *J. Biol. Chem.* **282**, 12164–12175 (2007).

Chapter 12

Micromanipulation, Micro-Injection Microscopes and Systems for ICSI

Steven D. Fleming

Introduction

In the context of assisted reproduction technology (ART), micromanipulation is essentially microsurgery and manipulation of gametes and embryos under high magnification by hand alone. It is believed that the concept of manipulating cells under magnification originated during the eighteenth century, in the form of simple microscope-mounted needles [1]. Nevertheless, it was not until the mid-late nineteenth century that scientific reports of investigators using dissecting microscopes for micro-injection began to appear, with Schmidt being recognized as one of the pioneers of this approach to biomedical research [2]. However, the first studies of oocyte and embryo micromanipulation did not occur until the middle of the twentieth century [3]. Successful mammalian fertilization following intracytoplasmic sperm injection (ICSI) was first demonstrated in the hamster [4], and the first human pregnancies following ICSI were reported in 1992 [5]. Clearly, this breakthrough in the alleviation of male factor infertility would have been impossible without the development of sophisticated micromanipulation equipment. Furthermore, various applications of such equipment have proven fundamental to the reproductive potential of subfertile couples and the genetic health of their offspring.

Prototype micromanipulators were designed during the 1920s by pioneers such as Chambers, De Fonbrune, Emerson, May and Taylor. At that time, Leitz (Wetzlar, Germany) was one of the leading manufacturers of microscopes, the company then being managed by Ernst Leitz, who had previously founded Leica Camera AG in 1914. However, it was not until 1986 that Leitz changed its name to Leica. The original Leitz joystick micromanipulators, released in 1952, were built to last and had a high mass to reduce interference from external vibration, some remaining in operation today. In fact,

micromanipulation of human gametes was originally performed using mechanical Leitz micromanipulators [6]. Research Instruments (RI; Falmouth, UK) was established by Mike Lee and Vince Grispo in 1962 and released a triple axis, single lever mechanical micromanipulator in 1964. In response to a request from Dr Simon Fishel, RI began adapting micromanipulators for use in ART during the 1980s. Narishige Scientific Instrument Laboratory (Tokyo, Japan) was established by Eiichi Narishige in 1958, with the first single axis hydraulic micromanipulator being released in 1969. In the early 1980s, a triple axis hydraulic micromanipulator was manufactured so that microsurgery could be performed properly, with Narishige Co. Ltd. subsequently being established as a separate company from Narishige Scientific in 1985. Eppendorf (Hamburg, Germany) was founded by Heinrich Netheler and Hans Hinz in 1945. The company began designing micromanipulation equipment in 1982 in response to a request from the European Molecular Biology Laboratory for a device capable of injecting femtoliter volumes into living cells, with the first prototype being tested in 1984. This prototype was subsequently allied to joystick-controlled stepper motors in 1988. Hence, it is apparent that the rapid evolution of micromanipulation equipment during the 1980s laid the way for successful application of ICSI during the 1990s.

Modern micromanipulators have a low mass, requiring some form of isolation such as an anti-vibration table. Other important features of various micromanipulation systems include their ergonomics, their reliability during use and their ease of maintenance and troubleshooting [7]. Further considerations include the ability to maintain sterility and physiological temperature during micromanipulation, which can be mitigated by their adaptability for integration into laminar flow workstations and high-efficiency particulate-air-filtered biological cabinets. The purpose of this chapter is not to review all the makes of microscopes and micromanipulators that have been produced, rather it is to bring readers up to date with the very latest models available from the major manufacturers and, furthermore, to provide a glimpse into possible future technical innovations in ICSI.

Inverted Microscopes and Anti-Vibration Systems

The efficiency of ICSI depends on two vital pieces of equipment that make it possible to view and manipulate the gametes clearly, these being an inverted microscope and an anti-vibration system. Good ergonomics are also desirable, as is the ability for an inverted microscope to be mounted within a laminar flow workstation or biological cabinet. The inverted microscope needs to be adaptable to the major types of micromanipulator systems and of sufficiently high quality that it features a robust and stable stand, free of vibration, and has sufficient ports to enable attachment of a camera and laser. Essentially, all of the common micromanipulation systems can be adapted for use with various inverted microscopes from the big four companies: Leica, Nikon, Olympus and Zeiss (Table 12.1). Furthermore, inverted microscopes need to incorporate high-quality optics providing a large field of view (FOV) with a magnification range of 40–400×, modulation contrast, a condenser with a long or ultra-long working distance, ease of ICSI dish handling and a heated stage capable of maintaining physiological temperature which should, ideally, be flush with the mechanical stage. Nomarski interference contrast or differential interference contrast (DIC) optics, invented by Georges (Jerzy)

Nomarski in 1952, were originally used for ICSI but have mostly been superseded by Hoffman modulation contrast (HMC) optics, invented by Robert Hoffman in 1975. Although DIC can be used with plastic ICSI dishes, it was optimized for glass dishes, whereas HMC is better suited to plastic dishes as it is not affected by their polarizing effect. In 1996, Carl Zeiss introduced the "Varel" system and the "big four" have since developed their own variants of DIC and HMC including Leica's integrated HMC (iMC), Nikon's advanced modulation contrast (NAMC), Olympus' relief contrast (RC) and Zeiss' PlasDIC and improved HMC (iHMC). In recent years, coinciding with the rapid expansion of ART worldwide, the "big four" have developed inverted microscope models that are particularly suited to ICSI within a clinical setting, as discussed in the following sections.

Leica

Leica's DMi8 inverted microscope has a modular design, allowing either manual or motorized operation (www.youtube.com/watch?v=XIIfD9WgaLw) plus alignment with a manipulator via a digital interface. It is designed to provide direct access for a laser system to the infinite light path via its "infinity port" and also has three camera ports. It incorporates Leica's microscope stage automatic thermo-control system within a three-plate stage and a condenser for modulation contrast of objective lenses in the magnification range, 5–63×. Push button selection of different optical pathways allows for switching between DIC and Leica's iMC. Therefore, the DMi8 may be adapted for intracytoplasmic morphologically

Table 12.1 Micromanipulator compatibility with commonly available microscopes

	Eppendorf TransferMan® 4 m	Narishige Takanome™	Research Instruments Integra 3™
Leica microscopes	DMI3000B, 3000 M, 4000B, 5000B, 5000 M, 6000B; DMIRBE; HC; DMi8; DMIRE2; DMILED	DMI3000B, 4000B, 6000B; DMi8	DMI3000B, 4000B, 6000B; DMIRB; DMi8; DMIL
Nikon microscopes	Eclipse Diaphot 200, 300; Eclipse Ti-E, Ti-U, Ti-S; TE200; TE300; TE2000; Eclipse Ts2 R; Eclipse Ti2-E, Ti2-A, Ti2-U	Eclipse TE2000; Eclipse Ti; Eclipse Ts2 R; Eclipse Ti2	TMD; Eclipse Diaphot 200, 300; Eclipse Ti; TE200; TE300
Olympus microscopes	IX50; IX51; IX53; IX70; IX73; IX80; IX81; IX83	IX70; IX71; IX73; IX83	IMT2; IX50; IX51; IX53; IX70; IX71; IX73; IX81; IX83
Zeiss microscopes	Axiovert 200; Axio Observer A1, D1, Z1, 3, 5, 7; Axio Vert A1	Axiovert 200; Axio Observer; Axio Vert A1	Axiovert 40, 100, 200; Axio Observer; Axio Vert A1

selected sperm injection (IMSI), using a glass-bottomed dish and glass heated stage, DIC and 100× objective lens with a high numerical aperture combined with additional optical magnification, resulting in >8000× magnification via a liquid crystal display screen.

Nikon

Nikon's Eclipse Ti2 and Ts2 R inverted microscopes have been especially designed for research and clinical applications, respectively. They have a variable inclination eyepiece tube for ergonomics plus a wide 25 mm FOV and an imaging port with a large 25 field number. Glass heated stages are typically supplied by Tokai Hit Co Ltd (Shizuoka, Japan). The Ti2 is available as a motorized (Ti2-E) or manual (Ti2-A) model, the former employing a motorized condenser and nosepiece with joystick stage control, the latter having imaging capability for laser applications. In addition to the plastic-compatible NAMC, which provides pseudo-three-dimensional images with a shadow-cast appearance, DIC optics is available throughout the magnification range. Furthermore, an intermediate magnification switching function enables viewing at two different magnifications via a 1.5× frontal extra tube lens without having to change objective lenses. The Ts2 R has a compact ergonomic design and small footprint, allowing it to be easily fitted within a laminar flow workstation or biological cabinet. It also features a newly developed pseudo-relief contrast system called "Emboss," which is compatible with both glass and plastic dishes. Emboss provides a sharper image within the focal plane, which allows accurate observation of the meiotic spindle, and is a cheaper alternative to NAMC, which provides a greater sense of depth.

Olympus

Olympus' IX3 series inverted microscopes (www.youtube.com/watch?v=ls7NHOsoDVQ), including the IX-73, are available as manual or semi-motorized microscopes, the latter designed to speed up ICSI workflow. They can be easily upgraded for meiotic spindle observation using an integrated automated polarization technique, and for motile sperm organelle morphology examination (MSOME) using DIC optical elements and slider plus polarizer attachment. Push-button

selection of the different observation methods enables rapid transition between DIC for MSOME, spindle localization for ICSI and RC for sperm immobilization and IMSI. Similar to Nikon, smooth zooming with any given objective lens is possible using an adjustment lever with 1×, 1.6× and 2× magnification.

Zeiss

Zeiss' inverted microscopes, including the Axio Vert A1 (www.youtube.com/watch?v=yRCw6nQvz4M) and Axio Observer series, are available as manual and/or motorized models, respectively, and are compatible with all commonly available micromanipulators. The Axio Vert A1 is a compact inverted microscope, particularly suitable for fitting into a laminar flow workstation or biological cabinet. In addition to DIC and iHMC, Zeiss have a modified form of DIC (PlasDIC) that is also optimized for use with plastic dishes, making the system easy to switch between observation methods for different procedures, also giving the operator choice between iHMC and PlasDIC for ICSI. Similar to other manufacturer's inverted microscopes, Zeiss' ergo-tube allows tilting of the eyepieces for more ergonomic use.

Anti-Vibration Systems

Despite the high quality of inverted microscopes designed for ART, vibration remains a problem that is experienced universally. Regardless of where the micromanipulators are mounted upon the inverted microscope, the body of the microscope will transmit external vibrations reaching the table on which it is mounted, observed as a shaking of the injection micropipette, unless some form of anti-vibration device is placed between the two. Typically, ICSI rigs are most sensitive to vibrations within the vertical axis, but vibrations within the horizontal axis may also present a problem. These vibrations may originate externally, from vehicles and trains, within the laboratory itself, or from another room or floor of the building; for example I have observed rhythmic vibration of the injection micropipette in synchrony with a hospital's power plant engine situated on a lower floor of the building. Simple homemade solutions, such as squash or tennis balls placed between the inverted microscope and the table, have limited ability to absorb vibrations and, therefore, various commercially available devices have been manufactured to better solve the problem (Table 12.2). These

Table 12.2 Some commercially available anti-vibration devices

Device	Manufacturer/distributor	Mode of operation
Active Vibration Isolation table	Accurion	Active
AMC-1 Microscope Platform	Speirs Robertson	Passive
AMC-12/12S/13 Platforms	ProSciTech	Active and passive
Anti-Vibration Pads	Eppendorf	Passive
Anti-Vibration Table	IVFtech	Active and passive
AVT-I	Esco	Passive
Cell-Tek Anti-Vibration Plate	Tek-Event	Passive
CleanBench Aktiv Lab Table	TMC	Active
CleanBench Laboratory Table	TMC	Passive
K-Systems AV1	CooperSurgical	Passive
Origio TMC 63–500	CooperSurgical	Passive
Vistek Anti-Vibration Platform	Newport	Passive

range from simple, relatively cheap, passive air-filled plates to sophisticated, relatively expensive, active electronic tables. In this respect, it is known that pneumatic isolation chambers perform well and that isolation of vibration is optimal when the weight of the ICSI rig is at or close to the maximum load of the anti-vibration system.

Siting and Installation of Micromanipulation Rigs

Placement of Micromanipulation Rigs Within the Laboratory

It is preferable to site micromanipulation rigs along an interior wall, a safe distance away from areas of high staff traffic such as corridors and doorways, although effective anti-vibration systems will mitigate those effects to some extent. On the other hand, an important aspect of risk management is minimizing the distance between related pieces of equipment, such as incubators, workstations and ICSI rigs. Some IVF units have addressed this risk by designing their embryology laboratory in a modular fashion with multiple self-contained "work pods" that incorporate incubators, narrow workstations and ICSI rigs all within a small area restricted to use by only one or two embryologists [8]. Furthermore, as temperature maintenance is a crucial requirement for ICSI, it is vital that the heated stage of the inverted microscope be protected from any cooling drafts such as those

that can be generated by the heating, ventilation and air-conditioning (HVAC) vents mounted in the ceiling overhead. In this respect, there are various options including placing the ICSI rig on an anti-vibration table that is not directly beneath an HVAC vent, and placing it onto an anti-vibration table integrated into a low vibration laminar flow workstation (Figure 12.1) or onto an anti-vibration pad within a biological cabinet (Figure 12.2). Performing ICSI "in the open" is perfectly acceptable, providing the embryology laboratory meets certified clean room standards whereas performing it within a workstation is preferable if the laboratory fails to meet such standards. There should be sufficient space to house an ICSI rig within most workstations, although some may need to be specially adapted for micromanipulation, with a small aperture in the front window through which the eyepieces of the inverted microscope can project. However, it should be appreciated that laminar airflow also has a cooling effect and, therefore, the heated stage needs to be calibrated using a thermocouple placed into a media micro-drop within an ICSI dish overlaid with oil to determine the temperature setting required to achieve a temperature of 37°C within the dish under typical working conditions. Furthermore, although biological cabinets provide excellent control of temperature, it should be noted that they are less effective than workstations at maintaining aseptic conditions and are less easy to disinfect and, therefore, keep free of microbial contamination, especially should they be humidified.

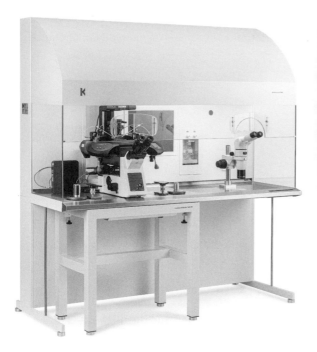

Figure 12.1 Workstation with integrated anti-vibration table. (A black and white version of this figure will appear in some formats. For the color version, please refer to the plate section.)

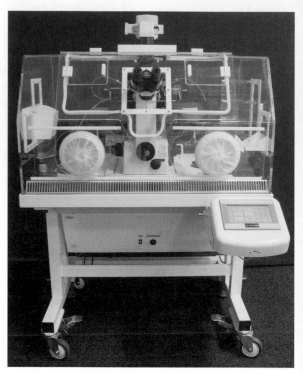

Figure 12.2 Biological cabinet with integrated anti-vibration pad. (A black and white version of this figure will appear in some formats. For the color version, please refer to the plate section.)

Installation and Validation of Micromanipulation Rigs

Installation of micromanipulators and micro-injectors is usually performed by a company's representative or distributor, although sometimes the purchaser is obliged to carry out this task. In either instance, it is wise for an experienced embryologist to supervise the process to avoid errors in installation that can otherwise occur; for example micromanipulators may not be firmly fitted to the microscope stand, resulting in vibration, or micromanipulator motors may be fitted the wrong way round, causing them to drive the micropipette towards, rather than away from, the microscope stage when the 'home' function is selected (I have witnessed both errors in the past, having to refit the micromanipulators myself to rectify those problems). Fortunately, most companies provide very good installation instructions these days, in written and/or video format, and provide excellent after-sales troubleshooting support. An important aspect of equipment installation is documented validation that the installation was performed safely and correctly, according to manufacturer's recommendations, and that it subsequently functions according to manufacturer's specifications. Furthermore, a schedule of routine

calibration and preventative maintenance should be devised and documented to ensure ongoing reliability of the equipment and reproducibility of ICSI results. An inventory of spare parts should be made on a regular basis to ensure their availability when and if required, and back-up equipment should be available in the event of unexpected failure of a micromanipulator or micro-injector. Ideally, each IVF unit would have their own back-up ICSI rig or, failing that, have a mutually beneficial arrangement in place with another nearby IVF unit and/or their distributor to supply replacement equipment if required at short notice.

Mechanical Micromanipulation Systems

Mechanical micromanipulators are directly controlled using joysticks, the principle behind such design philosophy being that direct, proportional movement enables greater control, while requiring minimal routine maintenance and servicing because of the simplicity of the mechanical components. The original Leitz micromanipulators were purely mechanical systems based on high-quality, solid engineering, and were renowned for their smoothness of action, it being possible to alter the degree of resistance to joystick movement in the x- and y-axes. Likewise, the micromanipulators manufactured by RI are also purely mechanical, with extremely smooth movement in all three axes. Historically, Leitz micromanipulators were the preferred choice of many transgenics laboratories, whereas RI micromanipulators have been developed primarily for clinical use in micromanipulation, including ICSI [9].

The RI Micromanipulation System

RI's latest model of micromanipulator is the Integra 3™ (Figure 12.3). It is different from most other micromanipulators in that, rather than being adapted to the mechanical stage of a specific microscope, it comes with its own mechanical heated stage that has been custom-designed purely for micromanipulation procedures (www.youtube.com/watch?v=e_ukn4PwDro), each turn of the XY control moving the stage plate by 28 mm with up to 40 mm full travel. Indeed, one of the issues confronting an ICSI operator is what type of heated stage to employ in conjunction with their choice of inverted microscope. Traditional metal heated stages with a central hole for the light path of the inverted microscope are evidently incapable of maintaining

physiological temperature at their center. To some extent glass heated stages overcome this problem, but are undermined by the "heat-sink" effect of the underlying metal objective lens, which draws heat away from the stage, resulting in variable heating across its surface. With the Integra 3™, RI have addressed this "heat-sink" problem by incorporating a fan-heater system, called Thermosafe™, that directs precisely warmed heated air between the heated stage and objective lens, thereby maintaining uniform physiological temperature across the entire bottom surface of the ICSI dish. Monitoring of the heated stages is an integral feature of Thermosafe™, with an audible and visible alarm being activated should the temperature drift outside of the set point. Either side of the mechanical stage of the Integra 3™ there are two large built-in touch-screen displays. The one on the right enables independent four-channel temperature control, which is accurately calibrated to within 0.1°C of the selected set-point, and has a stopwatch and counter (Figure 12.4), useful for ICSI quality control. An integrated linkage with RI Viewer software for recording photos and videos is available on the left-hand touch-screen display. Below the heated stage, there is a motion sensor light-emitting diode, which makes it easier to view and select the desired objective lens.

Both fine and coarse control of the manipulators is incorporated into one compact unit, with coarse control levers projecting above and fine control joysticks hanging below the heated stage (Figures 12.3 and 12.5). For those admirers of the classic TDU500 micromanipulator, longer fine control hanging joysticks are available as an optional extra. Green electronic height

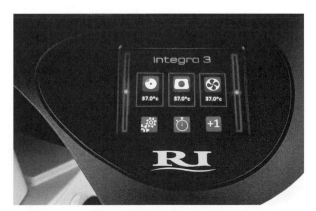

Figure 12.3 RI Integra 3™. (A black and white version of this figure will appear in some formats. For the color version, please refer to the plate section.)

Figure 12.4 Touchscreen display of the RI Integra 3™. (A black and white version of this figure will appear in some formats. For the color version, please refer to the plate section.)

indicators that help establish the midpoint range of the fine manipulators are present on each side of the right-hand touch-screen display (Figure 12.4), with an audible and visible warning alarm sounding should the limit of travel be imminent. The manipulators control the PL3 tool-holders, which incorporate one-touch "home" and one-touch angle adjustments of the micropipettes. Micropipettes can be accurately adjusted for a range of micropipette bend angles, from 16° to 43° using a single calibrated screw (Figure 12.5). Furthermore, adjustments can be made "on-the-fly" as the position of the micropipette tip remains constant whenever the micropipette angle is adjusted. The PL3 tool-holders support RI's MPH micropipette holders, which can be either clipped into place or more gently slid into place using the MPH axial drive screw. Together, the PL3 and MPH holders enable easy and rapid set-up of the micropipette via vertical, axial and

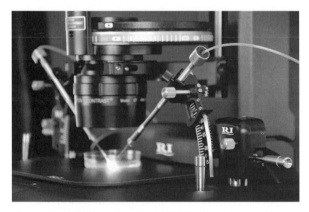

Figure 12.5 RI PL3 tool-holder and MPH micropipette holder. (A black and white version of this figure will appear in some formats. For the color version, please refer to the plate section.)

rotational movements. Micropipette set-up is further facilitated using the 4× objective lens with built-in spacer, supplied by RI, which enables alignment of the micropipettes 14 mm above the heated stage. A double tool-holder is also available from RI for those practitioners who still elect to use acid Tyrode's, rather than a laser, for zona drilling and embryo biopsy.

Screw-actuated syringes (SAS™) with a characteristic inverted mushroom design are the micro-injectors supplied by RI as standard with the Integra 3™ (Figure 12.6). An extra smooth, special edition, chrome version (SAS-SE™) is often preferred by ICSI operators and is available from RI as an optional extra (Figure 12.6). As their design incorporates a heavy stable circular base, they have a small "footprint" and they are able to generate high aspiration pressure, having a capacity of 2 mL. They come supplied with hard polythene tubing for connection to the MPH micropipette holders. The pressure release button situated on top of the SAS enables rapid equilibration of pressure for stabilizing capillary flow. RI also supply a quick-fill micrometer-actuated sealed oil syringe (SOS™) mounted on a sturdy, non-slip base (Figure 12.6).

The Integra 3™ is supplied largely preassembled within a purpose-built dispatch case and, therefore, installation onto an inverted microscope is a quick and simple process. If required, installation manuals/troubleshooting guides may be downloaded from the company's website (https://fertility.coopersurgical.com/products/integra-3/) and a dedicated technical support department is on-hand via telephone and/or email to assist with any queries regarding installation or operation of the Integra 3™.

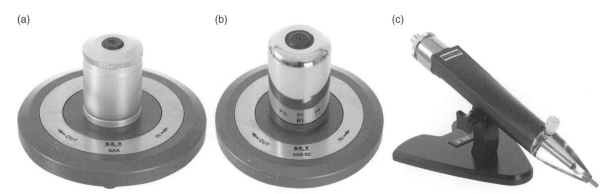

Figure 12.6 (a) RI SAS™,(b) SAS-SE™ and (c) SOS™ screw-actuated syringes. (A black and white version of this figure will appear in some formats. For the color version, please refer to the plate section.)

Hydraulic Micromanipulation Systems

Hydraulic micromanipulators are based on the concept of remotely controlling movement of a "slave" drive unit in three axes by the movement of a "master" control unit via hydraulic flow lines connecting the two units. In essence, movements of a joystick push a short rod into the diaphragm of a master cylinder, displacing hydraulic oil from the diaphragm of the slave cylinder, which pushes a rod attached to a slide of the drive unit on the head-stage by an equal amount. The remote nature of the joystick allows individual positioning to suit the preference of each ICSI operator and avoids direct transmission of vibration to the microscope as a result of any unintended hand movements. The application of hydraulic micromanipulators to ICSI originated at the Dutch-Speaking Free University of Brussels (AZ-VUB), now known as UZ, following a joint venture to develop a three-axis, oil-hydraulic, joystick-controlled micromanipulator by Nikon and Narishige [7,10].

The Narishige Micromanipulation System

Narishige's latest model (MTK-1) of micromanipulator is called the Takanome™ (Figure 12.7). The MTK-1 is a four-axis hanging joystick oil-hydraulic micromanipulator, the name Takanome™ being derived from the Japanese metaphor for a hawk locking on to its target (https://www.youtube.com/watch?v=-pXhEj9klZk&t=46s). The fourth axis (T-axis) enables hydraulic adjustment of the position of the micropipette towards or away from the heated stage using a coarse control knob mounted on the pillar of the control unit adjacent to the hanging joystick (Figure 12.8). This feature is extended by the slider mechanism of the micropipette tool-holder, which provides one-touch retraction of the micropipette to its "home" position and one-touch return to its "working" position (Figure 12.9). Together, the slider and T-axis control obviate any requirement for an electrically driven coarse manipulator, making the system simpler to install and less cluttered with unnecessary additional control units and electrical cables. Furthermore, they make micropipette exchange a quicker and safer process. As with previous models, the MTK-1 control unit may be securely placed wherever desired by attaching it to a metal baseplate via a switch that activates the magnetic stand of the hanging joystick. Furthermore, the height of both the joystick stand and the joystick itself are adjustable. With respect to the joystick, a movement ratio adjustment ring regulates the amplitude and a tension adjustment ring regulates the sensitivity of its movement. Above the joystick there are three graduated rotating knobs that control movement in the x- and y-axes, and at the base of the joystick there is a single graduated knob that controls movement in the z-axis (Figure 12.8). Their presence enables fine movements to be made free of any joystick control that might otherwise fail to maintain the micropipette

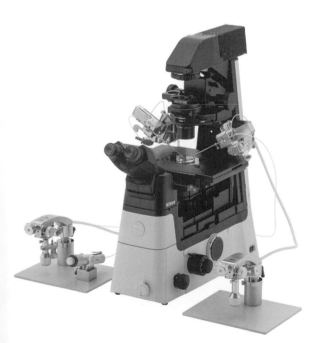

Figure 12.7 Narishige Takanome™ MTK-1. (A black and white version of this figure will appear in some formats. For the color version, please refer to the plate section.)

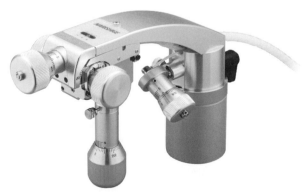

Figure 12.8 Narishige Takanome™ MTK-1 control unit. (A black and white version of this figure will appear in some formats. For the color version, please refer to the plate section.)

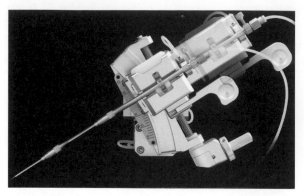

Figure 12.9 Narishige Takanome™ MTK-1 drive unit. (A black and white version of this figure will appear in some formats. For the color version, please refer to the plate section.)

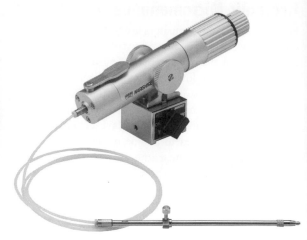

Figure 12.10 Narishige IM-11–2 pneumatic injector. (A black and white version of this figure will appear in some formats. For the color version, please refer to the plate section.)

within the same focal plane, ensuring that an ICSI pipette moves into an oocyte in a very straight line. The micropipette tool-holder simply clips into its attachment connected to the drive unit and its angle may be adjusted from 15° to 40° without affecting the position of the micropipette tip, which allows adjustments to be made "on-the-fly" (Figure 12.9).

Narishige supplies both oil and pneumatic (air) injectors. Their latest model (IM-9B) of oil injector may be securely placed onto a metal baseplate via a switch that activates its magnetic stand. Likewise, their latest models (IM-11–2 and IM-12) of higher-pressure pneumatic injectors may also be securely placed onto a metal baseplate and incorporate a pressure relief valve on top of the syringe barrel (Figure 12.10). Together with an adjustable syringe volume, fine and coarse control knobs allow variable control of the speed and strength of pressure applied to the IM-11–2 pneumatic injector (www.youtube.com/watch?v=RSKQ78lVb6Q). For the holding micropipette, there is the option of fitting a space-saving model (IM-HD1T) of pneumatic injector which is attached to the joystick (Figure 12.11). This novel arrangement enables concurrent control of both holding micropipette position and aspiration, the IM-HD1T also incorporating a pressure relief valve (https://www.youtube.com/watch?v=9Ip6K1MTKA4).

In the past, assembly and installation of Narishige micromanipulation rigs could be a daunting proposition for some practitioners [7]; however, with pre-assembly and rationalization of micromanipulator design, installation of the Takanome™ MTK-1 micromanipulator is now a simple task (www.youtube.com/watch?v=-pXhEj9klZk&t=46s). It is important to site

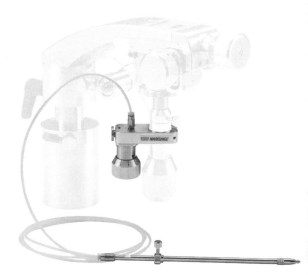

Figure 12.11 Narishige IM-HD1T pneumatic injector. (A black and white version of this figure will appear in some formats. For the color version, please refer to the plate section.)

the micromanipulation rig away from sources of ultraviolet (UV) light, such as sunlight and UV sterilization, as exposure to UV adversely affects the condition and function of the hydraulic oil. Narishige also recommends sending in devices for servicing should the appearance of the hydraulic lines change from their light blue color, when new, to yellow or reddish-brown. It is also recommended that the drive units be moved almost their entire distance several times each year to prevent drying out of their lubrication grease.

Electronic Micromanipulation Systems

In contrast to mechanical and hydraulic micromanipulators, electronic micromanipulators rely on microprocessor control, there being no form of mechanical linkage between the control and motor units. With electronic micromanipulators, movements of the joystick are digitally encoded and transmitted to the head-stage via a microprocessor. Eppendorf pioneered the concept of electronic micromanipulators, collaborating with the Gamete & Embryo Research Laboratory at St Barnabas Medical Center in New Jersey on development of an electronic micromanipulator with proportional control suitable for ICSI [7].

The Eppendorf Micromanipulation System

Eppendorf's latest model of micromanipulator, the TransferMan® 4 m (Figure 12.12), combines an intuitive interface with unprecedented movement control [11]. Registered as a medical product, the TransferMan® 4 m is designed and manufactured for human reproductive medicine, whereas the TransferMan® 4 r model designation denotes that it is for research use only (www.youtube.com/watch?v=H8hhrrWSn8Y). The main components of the TransferMan® 4 m are the joystick control board (Figure 12.13) and the head-stage motor module

(Figure 12.14). Power and electrical connections to the motor module unit are located at the rear of the control board. The motor module comprises three individual precision stepper motors arranged at right angles to each other to control movement within the x-, y- and z-axes (Figure 12.14). The steps of each stepper motor are small and rapid enough to achieve smooth movement. The x-axis stepper motor incorporates an angle head with adjustable clamp, which supports the micropipette tool-holder, and a swivel joint which allows it to be swung out and away from the heated stage to facilitate micropipette replacement (Figure 12.14). The joystick sits towards the back of the control board, both proportional and dynamic movement movements in all three axes being possible at different speeds by virtue of DualSpeed™ technology (Figure 12.13). In dynamic mode, the position of the joystick determines the speed of stepper motor movement, the further it is moved the faster the micropipette travels. In proportional mode, however, the speed at which the joystick is moved is precisely replicated by the speed of stepper motor movement. The range of movement of the stepper motors is determined by selecting coarse, fine and extra-fine modes on the control board, with the selection dial on the left-hand side of the control board enabling adjustment of the range within each mode (Figure 12.13). Moving the joystick within its central range permits fine

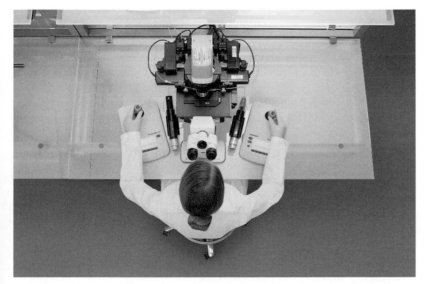

Figure 12.12 Eppendorf TransferMan®
4 m © Eppendorf AG. (A black and white version of this figure will appear in some formats. For the color version, please refer to the plate section.)

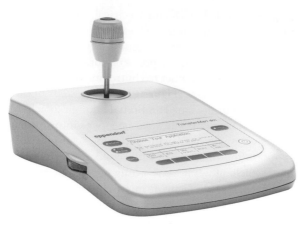

Figure 12.13 Eppendorf joystick control board © Eppendorf AG. (A black and white version of this figure will appear in some formats. For the color version, please refer to the plate section.)

control, whereas pressing the joystick against the outer black ring enables control similar to an auto-scroll function. Furthermore, range of movement is not limited by joystick travel as it may be uncoupled from the motor module by pushing down the button on top of it, allowing repositioning without interfering with the position of the micropipette. Different tool-holder positions can be saved via the control board, with rapid movement between saved positions being possible with either the push of a button or "double-click" of the joystick button. Indeed, positions saved by different operators may be recalled by them. In addition, there is a "home" button that can be pressed to rapidly withdraw the micropipette from the heated stage, which, when pressed again, returns it to its previous position (Figure 12.13). The control board software can also be programmed for specific applications such as ICSI, whereby a z-axis limit may be set to prevent micropipette damage and y-axis lockout can be applied to ensure any movement within the x-axis is maintained in a straight line.

Eppendorf supplies both air and oil manual injectors known as the CellTram® 4 air and oil, respectively (Figure 12.15). There is also a CellTram® Vario oil injector that provides very fine control. The transparent barrel of the CellTram® 4 oil injector makes it easy to check the oil level and for the presence of air bubbles, which might affect injector performance. Filling an Eppendorf micro-injector with oil is a simple process (www.youtube.com/watch?v=JQne1jUPq-g). Eppendorf also supplies a piezo-injector, which can be connected to the TransferMan® 4 m for piezo-ICSI, called the PiezoXpert® (Figure 12.16).

Electronic coupling of the two devices enables integration of the PiezoXpert® operating functions with micromanipulation control, piezo-impulses being transmitted directly to the piezo-micropipette. No service intervals for micromanipulators or injectors are prescribed by Eppendorf.

Advanced ICSI Technology

Over the past quarter century, ICSI has become a routine method and has been increasingly applied to both male and non-male factor patients. However, it remains an imperfect technique, with variability between ICSI operators in terms of rates of fertilization and viability of oocytes following injection. For these reasons, there is interest in advances in technology such as piezo-ICSI, robotic ICSI and ICSI using photonic micropipettes.

Piezo-ICSI

The most commonly used equipment for piezo-ICSI is that supplied by Prime Tech (Figure 12.17). The control unit operates the piezo-micromanipulator drive unit, which is attached to the micropipette toolholder (Figure 12.18). Piezo-ICSI relies on ultrafast submicron forward momentum of ultrathin flat-tipped micropipettes in response to piezo-pulses that result in submicron negative pressure at the pipette tip. Consequently, the technique avoids deformation of the zona pellucida (ZP) and aspiration of ooplasm, resulting in improved oocyte viability and increased fertilization rates [12]. Nevertheless, the piezo-pulses do result in a core of the ZP being removed and having to be discarded. Also, the technique depends on priming the piezo-micropipette with either mercury or a colorless, non-toxic, water-insoluble, fully fluorinated liquid with a high specific gravity, called Fluorinert. Air or oil micro-injectors may be used for piezo-ICSI, although the technique fails should air bubbles be allowed to penetrate the oil [12].

Robotic ICSI

As currently performed, successful ICSI is highly operator-dependent and time-consuming. Therefore, automation of the ICSI technique has been investigated as a potential solution to these issues, although commercially available equipment has yet to be developed since the first report of robotic ICSI [13]. Specific orientation of the metaphase II oocyte does not appear to influence

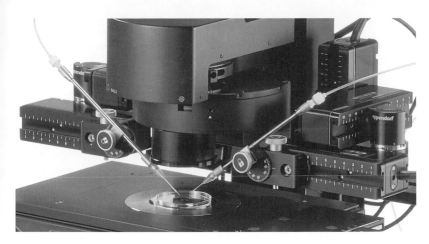

Figure 12.14 Eppendorf head-stage motor module © Eppendorf AG. (A black and white version of this figure will appear in some formats. For the color version, please refer to the plate section.)

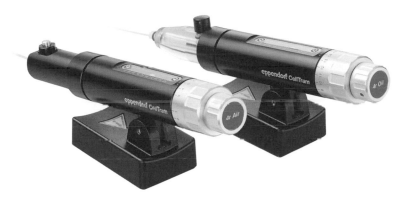

Figure 12.15 Eppendorf CellTram® 4 air and CellTram® 4 oil injectors © Eppendorf AG. (A black and white version of this figure will appear in some formats. For the color version, please refer to the plate section.)

fertilization rates and clinical outcomes [14–16], but damage to the meiotic spindle must nevertheless be avoided. Therefore, as the position of the meiotic spindle is expected to be adjacent to the extruded first polar body (PB), PB position recognition is essential for automated ICSI. A vision detection algorithm adaptable to commercially available inverted microscopes has been developed to achieve oocyte orientation in a relatively quick, reliable and computationally inexpensive manner that allows for morphological variance between oocytes and their PBs [17]. Successful oocyte activation and fertilization is dependent on tracking,

selection, orientation and rupture of the sperm plasmalemma, while avoiding damage to the sperm head. Recently, a tracking algorithm integrated with a visual servo control and motorized rotational microscope stage has been developed [18]. This automated system is capable of distinguishing a targeted sperm head from interfering spermatozoa and estimating sperm tail positions to actively adjust sperm orientation for immobilization with approximately 95% success, independent of either sperm velocity or direction of progression. It is likely that successful and reliable fully automated micro-injection will ultimately depend on

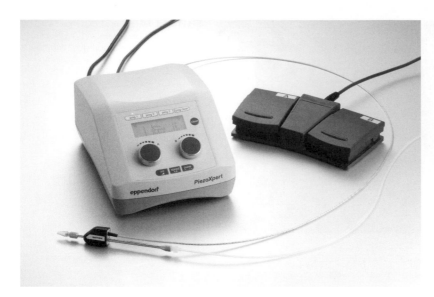

Figure 12.16 Eppendorf PiezoXpert® © Eppendorf AG. (A black and white version of this figure will appear in some formats. For the color version, please refer to the plate section.)

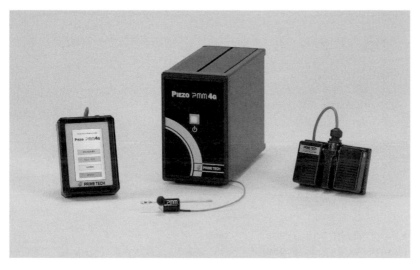

Figure 12.17 Prime Tech piezo PMM4G. (A black and white version of this figure will appear in some formats. For the color version, please refer to the plate section.)

integration of visual algorithms with servo-controlled inverted microscopes and piezo-ICSI.

Summary

Micromanipulation systems have gradually evolved to help improve clinical outcomes following ICSI; however, fertilization and survival rates remain largely operator-dependent. The advent of robotic ICSI is tantalizingly close but still to be realized in the clinical setting. Furthermore, it is possible that we will be able to assess gamete quality and fertilization during ICSI in future using bio-photonic

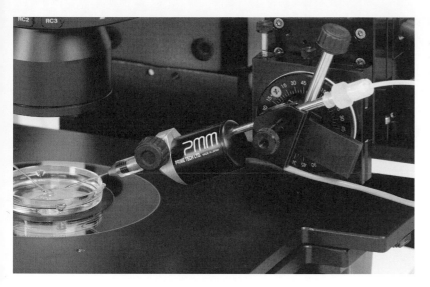

Figure 12.18 Prime Tech piezo drive unit. (A black and white version of this figure will appear in some formats. For the color version, please refer to the plate section.)

micropipettes for non-invasive imaging of molecular events. Indeed, the next steps in the evolution of ICSI hold great promise.

Acknowledgments

The author is extremely grateful to Lis Goulder and Stephen Bedser for supply of RI and CooperSurgical images, to Dieter Regel for supply of the Tek-Event image, to Yuki Narishige for supply of Narishige images, to Christian Haberlandt for supply of Eppendorf images and to Masaki Yasuda for supply of Prime Tech images.

References

[1] Malter, H.E. (2016). Micromanipulation in assisted reproductive technology. *Reproductive BioMedicine Online*, **32**, 339–347.

[2] Schmidt, H.D. (1864). On the microscopic anatomy, physiology and pathology of the human liver. *Confederate States Medical & Surgical Journal*, **1**, 49–54.

[3] Fishel, S., Timson, J., Green, S. *et al.* (1993). Micromanipulation. *Reproductive Medicine Review*, **2**, 199–222.

[4] Uehara, T. and Yanagimachi, R. (1976). Microsurgical injection of spermatozoa into hamster eggs with subsequent transformation of sperm nuclei into male pronuclei. *Biology of Reproduction*, **15**, 467–470.

[5] Palermo, G., Joris, H., Devroey, P. *et al.* (1992). Pregnancies after intracytoplasmic injection of single spermatozoon into an oocyte. *Lancet*, **340**: 17–18.

[6] O'Neill, C.L., Chow, S., Rosenwaks, Z. *et al.* (2018). Development of ICSI. *Reproduction*, **156**: F51-F58.

[7] Fleming, S.D. and King, R.S. (2003). *Micromanipulation in Assisted Conception: A users' manual and troubleshooting guide* – Cambridge: Cambridge University Press.

[8] Cooke, S. (2016). Low-risk laboratory management. In. *Organization and Management of IVF Units: A practical guide for the clinician*, ed. S.D. Fleming and A.C. Varghese, pp. 115–152. Cham: Springer Nature Switzerland AG.

[9] Fleming, S. and Pretty, C. (2019). Research Instruments micromanipulation systems. In. *In Vitro Fertilization: A textbook of current and emerging methods and devices*, Second Edition, ed. Z.P. Nagy, A.C. Varghese and A. Agarwal, pp. 455–463. Cham: Springer Nature Switzerland AG.

[10] Joris, H. (2019). Hydraulic micromanipulators for ICSI. In. *In Vitro Fertilization: A textbook of current and emerging methods and devices*, Second Edition, ed. Z.P. Nagy, A.C. Varghese and A. Agarwal, pp. 449–454. Cham: Springer Nature Switzerland AG.

[11] Nanassy, L. (2019). Eppendorf micromanipulator: setup and operation of electronic micromanipulators. In. *In Vitro Fertilization: A textbook of current and emerging methods and devices*, Second Edition, ed. Z.P. Nagy, A.C. Varghese and A. Agarwal, pp. 465–469. Cham: Springer Nature Switzerland AG.

[12] Hiraoka, K., Kawai, K., Harada, T. *et al.* (2019). Piezo-ICSI. In. *In Vitro Fertilization: A textbook of current and emerging methods and devices*, Second Edition, ed. Z.P. Nagy, A.C. Varghese and

A. Agarwal, pp. 481–489. Cham: Springer Nature Switzerland AG.

[13] Lu, Z., Zhang, X., Leung, C. *et al.* (2011). Robotic ICSI (intracytoplasmic sperm injection). *IEEE Transactions On Biomedical Engineering*, **58**, 2102–2108

[14] Nagy, Z.P., Liu, J., Joris, H. *et al.* (1995). The influence of the site of sperm deposition and mode of oolemma breakage at intracytoplasmic sperm injection on fertilization and embryo development rates. *Human Reproduction*, **10**, 3171–3177.

[15] Stoddart, N.R. and Fleming, S.D. (2000). Orientation of the first polar body of the oocyte at 6 or 12 o'clock during ICSI does not affect clinical outcome. *Human Reproduction*, **15**, 1580–1585.

[16] Woodward, B.J., Montgomery, S.J., Hartshorne, G.M. *et al.* (2008). Spindle position assessment prior to ICSI does not benefit fertilization or early embryo quality. *Reproductive BioMedicine Online*, **16**, 232–238.

[17] Saadat, M., Hajiyavand, A.M. and Bedi, A.S. (2018). Oocyte positional recognition for automatic manipulation in ICSI. *Micromachines*, **9**, 429.

[18] Zhang, Z., Dai, C., Huang, J. *et al.* (2019). Robotic immobilization of motile sperm for clinical intracytoplasmic sperm injection. *IEEE Transactions On Biomedical Engineering*, **66**, 444–452.

Chapter 13

Automation Techniques and Systems for ICSI

Changsheng Dai, Zhuoran Zhang, Guanqiao Shan, and Yu Sun

Introduction

Intracytoplasmic sperm injection (ICSI) is widely used for in vitro fertilization. It involves insertion of a single sperm into an oocyte by a sharp micropipette. As a clinical surgery at single cell level, it requires high dexterity, experience, and patience. Automation has enabled unprecedented capabilities to single cell manipulation, such as cell injection, transfer, and characterization. For ICSI, automation techniques could increase the efficiency and consistency of the operation, reduce cell damage, and relieve the labor on operators. This chapter reviews the techniques and systems required to achieve automated ICSI in the following sections.

Sperm analysis is important for selecting a single sperm in ICSI. The quality of the selected sperm contributes to ICSI outcome. Sperm are currently evaluated by motility and morphology, based on qualitatively manual observation. The use of automation techniques allows for quantitative and objective analysis of sperm

After identifying the appropriate sperm, the sperm needs to be immobilized by tapping its tail with a micropipette. In manual operation, sperm tail needs to be approximately perpendicular to the micropipette, imposing a constraint on which sperm can be immobilized. Recent advances in automation allows for the immobilization of sperm swimming in all directions regardless of tail orientation.

Aspiration of the immobilized sperm into a micropipette is usually achieved with a hydraulic pump. Precisely positioning the sperm within the micropipette is challenging because fluid flow at this microscale is highly nonlinear. To prevent large overshoot and sperm loss, automated aspiration of sperm has been developed including fluid dynamics and controller design.

Prior to sperm injection, the polar body needs to be rotated away from the injection site to protect the spindle. It is commonly implemented using a holding micropipette to repeatedly release and aspirate an oocyte, or using an injection micropipette to push on the oocyte. Automated methods for oocyte orientation control have been developed, using fluid flow, customized devices, and micropipettes.

The final section of this chapter discusses sperm injection. Robotic sperm injection was integrated with visual feedback and image processing for precise operation. Moreover, piezo drills were developed to reduce oocyte deformation and potential damage during injection.

Automated Sperm Analysis

Sperm Tracking for Motility Measurement

As defined by the World Health Organization (WHO), sperm motility parameters (curvilinear velocity, linearity, wobble, etc.) are all calculated based on sperm trajectories. Automated motility measurement is achieved by computer vision tracking to obtain sperm trajectories. In general, sperm tracking algorithms start with image segmentation to detect the positions of each sperm of the current image frame (time instance). Then a data association algorithm is applied to associate the data (position) of the same sperm in different frames (time instances) to obtain the trajectory. A clinical sperm sample contains a high number of sperm; therefore, one challenge of data association in sperm tracking is how to accurately distinguish/match each sperm during their intersections (cross-over) in close proximity.

Common algorithms for tracking multiple objects include the nearest neighbor (NN), global nearest neighbor (GNN), multiple hypothesis tracker (MHT), and joint probabilistic data association filter (JPDAF) [1]. The NN method always assumes the nearest measurement to the tracked sperm to be the correct association case. The GNN method assumes the association case that minimizes the global sum of pair-wise distance to be the correct association. The NN and GNN methods are easy to implement and can achieve real-time measurement, but do not accounts for the possibility of false association and would cause mismatch during sperm cross-over. The MHT method exploits the entire measurement history to estimate the state of each target and is generally more accurate than NN and GNN, but suffers from the rapidly growing memory with increasing time duration and the number of targets.

The JPDAF method is suitable for real-time tracking of multiple sperm because it uses only the current measurement to enumerate all association cases and update association probability. For the specific application of sperm tracking, the JPDAF method can be adapted by incorporating the sperm dynamics model to achieve a high tracking accuracy of 95.6% [2] (Figure 13.1).

Sperm Morphology Measurement

Sperm morphology is an important criterion for male infertility diagnosis and treatment. A normal sperm should have a smooth, generally oval head, a slender, regular midpiece, and a uniform tail, according to the WHO. Morphological normalcy is found to be correlated with fertilization rate and pregnancy outcomes [3].

A stained smear of semen is commonly used to examine sperm morphology, because of its higher contrast of head, midpiece, and tail. A variety of methods have been developed for stained morphology analysis. For example, Bijar *et al.* segmented sperm's acrosome, nucleus, and midpiece by a Bayesian classifier, and achieved accuracy over 90% [4]. However, fixation and staining destroys the sperm, rendering it not applicable for ICSI use.

For live sperm morphology analysis, an automated method based on Sobel edge detection and boundary finding was developed [5] (Figure 13.2 (a–d)). Although an accuracy of 88.1% was achieved for sperm head detection, this method suffers from high time cost (9 seconds for processing an image). Also, because of the contrast and resolution limit (under 40× objective), the method cannot be used to detect subcellular structures such as acrosome and nucleus.

For fine morphology analysis of sperm, automated non-invasive techniques were established [2]. Subcellular structures (such as acrosome, nucleus, and vacuole) were measured under 100× microscope objective without staining. The 100× microscope objective is commonly used in intracytoplasmic morphologically selected sperm injection (IMSI) for selecting sperm with normal fine morphology. Differential interference contrast (DIC) imaging is used to enhance contrast, but it has an inherent side illumination effect to cause inhomogeneous image intensity. As this poses difficulties to image processing, DIC image reconstruction is proposed to remove the side illumination effect. Image reconstruction is intrinsically a deconvolution process, and image smoothing is required in the process; however, the smoothing can cause a loss of subtle edge information, which reflects the subcellular structures of the sperm. To preserve the subtle edge information, total variation norm is introduced into the cost function for DIC image reconstruction, which can smooth the image while preserving the edges (Figure 13.2 (e, f)).

After removing the side illumination effect in DIC, image segmentation is performed to segment the

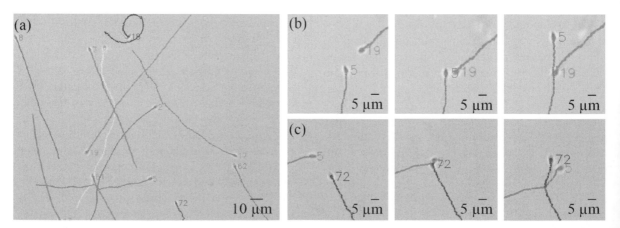

Figure 13.1 (a) Multiple sperm tracking using the JPDAF method. (b) The tracking of two sperm in close proximity. (c) The tracking of two sperm in intersection. Reproduced from [2]. (A black and white version of this figure will appear in some formats. For the color version, please refer to the plate section.)

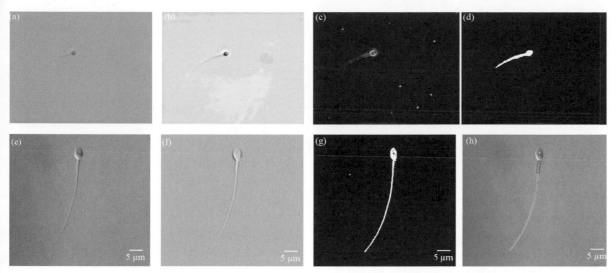

Figure 13.2 Live sperm morphology analysis. (a) Sperm image under 40× objective. (b) Denoising by wavelet transform. (c) Applying Sobel edge detection. (d) Sperm segmentation after median filter. Reproduced from [5]. (e) Sperm image under 100× objective and DIC imaging. (f) Image reconstruction to remove DIC side illumination effect. (g) Sperm segmentation by fuzzy c-means clustering. (h) Separation of head, midpiece, and tail, and the detection of vacuole. Reproduced from [2]. (A black and white version of this figure will appear in some formats. For the color version, please refer to the plate section.)

sperm from the background and further segment the head, midpiece, and tail. To accurately segment the sperm, fuzzy c-means clustering is used as this utilizes fuzzy set theory to segment low contrast objects. The head, midpiece, and tail are separated based on their difference in distance from their contours to the sperm centerline (Figure 13.2 (g, h)). Further, nucleus area, acrosome area, vacuole number, and area are measured. The measurement errors for morphology parameters are all less than 10%, compared to manual benchmarking.

Morphology analysis of live sperm is important to guide the selection of morphologically normal sperm for ICSI. As found by Dai *et al.*, of 50 sperm measured, only one will meet the WHO criteria of normality [2]. Automation in sperm analysis (motility and morphology measurement) holds potential for improving efficiency, consistency, and objectivity of sperm selection in ICSI.

Sperm Immobilization

Robotic Immobilization

In manual sperm immobilization, an embryologist controls a micropipette to tap a sperm tail against a substrate (e.g. the bottom of a petri dish) so that the motor proteins on the sperm tail are damaged (Figure 13.3 (a)). Manual immobilization follows a look-

and-move scheme, that is the embryologist first observes the entire field of view to choose a target sperm, then controls the micropipette to approach a moving sperm, and finally immobilizes the sperm. Because of the fast movement of a healthy sperm (>25 μm/s) and the small size of the sperm tail (<1 μm in diameter), manual manipulation has stringent skill requirements, demanding the reduction of human involvement and automated robotic immobilization.

To tackle these limitations, robotic sperm immobilization was developed [6]. In robotic immobilization, a petri dish containing a sperm sample is placed on a motorized microscopy stage (Figure 13.3 (b)). The robotic system uses computer vision to track the position of the sperm tail, then uses visual servo control to move the motorized stage to maintain the sperm tail at the center of the field of view. Here, visual servoing serves two purposes: to avoid sperm moving out of the field of view, and to ensure the success of micropipette tapping because the sperm tail is maintained at a fixed location (i.e. center of the field of view). Finally, the micropipette is controlled by a motorized manipulator to perform a sequence of motion to tap the sperm tail.

The target sperm to immobilize is selected by an embryologist who clicks on the target sperm within the field of view. This minimal human input allows the embryologist to exercise his/her expert knowledge

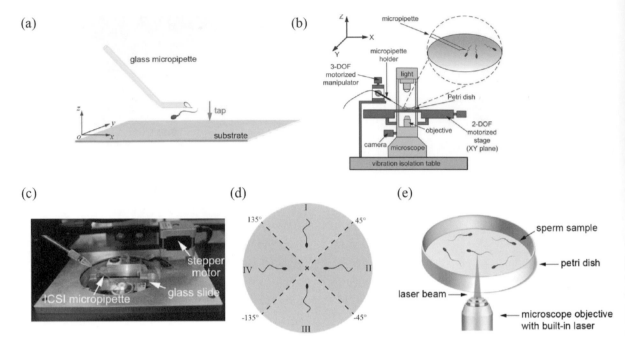

Figure 13.3 Robotic sperm immobilization. (a) Conventional manual immobilization uses a micropipette to tap the sperm tail against a substrate. Reproduced from [7]. (b) Schematic illustration of the robotic sperm immobilization system. Reproduced from [6]. (c) A rotational microscopy stage for actively adjusting sperm orientation to enable immobilization of sperm swimming in all directions. (d) Based on sperm head orientation, sperm swimming in all directions are classified into four quadrants for orientation adjustment. Reproduced from [7]. (e) Sperm immobilization using laser ablation. Reproduced from [8]. (A black and white version of this figure will appear in some formats. For the color version, please refer to the plate section.)

in sperm selection. The system then tracks the position of the sperm head and tail. Similar to that described in "Sperm Tracking for Motility Measurement" above, there may be interference to the target sperm by neighboring sperm (e.g. crossover). Furthermore, the sperm tail is unavoidably occluded by the micropipette during tapping. To address these problems, Zhang *et al.* developed a sperm tracker by adapting the probabilistic data association filter (PDAF) algorithm [7]. The tracker first tracks the spatial position of the sperm head, based on which the sperm tail position is estimated. The tracker also measures the sperm head orientation, which is the angle between the major axis of the sperm head and the horizontal axis of the image frame, to further distinguish sperm swimming in different directions. The sperm tail position is estimated by extending the major axis of the head. As micropipette tapping only occludes the sperm tail and the sperm head remains unaffected, the tracker ensures the position of the sperm tail is available throughout the immobilization process.

In terms of performance, the system achieved an accuracy of 1.08 μm for tail tracking, an average immobilization time of 6–7 seconds, and an overall immobilization success rate of 88.2% (based on experiments on 1000 sperm). The failure cases were mainly because the sperm changed its orientation (swimming direction) or swimming plane (z position) during immobilization. When sperm immobilization fails, the human operator can readily select the same sperm to attempt to immobilize it or select a different sperm for tracking and immobilization.

The major limitation of this robotic immobilization system was its incapability of immobilizing sperm swimming in all directions. Sperm with head orientation within [-135°,-45°] and [45°,135°] can be immobilized; however, sperm with orientation falling outside this interval were discarded for immobilization, because there was a high risk of tapping the sperm head and thus damaging its DNA. As shown in Figure 13.3 (d), only half of all sperm can be immobilized. The orientation limitation must be overcome if robotic sperm immobilization is to become clinically useful.

Techniques for Overcoming Sperm Orientation Limitation

Two robotic sperm immobilization techniques have been developed to enable the immobilization of sperm swimming in all directions: (1) adding a rotational microscopy stage to actively adjust sperm orientation (Figure 13.3 (c)), and (2) using a non-contact laser for sperm immobilization (Fig. 13.3 (e)).

The orientation limitation in conventional immobilization arises because both the manipulator and microscopy stage have only translational degrees of freedom. To change the relative orientation between the sperm and the micropipette, a rotational degree of freedom must be added either to the manipulator to adjust the orientation of the micropipette, or to the microscopy stage to adjust the orientation of the sperm. Zhang *et al.* used a motorized rotational stage integrated into the manipulation system [7]. As shown in Figure 13.3 (d), the system classifies each sperm into four quadrants based on their head orientations. Both translational and rotational control were performed via position-based visual servoing to orient a target sperm in quadrants II and IV into quadrant I or III. During the rotational stage, coordinate transformation was used to compensate for sperm motion to bring the sperm back into the center of field of view after active orientation adjustment. The system achieved a consistent immobilization success rate of 94.5%, independent of sperm swimming directions.

Another option for immobilization is to use a non-contact laser to ablate the motor proteins in the sperm tail. An infrared laser is commonly used in IVF clinics, such as for assisted embryo hatching and biopsy of preimplantation embryos. Manual immobilization using laser ablation was attempted in the early 2000s but not widely adopted in clinics because of the poor positioning capability in manual operation. It is challenging for embryologists to align the laser spot with the fast-moving sperm tail, and falsely firing laser pulses near the sperm head would induce undesired temperature rise (up to 150°C), which could damage the sperm DNA. Zhang *et al.* developed a robotic system with a visual servo controller with feedforward compensator to position the sperm tail to the laser spot (Figure 13.3 (e)) [8]. The feedforward compensator predicts and compensates for sperm motion and reduces positioning errors from 9.8 μm (without compensator) to 1.7 μm (with compensator). By quantitatively testing different laser energy levels on 900 sperm, the system achieved a consistent 100% immobilization success rate. Further DNA analysis confirmed that the technique did not induce extra damage to sperm DNA, confirming its safety for clinical use.

Sperm Aspiration

To perform sperm aspiration for clinic ICSI, a micropipette is first moved to the target immobilized sperm. By changing the piston position of a hydraulic pump, a small negative pressure is applied to the micropipette tip to aspirate the sperm into the micropipette. Once the sperm enters the micropipette, the operator must quickly apply a positive pressure to stop the sperm movement so that it does not move too far into the micropipette and disappear. To position a sperm to a desired location inside the micropipette, the operator must repeatedly adjust the application of negative and positive pressure. Because of the small volume of a single sperm (picoliter), the operator must be highly skilled manual sperm aspiration to avoid sperm loss and long operation time.

System Dynamics for Sperm Aspiration

To analyze the dynamics of sperm motion inside a micropipette, the aspiration system is modeled as shown in Figure 13.4. As the mass of a sperm is negligible, there is no relative motion between the sperm and the flow surrounding it. Here, only the fluid dynamics inside the micropipette is discussed.

The chamber diameter of the syringe pump used in clinics is at the millimeter scale, and the diameter of the ICSI micropipette is ~5 μm. In fluid mechanics, when a viscous liquid (i.e. sperm medium) flows from a large channel (e.g. a petri dish) into a micropipette tip having a cross-section at the micrometer scale, pressure changes abruptly because of the viscous effect. Corresponding to the pressure change is a strong density change, resulting in oil compression and elastic deformation of the connecting tube [9]. Therefore, when aspirating a sperm using a micropipette, the sperm medium volume change inside the micropipette tip is much smaller than the oil volume change caused by the piston

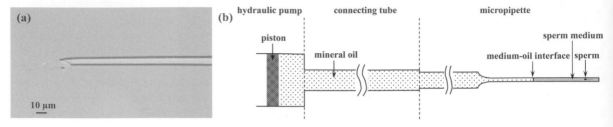

Figure 13.4 (a) Sperm aspiration and (b) schematic of a general sperm aspiration setup. Reproduced from [9].

movement of a hydraulic pump. This effect enables manual aspiration of a sperm with a volume of ~1 pL. To enhance this effect for facilitating aspiration control, the sperm medium is usually mixed with PVP at 1:2 in clinical ICSI to increase the medium viscosity.

When the viscous sperm medium moves inside the micropipette, damping caused by the viscosity of the medium depends on the medium length and speed, which keeps changing during sperm aspiration. This varying damping leads to system nonlinearity and degrades the control performance of sperm aspiration. It is also the main reason for limitation of the accuracy of manual aspiration, increasing the demand for automated aspiration control.

Robotic Control Methods

To improve the success rate and accuracy of sperm aspiration and reduce the time cost, robotic systems have been developed to perform sperm aspiration. In sperm aspiration, nonlinearity is mainly caused by the varying damping when medium carrying the sperm moves inside the micropipette. To address this issue, a control method was developed [10], robust to the variation in system damping. Compared with traditional proportional-derivative (PD) control, it achieved a high success rate of 98% with positioning accuracy of ±0.625 μm and average settling time of 10 seconds. Recently, a model-based adaptive control method was developed [9]. This method can effectively compensate for the sperm position error by estimating the time-varying system damping in real time. With this method, the settling time was reduced to 6 seconds. Other control methods, such as optimal control, have only been demonstrated for aspirating large-sized cells (e.g. embryos), with the aim of aspirating single cells with a minimum volume of excess medium [11].

These robotic techniques could potentially contribute to better outcomes in clinical ICSI. Robotic operation can complete the sperm aspiration process in a shorter time period. In addition, as the volume injected into the oocyte is critical, robotic aspiration is able to accurately position the sperm at the micropipette tip to reduce the medium volume deposited into an oocyte. With robotic techniques, sperm aspiration can be performed with high success rate and high accuracy, within a short time.

Oocyte Orientation Control

Before sperm injection in ICSI, the polar body of an oocyte should be rotated to the 6 or 12 o'clock orientation to prevent damage to the oocyte spindle during cell penetration. Rotation of an oocyte can be performed manually using a holding micropipette to repeatedly release and aspirate the oocyte or using an injection micropipette to push the oocyte; however, as the manual approach is empirical and inconsistent, automated techniques have been developed to achieve cell orientation control.

Polar Body Detection

The first step in oocyte orientation control is to detect the polar body. Automatic polar body detection has been developed using traditional image processing such as image thresholding and edge detection. However, these methods are not effective in accommodating variances in size and shape of polar bodies.

Deep learning has been used for robust polar body detection [12], with the advantage that it can automatically learn visual features from raw images. The deep neural networks are composed of convolutional layers, max pooling layers, and fully connected layers (Figure 13.5). A total of 1000 polar body images were collected to train the deep neural networks. In an input image, the pixel at the center of the polar body is manually labeled as 1 while other pixels are labeled as 0. The training set consists of square patches of the input images labeled with the same class as their central pixels. As the training set contains images of polar bodies with different sizes and shapes, deep learning-based polar body detection has robustness to variances in size and shape.

When an image is input to the trained deep neural networks, a probability map is generated, representing the probability of the polar body's presence in the image. The position with maximum intensity exceeding the pre-set threshold is determined to be the position of the polar body (Figure 13.5). If no position has intensity higher than the pre-set threshold, the polar body is assumed not to be present in the image, and out-of-plane orientation control is required to search for the polar body.

To evaluate deep neural networks' performance on polar body detection, 300 additional images were captured on different polar bodies from those in training set. The deep learning-based polar body detection achieved an accuracy of 97.6%, much higher than the accuracy by traditional image processing (~90%). The required time for detection of a polar body is 0.2 second (Intel i7 processor, Nvidia GTX1080 GPU).

Flow-Based Orientation Control

Oocyte orientation control can be achieved by accurately controlling the fluid flow. The advantage of manipulation using fluid flow is non-contact on the cell, potentially reducing cell damage. In a three-dimensional cell rotation strategy, fluid flow was generated from the holding micropipette and adjusted by a glass syringe mounted on a motorized linear stage [13]. The polar body was tracked by the method of optical flow to provide visual feedback, then a proportional differential controller was designed to regulate flow rate for visual servo control of cell orientation (Figure 13.6 (a–d)). The system achieved an orientation accuracy of 1.9° and an average speed of 22.8 s/cell.

Fluid flow was also generated by vibration: a microchip patterned with micropillars was subjected to vibration, and local whirling flow was induced around the micropillars to achieve oocyte rotation (Figure 13.6 (e, f)) [14]. This method achieved average rotation speed of 64°/s. Another work used the vibration of a magnetically driven oscillation tool to generate local streamlines (Figure 13.6 (g)) [15]. These flows can be tuned by the actuator's vibration to control the oocyte's rotation direction and speed.

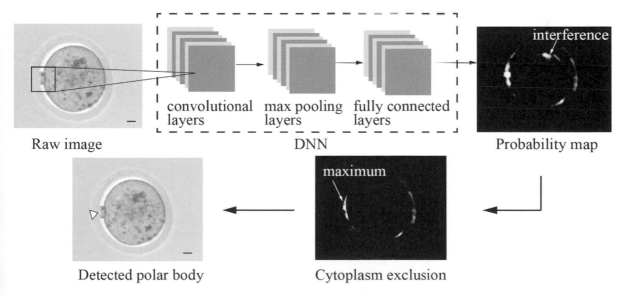

Figure 13.5 The deep neural networks are composed of convolutional, max pooling, and fully connected layers. The output of the networks is a probability map showing the presence possibility of the polar body. By finding the maximum in the probability map, the position of the polar body is determined. Reproduced from [12].

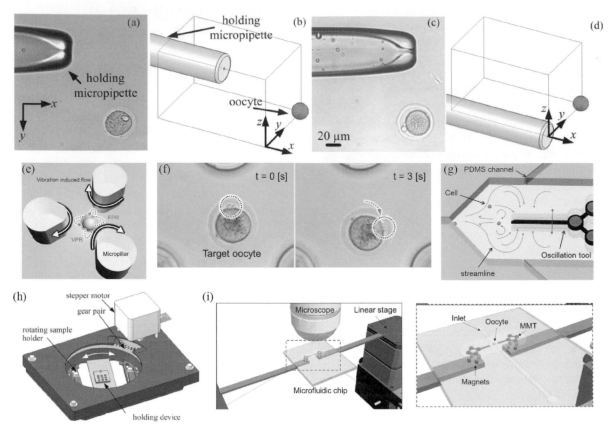

Figure 13.6 Oocyte orientation control using fluid flow and customized devices. (a, b) In-plane and (c, d) out-of-plane orientation control by the flow from the holding micropipette. Reproduced from [13]. (e, f) 3D oocyte rotation by the local whirling flow induced around the micropillars. Reproduced from [14]. (g) Oocyte rotation by local streamline generated by a magnetically driven oscillation tool. Reproduced from [15]. (h) Motorized rotational stage for 2D orientation control. Reproduced from [16]. (i) Magnetically driven microtools controlled to push an oocyte for 3D rotation of oocytes. FPR, focal plane rotation; VPR, vertical plane rotation; PDMS, polydimethylsiloxane; MMT, magnetically driven microtool. Reproduced from [17]. (A black and white version of this figure will appear in some formats. For the color version, please refer to the plate section.)

However, the rotation accuracy was susceptible to flow inertia and the cell position within the fluid flow.

Device-Driven Orientation Control

Several customized devices have also been developed to achieve oocyte orientation control. A motorized rotational stage was built and the motion from a stepper motor was transmitted to the cell holding device by gear pair (Figure 13.6 (h)) [16]. While a cell is not at the rotation center, the rotation of the stage would move the cell out of the microscope's field of view. To compensate for rotation-induced translation, an image-based proportional-integral-derivative (PID) visual servo controller was designed to keep the cell within the microscope field of view during stage rotation. However, the rotational stage cannot perform out-of-plane oocyte orientation control.

Magnetically driven microtools were developed for 3D rotation of oocytes [17]. The microtools were actuated by permanent magnets mounted on linear motion stages (Figure 13.6 (i)). The microtools were controlled to push an oocyte for orientation control based on computer vision tracking of the oocyte, and had an orientation error of 7°. However, these customized devices alter the standard setup in clinics, and inevitably disturb the conventional clinical workflow.

Orientation Control Using Micropipette

Use of micropipettes is common in clinics to rotate an oocyte. A holding micropipette is used to aspirate the oocyte, and an injection micropipette is used to push the oocyte to rotate it. But it is difficult to constrain cell deformation in manual cell rotation, and large deformation may risk damaging the oocyte. Robotic rotation based on the minimal force to rotate an oocyte was developed [18]. However, the force analysis was based on a spherical model, and, as most oocytes are elliptical in shape, this approach caused large cell deformation (11.7 μm). Additionally, it did not take into account cell variances in mechanical parameters such as Young's modulus and friction coefficient between a cell and a micropipette; thus, cell rotation failed when insufficient force was applied to the oocyte.

To accommodate variances in shape and mechanical parameters of oocytes, robotic cell orientation control was developed by including such variances in modelling and path planning [12]. Thus, a cell is effectively rotated while consistently maintaining minimal cell deformation. An elliptical model was used in force analysis to determine the required minimal force to rotate an oocyte. The force was then translated into the micropipette indentation by a contact mechanics model. The manipulation path of the robot was formulated by connecting the indentation position on the oocyte. To compensate for variations in mechanical properties of oocytes, an optimal controller was developed to update micropipette indentation based on a cost function of cell deformation and orientation error. By minimizing the cost function, both cell deformation and orientation error were minimized. The robotic oocyte orientation process by micropipettes is illustrated in Figure 13.7. The system achieved orientation control with an orientation error of 0.7° and maximum oocyte deformation of 2.70 μm, significantly less than those in manual operation. The time cost of rotating an oocyte was 10–15 seconds, comparable to that in manual operation.

Sperm Injection

Automated Injection

In clinical ICSI, a sperm is aspirated into a micropipette and injected into an oocyte. To perform sperm injection, an oocyte is held by a holding micropipette, an injection micropipette first approaches the oocyte then quickly penetrates the zona pellucida and oolemma. To ensure that the oolemma is penetrated, a small negative pressure is applied to the injection micropipette tip to aspirate the cytoplasm and break the oolemma. A small positive pressure is then applied to the tip to deposit the sperm into the oocyte.

The first robotic ICSI system was reported in 2011 [19]. The system was able to detect the position and profile of an oocyte by computer vision and used it as feedback to control the injection position and depth of the ICSI micropipette (Figure 13.8 (a)). This robotic ICSI system performed complete ICSI procedures

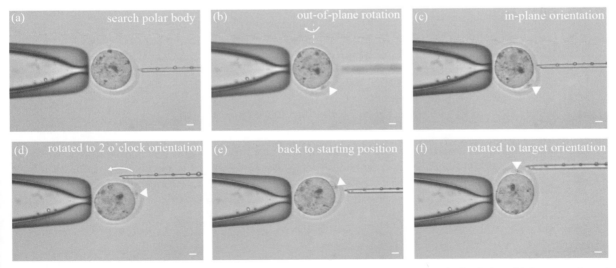

Figure 13.7 Robotic oocyte orientation control by micropipettes. (a) Polar body was not present in the focal plane. (b) System performed out-of-plane orientation control, searched for the polar body, and rotated it into the focal plane. (c–f) In-plane orientation control was followed by the system to rotate the polar body toward the target orientation of 12 o'clock. Reproduced from [12].

using a hamster oocyte–human sperm model with a success rate of 90.0% and a survival rate of 90.7% (n = 120). Using computer vision, it was difficult to identify the penetration of oolemma by the injection micropipette. To address this challenge, micro-electromechanical systems (MEMS) and piezoresistive force sensors can be attached to the micropipette to measure the force change on it during penetration. However, these force sensors can only identify the time instance of oolemma breakage, and cannot reduce the deformation of the oocyte caused by indentation of the injection micropipette.

Less Invasive Oocyte Penetration

Oocytes usually suffer from large deformation during sperm injection. Large deformation can lead to spindle dislocation or damage, and can also increase the internal pressure of the oocyte and contribute to oocyte degeneration [20]. Moreover, negative pressure needs to be applied by the injection micropipette to break the oolemma. However, once the oolemma is broken, a portion of cytoplasm is inevitably aspirated into the micropipette and needs to be deposited back to the oocyte along with the sperm. As the cytoskeleton plays an important role in cell signaling, division, and intra-cellular transport, cytoplasm aspiration can cause cell damage as the oocyte's cytoskeleton is locally disrupted.

To reduce cell damage during injection, piezo drills were developed using piezoelectric actuators to generate micropipette vibration. With the micropipette's vibrating motion, the oocyte can be penetrated with small deformation and without cytoplasm aspiration. Although not yet widely adopted by clinics, piezo drills have been used in human ICSI, and

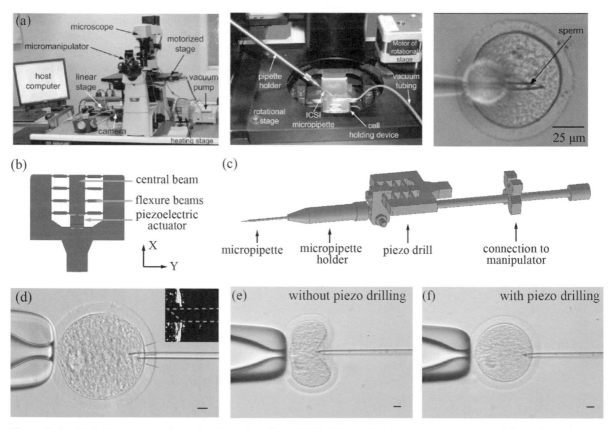

Figure 13.8 (a) Robotic sperm injection system. Reproduced from [19]. (b–f) Piezo drill developed to reduce oocyte deformation and prevent cytoplasm aspiration. (b) Flexure beams as lateral constraints to guide the micropipette motion along the axial direction, without the use of damping fluid such as mercury. (c) Eccentric configuration to be compatible with clinical setup. (d) Automated detection of membrane breakage to minimize the time delay between cell penetration and piezo stoppage. Motion history image of the membrane is shown in the inset. (e, f) Hamster oocyte penetration without and with piezo drilling. Reproduced from [23]. (A black and white version of this figure will appear in some formats. For the color version, please refer to the plate section.)

achieved higher rates of fertilization, blastocyst formation, pregnancy, and live birth than without piezo drilling [20,21].

However, existing piezo drills suffer from detrimental large lateral vibration, which is perpendicular to the penetration direction. To reduce undesired lateral vibration, damping fluid such as mercury and Fluorinert is filled into the micropipette [21], which raises biosafety concerns. A few piezo drills were developed to circumvent the use of damping fluid by placing piezoelectric actuators concentrically behind the micropipette. However, they require a customized micropipette holder, thus altering the standard ICSI setup.

To reduce lateral vibration and prevent the use of damping fluid, flexure beams were used as lateral constraints in a piezo drill (Figure 13.8 (b)) [22]. The flexure beams allow for lower stiffness along the axial direction (3.5 N/μm) than along the lateral direction (>200 N/μm), thus guide the micropipette motion along its axial direction. Moreover, an eccentric design was used by mounting the piezo drill beside the standard micropipette holder [23], which enables compatibility to the standard clinical setup (Figure 13.8 (c)).

To further reduce cell damage, membrane breakage was automatically detected to minimize the time delay between cell penetration and piezo stoppage [23]. Membrane breakage was distinguished by its backward motion because of tension release after penetration. Motion history imaging was used to enhance the membrane motion by accumulating its motion over a period of time (Figure 13.8 (d)). For penetrating hamster oocytes, this piezo drill system achieved cell deformation of 5.68 μm, significantly less than the deformation of 54.29 μm without piezo drilling (Figure 13.8 (e, f)). Automated membrane breakage detection reduced the time delay of vibration stoppage after penetration to 0.51±0.27 second, significantly less than 2.32±0.98 seconds in manual operation.

Summary

Significant technical advances have been made to automate ICSI procedures: quantitative sperm analysis, robotic sperm immobilization and aspiration, oocyte orientation control with minimal deformation, and less invasive sperm injection. This chapter provided an introduction to the developed and emerging techniques for automated ICSI. These techniques hold promise for increasing efficiency and consistency of ICSI, reducing cell damage and improving ICSI outcome.

Further efforts in developing automation techniques are required to achieve higher consistency and lower cell damage. The directions of future development include: (1) to be compatible with standard setup for easy integration into clinics without disturbing clinical workflow; (2) to be minimally invasive to cells (e.g. reducing oocyte deformation and exposure time to ambient environment); and (3) to be clinically validated for safety and efficacy. Existing automation techniques have been mostly tested with animal models and are yet to be tested on human cells in IVF clinics. The readiness of automation techniques for translation to clinical use will be achieved by clinical trials and validation.

References

[1] Amann RP, Waberski D. Computer-assisted sperm analysis (CASA): capabilities and potential developments. *Theriogenology* 2014; 81: 5–17.

[2] Dai C, Zhang Z, Huang J, *et al*. Automated non-invasive measurement of single sperm's motility and morphology. *IEEE Transactions on Medical Imaging* 2018; 37: 2257–2265.

[3] Bartoov B, Berkovitz A, Eltes F, *et al*. Real-time fine morphology of motile human sperm cells is associated with IVF-ICSI outcome. *Journal of Andrology* 2002; 23: 1–8.

[4] Bijar A, Benavent AP, Mikaeili M. Fully automatic identification and discrimination of sperm's parts in microscopic images of stained human semen smear. *Journal of Biomedical Science and Engineering* 2012; 5: 384–395.

[5] Ghasemian F, Mirroshandel SA, Monji-Azad S, Azarnia M, Zahiri Z. An efficient method for automatic morphological abnormality detection from human sperm images. *Computer Methods and Programs in Biomedicine* 2015; 122: 409–420.

[6] Leung C, Lu Z, Esfandiari N, Casper RF, Sun Y. Automated sperm immobilization for intracytoplasmic sperm injection. *IEEE Transactions on Biomedical Engineering* 2010; 58: 935–942.

[7] Zhang Z, Dai C, Huang J, *et al*. Robotic immobilization of motile sperm for clinical intracytoplasmic sperm injection. *IEEE Transactions on Biomedical Engineering* 2018; 66: 444–452.

[8] Zhang Z, Dai C, Wang X, *et al*. Automated laser ablation of motile sperm for immobilization. *IEEE Robotics and Automation Letters* 2019; 4: 323–329.

[9] Shan G, Zhang Z, Dai C, *et al.* Model-based robotic cell aspiration: tackling nonlinear dynamics and varying cell sizes. *IEEE Robotics and Automation Letters* 2019; 5: 173–178.

[10] Zhang XP, Leung C, Lu Z, Esfandiari N, Casper RF and Sun Y. Controlled aspiration and positioning of biological cells in a micropipette. *IEEE Transactions on Biomedical Engineering* 2012; 59: 1032–1040.

[11] Zhang Z, Liu J, Wang X, *et al.* Robotic pick-and-place of multiple embryos for vitrification. *IEEE Robotics and Automation Letters* 2016; 2: 570–576.

[12] Dai C, Zhang Z, Lu Y, *et al.* Robotic manipulation of deformable cells for orientation control. *IEEE Transactions on Robotics* 2020; 36: 271–283

[13] Leung C, Lu Z, Zhang XP, Sun Y. Three-dimensional rotation of mouse embryos. *IEEE Transactions on Biomedical Engineering* 2012; 59: 1049–1056.

[14] Hayakawa T, Sakuma S, Arai F. On-chip 3D rotation of oocyte based on a vibration-induced local whirling flow. *Microsystems and Nanoengineering* 2015; 1:15001.

[15] Hagiwara M, Kawahara T, Arai F. Local streamline generation by mechanical oscillation in a microfluidic chip for noncontact cell manipulations. *Applied Physics Letters* 2012; 101: 074102.

[16] Liu X, Lu Z, Sun Y. Orientation control of biological cells under inverted microscopy. *IEEE/ASME Transactions on Mechatronics* 2010; 16: 918–924.

[17] Feng L, Turan B, Ningga U, Arai F. Three dimensional rotation of bovine oocyte by using magnetically driven on-chip robot. *IEEE/RSJ International Conference on Intelligent Robots and Systems* 2014; 4668–4673.

[18] Zhao Q, Sun M, Cui M, Yu J, Qin Y, Zhao X. Robotic cell rotation based on the minimum rotation force. *IEEE Transactions on Automation Science and Engineering* 2014; 12: 1504–1515.

[19] Lu Z, Zhang X, Leung C, Esfandiari N, Casper RF, Sun Y. Robotic ICSI (intracytoplasmic sperm injection). *IEEE Transactions on Biomedical Engineering* 2011; 58: 2102–2108.

[20] Yanagida K, Katayose H, Yazawa H, Kimura Y, Konnai K, Sato A. The usefulness of a piezo-micromanipulator in intracytoplasmic sperm injection in humans. *Human Reproduction* 1999; 14: 448–453.

[21] Hiraoka K, Kitamura S. Clinical efficiency of Piezo-ICSI using micropipettes with a wall thickness of 0.625 μm. *Journal of Assisted Reproduction and Genetics* 2015; 32: 1827–1833.

[22] Johnson W, Dai C, Liu J, *et al.* A flexure-guided piezo drill for penetrating the zona pellucida of mammalian oocytes. *IEEE Transactions on Biomedical Engineering* 2017; 65: 678–686.

[23] Dai C, Xin L, Zhang Z, *et al.* Design and control of a piezo drill for robotic piezo-driven cell penetration. *IEEE Robotics and Automation Letters* 2020; 5: 339–345.

Germline Nuclear Transfer Technology to Overcome Mitochondrial Diseases and Female Infertility

Mao-Xing Tang, Annekatrien Boel, Paul Couke, and Björn Heindryckx

Introduction

Mitochondria are crucial energy-generating organelles within eukaryotic cells mainly responsible for producing ATP through oxidative phosphorylation (OXPHOS). Mitochondria possess their own genome, mitochondrial (mt)DNA, which exhibits exclusively maternal inheritance. Similar to nuclear (n)DNA mutations, mtDNA mutations can also cause a broad range of mitochondrial disorders, which reportedly affect approximately 1 in 5,000 individuals. To date, no curative treatments exist for patients with mitochondrial diseases. Preventing the transmission of mitochondrial diseases is therefore of utmost importance, particularly for families affected by the most severe mtDNA-associated disorders. Here, we will focus on recently developed methodologies in assisted reproductive technology that are being used to circumvent mother-to-child transmission of mtDNA diseases. Moreover, we will discuss the applicability of these novel technologies to overcome certain female infertility indications.

Mitochondrial DNA and Mitochondrial DNA Diseases

In mammals, mtDNA is a tiny circular molecule, 16.6 kb in humans and 16.2 kb in mice. Unlike nDNA encoding more than 20,000 genes, mtDNA encodes for only 37 genes, including 13 mRNAs, 22 tRNAs and 2 rRNAs, which are mainly required to provide a functional OXPHOS system. Different cell types harbor varying numbers of mtDNA molecules, which is primarily dependent on the cell's demand for ATP production. Specifically, a somatic cell possesses a few hundred to a few thousand mtDNA molecules, while a mature oocyte contains 100,000 to 600,000 mtDNA copies [1]. Pathogenic mutations in the mtDNA can disrupt the OXPHOS system, ultimately leading to mtDNA diseases, with severity ranging from mild to life-threatening. Notably, mtDNA mutations can be present in a homoplasmic form (all mtDNA copies are affected), but mostly manifest in a heteroplasmic form (mixture of wild-type and mutated mtDNA). The severity of mtDNA disease is determined by the level of heteroplasmy (proportion of mutated to wild-type mtDNA, known as the mutation load), with higher levels of mtDNA mutation frequently being associated with more severe clinical symptoms. Generally, the threshold is thought to be 60–80%, but is variable depending on different tissues and the specific mtDNA mutation.

Predicting the risk of transmitting the disease from affected mothers to children is complex because of the so-called mitochondrial genetic bottleneck. This bottleneck involves a dramatic decrease in mtDNA copies during female germline development, with transmitting a small number of mtDNA molecules in primordial germ cells, the precursor cells of the gametes, which leads to a rapid shift in mtDNA heteroplasmy both within and between the generations [2]. This means that women who carry few mutated mtDNA copies can still produce oocytes with a very high mutation load, resulting in severe mitochondrial diseases. This highlights the need for novel approaches to prevent the transmission of mtDNA diseases from the mother to the next-generation.

Germline Nuclear Transfer to Prevent Mitochondrial DNA Diseases

While prenatal diagnosis (PND) or pre-implantation genetic diagnosis (PGD) can be applied to overcome mtDNA diseases by selecting fetuses or embryos with low or no mutation loads, they are not suitable for women harboring a high mutation load or a homoplasmic mtDNA mutation. In such cases, mitochondrial disease transmission may currently be prevented by applying germline nuclear transfer (NT). This is a novel in vitro fertilization (IVF)-based technique, also known as mitochondrial donation or mitochondrial replacement therapy, which involves the transfer of nuclear genome from an oocyte or zygote carrying mtDNA mutations to an enucleated donor oocyte or zygote with wild-type mtDNA. Evaluation of efficiency and safety of this new reproductive technology is paramount. Assessment of the level of mtDNA carry-over (karyoplast-derived mtDNA), as well as the effects on subsequent generations, for example the consequences of a mismatch between nuclear and mtDNA genotypes, is a necessity. Until now, different forms of NT have been investigated for circumventing mtDNA diseases, such as maternal spindle transfer (ST), pronuclear transfer (PNT) and polar body transfer (PBT) (see Figures 14.1 and 14.2).

Currently, the Human Fertilisation and Embryology Authority (HFEA) has granted approval for clinical application of PNT or ST to prevent mtDNA diseases to one IVF clinic in the United Kingdom. Also, a number of other countries (e.g. Greece, Ukraine and Mexico) have applied the NT technology to overcome either mitochondrial diseases or certain female infertility indications.

Spindle Transfer

The ST technique involves removing the metaphase II (MII) spindle-chromosome complex, and transferring it to an enucleated donor MII oocyte, followed by fertilization of the reconstructed oocyte (see Figure 14.1). This technique was pioneered in animal models (including Rhesus monkeys and mice), demonstrating the feasibility, safety and efficacy of the ST protocol, reflected by high blastocyst formation rates, healthy live births and minimal levels of mtDNA carry-over [1,3].

During recent years, the NT technology has been optimized in the human with some breakthrough papers focusing on the efficiency and safety of the technology. The first studies of human ST confirmed promising blastocyst rates of the reconstructed embryos comparable to controls, and low levels of mtDNA carry-over in ST blastocysts as well as within their derived human embryonic stem cell (hESC) lines [4,5]. Similar observations were also made in recent human studies, both revealing consistently undetectable or low levels of karyoplast-derived mtDNA in most hESC lines derived from ST blastocysts [6,7]. However, a limited number of hESC lines showed an increase in karyoplast-derived mtDNA during extended culture. In certain hESC lines, this involved

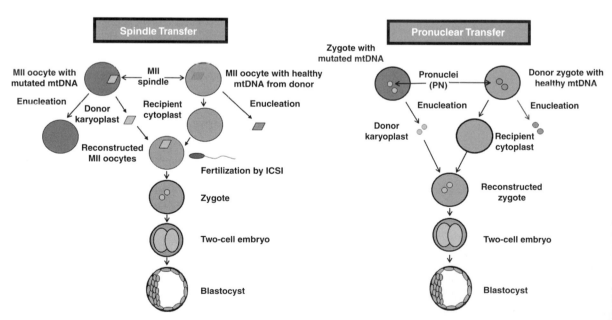

Figure 14.1 Diagrams outlining the procedures of spindle transfer (ST) and pronuclear transfer (PNT). The ST technique involves removing the metaphase II (MII) spindle-chromosome complex, and transferring it to an enucleated donor MII oocyte, followed by fertilization of the reconstructed oocyte. The method of PNT involves the removal of both pronuclei (PN) from a zygote and transferring them into an enucleated recipient zygote. (A black and white version of this figure will appear in some formats. For the color version, please refer to the plate section.)

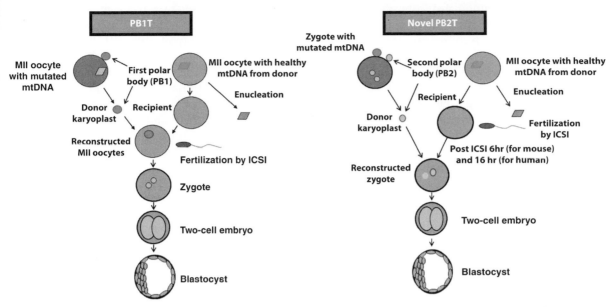

Figure 14.2 Diagrams outlining the procedures of first polar body transfer (PB1 T) and novel second polar body transfer (PB2 T). The PB1 T technique involves removal of PB1 from a MII oocyte, followed by transfer to an enucleated MII oocyte and fertilization of the reconstituted oocyte. The novel PB2 T approach, as described in the study by Tang *et al.* [17], circumvents the problem of distinguishing the female and male pronuclei, whereby the MII oocyte is first enucleated, followed by fertilization via ICSI. This oocyte then serves as the recipient for the transfer of the PB2 genome from a donor zygote. (A black and white version of this figure will appear in some formats. For the color version, please refer to the plate section.)

a transient increase followed by a decrease in the levels of mtDNA carry-over [6], while in others, a complete reversion to the karyoplast-derived mtDNA haplotype (homoplasmy) was reported [7]. Nevertheless, these results should be cautiously interpreted, based on the consideration that the pattern of mtDNA segregation in hESC lines may differ from the situation in vivo and the artificial character of hESC lines. To date, there is only one report on the successful clinical application of ST using human MII oocytes to prevent transmission of mtDNA disease, leading to a live human birth [8]. This study included a 36-year-old woman carrying a pathogenic mtDNA mutation (m.8993 T>G), which is known to cause Leigh syndrome. This patient experienced four miscarriages and two children who died as a result of a high mtDNA mutation load (>95%). The results revealed that after ST, the mtDNA mutation load in the ST blastocyst selected for embryo transfer was 5.73% on average, while the mutation load in several neonatal tissues was 1.60 ± 0.92% on average [8]. This study supports the efficiency of ST to reduce the transmission of pathogenic mtDNA mutations.

Overall, although the levels of mtDNA carry-over in stem cell lines or the neonatal tissue were shown to be low, it remains unclear whether the mutant mtDNA accumulates in various tissues and/or drifts to the karyoplast-derived mtDNA haplotype during development of resultant offspring. Therefore, long-term follow-up of children born after NT is of great importance.

Pronuclear Transfer

The method of PNT involves removal of both pronuclei (PN) from a zygote and transfer to an enucleated recipient zygote (see Figure 14.1). Similar to ST, the PNT protocol was initially developed using animal models, such as different strains of mice containing distinct nuclear and mtDNA genotypes and mito-mice harboring a large mtDNA deletion [9,10]. These animal studies experimentally demonstrated the feasibility of the PNT technique, revealing normal developmental potential of reconstituted zygotes, reducing transmission of mtDNA variants and the birth of healthy offspring [1].

Recent studies have focused on optimization of the PNT technology using human oocytes. A previous proof-of-concept study, performing PNT using human abnormally fertilized (1 PN or 3 PN) zygotes, showed successful reduction of the levels of mtDNA carry-over to <2% on average. Still, a lower blastocyst formation rate was observed after PNT in comparison to unmanipulated controls [11]. This might be attributed to the abnormal nature of the recipients (abnormally fertilized zygotes) used in this study. The PNT procedure was further improved using normally fertilized (2 PN) human zygotes [12]. In the latter study, the PNT protocol was further refined, mainly including a modification in the timing, with PNT being performed shortly after meiosis II completion (around 8 hours post-ICSI, early PNT) rather than before the first mitosis (around 16 hours post-ICSI, late PNT). This adapted methodology was shown to be highly beneficial in terms of blastocyst formation, with a concomitant minimal carry-over in generated blastocysts. Importantly, early PNT blastocysts did not show significant differences in aneuploidy rates and global gene expression, in comparison to unmanipulated controls. Notably, it was also observed that in one out of five hESC lines derived from early PNT blastocysts, the level of karyoplast-derived mtDNA was progressively elevated during culture despite an initial minimal carry-over during pre-implantation development [12]. Using human in vitro matured (IVM) oocytes, Wu *et al.* further shortened the timing of PNT by transferring female pre-pronuclei (PPN) at 3.5–4 hours after fertilization (via ICSI) [13]. This refined protocol, termed PPN transfer (PPNT), also resulted in high blastocyst rates similar to unmanipulated ICSI controls and a low degree of mtDNA carry-over in PPNT blastocysts. Importantly, in all hESC lines derived from PPNT blastocysts, the mtDNA carry-over did not increase through their long-term proliferation and differentiation. Taken together, PNT has the potential to greatly reduce the risk of transmission of mtDNA diseases.

Polar Body Transfer

Unlike meiotic spindle and zygotic PN, the first and second polar bodies (PB1 and PB2) are small structures extruded from oocytes and zygotes during the first and second asymmetric meiotic divisions, respectively, which are known to harbor low amounts of mitochondria and contain the same chromosome number and developmental capacity as their counterparts (meiotic spindle and female PN, respectively). PB1 transfer (PB1 T) involves removal of PB1 from a MII oocyte, followed by transfer to an enucleated MII oocyte and fertilization of the reconstituted oocyte (see Figure 14.2). Conventional PB2 transfer (PB2 T) involves the removal of PB2 from a zygote

followed by transfer to a recipient zygote with the female PN removed. Previous mouse studies have confirmed the ability of both PB1 T and PB2 T to produce developmentally competent embryos and generate live offspring [1]. Interestingly, both PB1 T and conventional PB2 T resulted in undetectable or very low levels (<2%) of mtDNA carry-over when compared to ST (~6%) and PNT (~24%) [14].

Having demonstrated the feasibility of PBT in animal models, this technology has also been proposed to prevent the transmission of human mtDNA mutations. Using donated human in vivo matured MII oocytes, Ma *et al.* (2017) revealed that reconstructed oocytes following PB1 T were capable of normal fertilization (by ICSI) at a comparable rate to unmanipulated controls, but their blastocyst formation capability and the efficiency of hESC derivation from PB1 T blastocysts was reduced. No significant difference regarding aneuploidy rates (in PB1 T blastocysts) and gene expression (in hESCs derived from PB1 T blastocysts) was observed when compared to controls [15]. To improve the efficiency of PB1 T, the protocol was further optimized using human IVM oocytes in another study [16]. The optimized protocol involves transfer of PB1 to an intact recipient MII oocyte, followed by removal of PPN and PB2 of the recipient oocyte at 3.5–4 hours after ICSI. This study revealed that optimized PB1 T could efficiently support onward development of reconstructed oocytes and the generation of hESCs. Importantly, the PB1 T blastocysts and their derived hESCs exhibited a low degree of mtDNA carry-over (<0.5% on average) [16].

The conventional PB2 T remains more challenging because it involves identification and removal of the female PN. Particularly in the human zygote, it is very difficult to distinguish the male from the female PN. To avoid this obstacle, a recent study reported that using human IVM oocytes, the PB2 T procedure was refined by transfer of PB2 from a donor zygote (6–7 hours post-ICSI) to a recipient zygote with female PPN and PB2 removed (3.5–4 hours post-ICSI) [16]. This refined procedure led to a blastocyst rate comparable to ICSI controls and a minimal level of mtDNA carry-over in both PB2 T blastocysts and their derived hESCs. More recently, Tang *et al.* successfully developed a novel method of PB2 T and verified its feasibility in both human IVM and *in vivo* matured oocytes [17]. This novel optimized PB2 T approach circumvents the problem of distinguishing the female and male pronuclei, whereby the MII oocyte is first enucleated, followed by fertilization via ICSI (see Figure 14.2). This oocyte then serves as the recipient for the transfer of the PB2 genome from a donor zygote. Consequently, both PB1 T and PB2 T may be a promising approach to overcome mtDNA diseases.

Safety Concerns Regarding Clinical Use of NT

An essential safety concern with NT arises from the currently reported phenomenon of heteroplasmic mtDNA drift/reversion [7]. As mentioned above, when ESC lines were derived from ST or PNT blastocysts in heteroplasmic mouse models or in human, it was observed that in a minority of these lines, mtDNA carry-over increases with passaging, even reaching 100% (homoplasmy) [2,12]. The reasons underlying this phenomenon are still poorly understood. It must be cautiously interpreted on the basis of the possibility that this phenomenon is only a trait of pluripotent stem cell biology. Moreover, because of the temporary existence of the pluripotency during in vivo embryo development, the relevance of ESCs as a post-implantation model remains obscure [1]. Nevertheless, long-term monitoring of children born following NT is paramount.

In addition, there is another major safety issue in relation to mtDNA-nDNA incompatibility after NT, leading to the recommendation of nuclear-mitochondrial match between the patient and oocyte donors in clinical applications of NT [18]. However, the evidence on the harmful effects of mtDNA-nDNA incompatibility after NT in humans is still controversial [19,20]. Specifically, the meta-analysis study of Dobler et al. was mostly based on the published data from invertebrate and vertebrate animal models. In this study, using statistical models, biomedical evidence from vertebrate studies showed that NT was safe for clinical use, whereas biological evidence from invertebrate studies revealed that NT might modify the organismal phenotypes after long-term breeding and crossing different nuclear and mtDNA backgrounds [20]. Another study reported that approximately 45% of human individuals carry heteroplasmic mtDNA variants, and their transmission is affected by the mother's nuclear genetic background. This leads to a hypothesis regarding potential haplotype mismatching related to NT in humans [18]. Rishishwar et al. further performed

analysis using human population genome data with divergent genetic distance, revealing that mitochondrial and nuclear genomes from divergent human populations can co-exist within healthy individuals, indicating that mismatched nDNA-mtDNA combinations are not deleterious in humans [21].

Germline NT and Other Methodologies for Overcoming Female Infertility

In the IVF clinic, reproductive aged women, particularly those aged over 35 years, often constitute a challenging population of infertility patients. This is mainly because ovarian ageing, resulting in decline in both quality and quantity of the oocytes. The poor oocyte quality in ageing women has been shown to be associated with cytoplasmic deficiencies and mitochondrial dysfunction, which have a negative impact on the ATP supply to support the oocyte maturation and subsequent embryo development. Accordingly, besides the use for avoiding mtDNA diseases, NT has currently been proposed as a novel reproductive approach to overcome certain forms of infertility disorders. The rationale of the NT treatment is that replacing a low-quality cytoplasm with a competent one by means of NT may enhance the oocyte competence, with the expectation of improving embryonic development. Nevertheless, this experimental treatment continues to be debated because of the lack of validation studies, also in animals. Zhang et al. reported on a 30-year-old woman, experiencing two IVF cycle failures because of embryo arrest at two-cell stage, who successfully became pregnant after PNT treatment, but without any live birth [22]. In some other countries (Ukraine and Greece), successful pregnancies were established by NT for some female-related indications, but these outcomes have not yet been published in peer-reviewed journals. Additionally, using a mouse model of reproductive ageing and embryonic developmental arrest, an ongoing study by our group reveals that both PNT and ST in mice may rescue poor embryo development associated with advanced maternal age and early embryo arrest (unpublished data).

Other methodologies have also been explored to improve oocyte competence. Previously, cytoplasm transfer (CT) was used for oocyte rejuvenation, to improve IVF outcomes. This method involves injecting a limited portion of cytoplasm (around 5%) from a competent oocyte to an incompetent one.

Nevertheless, the benefit and safety of this approach remains unclear because of certain abnormalities observed in the resultant children. Alternatively, the methodology of mitochondrial supplementation was claimed to enhance oocyte competence, termed "Autologous Germline Mitochondrial Energy Transfer" (AUGMENT). Unlike CT, this technique involves isolation of autologous mitochondria, followed by injection into the patient's oocytes along with ICSI. The autologous mitochondria can be obtained from oogonial stem cells or oocyte precursor cells present in a patient's ovaries. Nonetheless, it is difficult to confirm the efficacy of this technique because of the limited number of patients treated and the controversy regarding the existence of oogonial stem cells. A recent study indicated that AUGMENT therapy did not improve embryo quality in infertile women with a problem of multiple IVF failures [23]. Therefore, future studies aiming at the development of NT technology for treating infertile women are still required.

Conclusions and Perspectives

Animal and human studies support the efficient use of NT technology to prevent mitochondrial diseases. Although NT is capable of greatly reducing the transmission of mtDNA mutations, it cannot guarantee complete absence of mutated mtDNA copies following treatment. Nevertheless, the carry-over is within the safety margin used for PGD, as <18% carry-over should not lead to any clinical symptoms. Currently, eliminating karyotype-derived heteroplasmic mtDNA may be possible using genome editing technologies, such as CRISPR/Cas9, mitochondrially targeted zinc finger nucleases (mtZFNs) or mitochondrially targeted transcription activator-like effector nucleases (mitoTALENs), or by mitophagy induction.

Further improvements in the NT methodologies and further insight into the molecular mechanisms of heteroplasmic mtDNA reversion and mtDNA-nDNA incompatibility after NT are also imperative. Finally, it is essential to note that scientific evidence to support the use of NT and other IVF-based techniques for infertility indications is still pending.

References

[1] Craven L, Tang MX, Gorman GS, De Sutter P, Heindryckx B. Novel reproductive technologies to prevent mitochondrial disease. *Hum Reprod Update* 2017; **23**(5): 501–19.

[2] Neupane J, Ghimire S, Vandewoestyne M, et al. Cellular heterogeneity in the level of mtDNA heteroplasmy in mouse embryonic stem cells. *Cell Rep* 2015; **13**(7): 1304–9.

[3] Tachibana M, Sparman M, Sritanaudomchai H, et al. Mitochondrial gene replacement in primate offspring and embryonic stem cells. *Nature* 2009; **461**(7262): 367–72.

[4] Tachibana M, Amato P, Sparman M, et al. Towards germline gene therapy of inherited mitochondrial diseases. *Nature* 2013; **493**(7434): 627–31.

[5] Paull D, Emmanuele V, Weiss KA, et al. Nuclear genome transfer in human oocytes eliminates mitochondrial DNA variants. *Nature* 2013; **493**(7434): 632–7.

[6] Yamada M, Emmanuele V, Sanchez-Quintero MJ, et al. Genetic drift can compromise mitochondrial replacement by nuclear transfer in human oocytes. *Cell Stem Cell* 2016; **18**(6): 749–54.

[7] Kang E, Wu J, Gutierrez NM, et al. Mitochondrial replacement in human oocytes carrying pathogenic mitochondrial DNA mutations. *Nature* 2016; **540**(7632): 270–5.

[8] Zhang J, Liu H, Luo S, et al. Live birth derived from oocyte spindle transfer to prevent mitochondrial disease. *Reprod Biomed Online* 2017; **34**(4): 361–8.

[9] Sato A, Kono T, Nakada K, et al. Gene therapy for progeny of mito-mice carrying pathogenic mtDNA by nuclear transplantation. *Proc Natl Acad Sci USA* 2005; **102**(46): 16765–70.

[10] Neupane J, Vandewoestyne M, Ghimire S, et al. Assessment of nuclear transfer techniques to prevent the transmission of heritable mitochondrial disorders without compromising embryonic development competence in mice. *Mitochondrion* 2014; **18**: 27–33.

[11] Craven L, Tuppen HA, Greggains GD, et al. Pronuclear transfer in human embryos to prevent transmission of mitochondrial DNA disease. *Nature* 2010; **465**(7294): 82–9.

[12] Hyslop LA, Blakeley P, Craven L, et al. Towards clinical application of pronuclear transfer to prevent mitochondrial DNA disease. *Nature* 2016; **534**(7607): 383–6.

[13] Wu K, Chen T, Huang S, et al. Mitochondrial replacement by pre-pronuclear transfer in human embryos. *Cell Res* 2017; **27**(6): 834–7.

[14] Wang T, Sha H, Ji D, et al. Polar body genome transfer for preventing the transmission of inherited mitochondrial diseases. *Cell* 2014; **157**(7): 1591–604.

[15] Ma H, O'Neil RC, Marti Gutierrez N, et al. Functional human oocytes generated by transfer of polar body genomes. *Cell Stem Cell* 2017; **20**(1): 112–9.

[16]   Wu K, Zhong C, Chen T, et al. Polar bodies are efficient donors for reconstruction of human embryos for potential mitochondrial replacement therapy. *Cell Res* 2017; **27**(8): 1069–72.

[17]   Tang M, Guggilla RR, Gansemans Y, et al. Comparative analysis of different nuclear transfer techniques to prevent the transmission of mitochondrial DNA variants. *Mol Hum Reprod* 2019; **25**(12): 797–810.

[18]   Wei W, Tuna S, Keogh MJ, et al. Germline selection shapes human mitochondrial DNA diversity. *Science* 2019; **364**(6442).

[19]   Eyre-Walker A. Mitochondrial replacement therapy: are mito-nuclear interactions likely to be a problem? *Genetics* 2017; **205**(4): 1365–72.

[20]   Dobler R, Dowling DK, Morrow EH, Reinhardt K. A systematic review and meta-analysis reveals pervasive effects of germline mitochondrial replacement on components of health. *Hum Reprod Update* 2018; **24**(5): 519–34.

[21]   Rishishwar L, Jordan IK. Implications of human evolution and admixture for mitochondrial replacement therapy. *BMC Genomics* 2017; **18**(1): 140.

[22]   Zhang J, Zhuang GL, Zeng Y, et al. Pregnancy derived from human zygote pronuclear transfer in a patient who had arrested embryos after IVF. *Reprod Biomed Online* 2016; **33**(4): 529–33.

[23]   Labarta E, de Los Santos MJ, Herraiz S, et al. Autologous mitochondrial transfer as a complementary technique to intracytoplasmic sperm injection to improve embryo quality in patients undergoing in vitro fertilization-a randomized pilot study. *Fertil Steril* 2019; **111**(1): 86–96.

147

Nuclear Transfer Technology and Its Use in Reproductive Medicine

Pasqualino Loi, Marta Czernik, Luca Palazzese, Pier Augusto Scapolo, Helena Fulka, and Josef Fulka Jr

Nuclear Transfer: A Unique Tool to Explore a Fundamental Biological Question

Nuclear transfer was devised as the "fantastic experiment" by Spemann, to explore the mechanism leading to cell differentiation during embryonic development. The assay devised the transfer of a diploid nucleus into a chromosome-depleted oocyte, to demonstrate that cell differentiation does not arise as a result of "gene" loss. Because of a lack of suitable equipment for gamete micromanipulation, the "fantastic experiment" remained in limbo for half a century, until British scientists were able to implement it to production of viable offspring [1]. The experiments established the principle of "nuclear equivalence" in differentiated cells, that is, each cell owns a complete genome, but transcribes a small fraction of it, according to its role in the body. Following these remarkable achievements in an amphibian model, developmental biologists started to repeat the experiment in mammalian species, with their efforts culminating in successful pronuclear transfer between mouse zygotes [2,3].

These studies demonstrated the complementary role played by the two parental genomes during development, establishing the fundamental principle of "genomic imprinting" [3]. Thus, nuclear transfer not only demonstrated the "totipotency of the genome of a somatic cell", but also helped to discover genomic imprinting, a new regulatory mechanism for gene expression involved in development, alteration of which can result in anything from a wide spectrum of pathologies, from mental diseases to cancer.

This progress in basic research was promptly adopted by reproductive biologists dealing with farm animal embryos. Their priority in the late 1980s was multiplication of selected genotypes, through manipulation of the reproductive performances in farm animals. The proof of principle of embryo multiplication through nuclear transplantation of embryonic cells was produced by Steen Willadsen [4]. Successful multiplication of sheep embryos through nuclear transplantation triggered a plethora of studies aiming at optimization of nuclear transfer procedures. The easy "reprogrammability" of the early embryonic cells, coupled with the cell cycle synchronization trick between donor nuclei and recipient cytoplasts (enucleated oocytes), and effective activation procedures rapidly optimized the efficiency of embryonic cell nuclear transfer [5,6]. From the use of embryonic derived cell lines [7] as nuclei donors to cells taken from an adult animal the next step was very close, and in 1997 scientists announced to the world the production of Dolly the sheep [8]. The long-sought goal was reached: the potential multiplication of "elite" animals was now possible. Paradoxically, the success acted like a boomerang for developmental biologists because the ethical implications arising from potential use for human reproduction caused a negative perception of cloning.

First Attempts to Produce "Artificial Gametes" Using Nuclear Transfer Of Somatic Cells

Shortly after the production of Dolly, experts in human assisted reproduction started to explore the possibility of producing "artificial gametes", by haploidizing somatic cells transferred into oocytes.

The production of artificial gametes, was, and still is, the ultimate challenge for human assisted reproduction. The research is advancing rapidly in the mouse aided by the large availability of EC cells lines expressing fluorescent-tagged primordial germ cell (PGCs) genes in these species (Chapter 16 provides an authoritative and updated view on the topics). However, the direct haploidization of somatic cells using the oocyte's meiotic machinery as an alternative approach to produce artificial gametes, still stands, and here we explain why.

Few studies have been published on the topic, prevalently in model organisms but also in humans, primarily with mature (metaphase II, MII), but sometimes even immature (germinal vesicle, GV) oocytes as recipients. MII oocytes were frequently used for haploidization of somatic cells with negative outcomes [9], but the few reports in which GV oocytes were used did not provide any better data. Embryonic cells failed to undergo chromosome condensation when fused with intact or enucleated immature oocytes, whose maturation was prevented by dibutyryl cyclic AMP (dbcAMP). Following release from the meiotic block, first polar bodies were extruded, but the metaphase plates were abnormal. The picture was even worse when somatic cell nuclei were fused into the above cytoplasts, with polar bodies rarely extruded, and those that managed to do so invariably contained abortive metaphase plates [10]. Thus, the overall outcome of the earlier studies ruled out the possibility of correctly haploidizing somatic cells following their transfer into GV or MII oocytes [11,12].

Our retrospective analysis of the published data identifies two major problems:

- incorrect chromosome segregation
- inadequate nuclear reprogramming.

Incorrect chromosome segregation. The first limit was acknowledged by the authors of the published papers, and to our understanding was not a surprise. MII oocytes were predominantly used as recipients for somatic cell nuclei [9,11,12]. Metaphase to telophase transition occurs rapidly following artificial activation of MII oocytes, therefore, it is plausible that correct recognition of centromere DNA by spindle components cannot take place during this short time frame.

The same problem might have occurred when immature, nucleated or enucleated GV oocytes were used. The major problem in this case could be found instead in the absence of nuclear remodeling in these oocyte/cell combinations. The lack of nuclear remodeling could have prevented correct chromosome pairing and/or centromere recognition by the microtubule in the oocyte's cytoplasm. The behavior of somatic nuclei injected into GV oocytes has been thoroughly described in the mouse [10]. The overall picture is that, generally, somatic nuclei injected into intact or enucleated GV oocytes did not even enter meiosis, and when they did, aberrant chromosome segregation took place [10].

Inadequate nuclear reprogramming. This point was not considered by the previous reports. Haploidization of a somatic cell is not the only requirement to make artificial gametes: the haploid set of chromosomes must be ready to become totipotent, just like the fertilizing spermatozoa. This means that the DNA must be provided to the oocyte in a format easily "readable" by the oocyte reprogramming machinery, and ready to contribute to a normal individual.

We are convinced that the generation of "artificial gametes" of both sexes might be conveniently obtained through the nuclear transfer of a somatic cell into an oocyte. The advantages of the "direct" production of gametes using nuclear transfers, versus the "canonical" way, described in Chapter 16, are summarized in Table 15.1.

Table 15.1 ES/IPCs PGCLCs versus direct production of gametes: pro and cons

ES/IPCs PGCLCs derived gametes	Gametes through somatic cell haploidization by nuclear transfer
Requires advanced laboratory skills (molecular/cell biology/embryology), out of reach for a standard IVF technical profile	Within reach of personnel skilled in micromanipulation, slightly more complex than executing ICSI
Weeks (mouse), perhaps months (human) of differentiation/culture in vitro required	48–72 hours
Likely occurrence of epigenetic abnormalities consequent of the multistep differentiation process/long-term culture	Time in culture minimal, similar to routine gamete and embryo culture Possibility of epigenetic abnormalities following nuclear transfer
Need for genetic manipulation (transgene integration)	None
Possible genetic mutation in source cells (IPCs)	Possible mutation in source cells (somatic)
High costs	Minimal additional cost: above standard IVF with ICSI

Recent knowledge gains in the somatic cell's nuclear behavior into GV oocytes along with progress achieved on "in vitro" nuclear reprogramming in differentiated nuclei, have rendered realistic the direct production of gametes through haploidization of somatic cells.

The induction of nuclear totipotency of the somatic cells, prior to, and preferably even after, nuclear transfer is of fundamental importance. In a series of experiments aiming at improving nuclear reprogramming (NR) in somatic cells to be used in somatic cell nuclear transfer (SCNT), we demonstrated that somatic nuclei could be remodeled into sperm-like structures by transient expression of protamine 1 [13]. Moreover, we also demonstrated that the nuclear protaminization was reversed on nuclear transfer, and that the frequency of development was higher in embryos produced by SCNT of protaminized cells [14]. Surprisingly, the nuclear remodeling was related to the sequence of the Prm1: human Prm1 compacted nuclei is a straight shape, just like human spermatozoa, whereas mouse Prm1 compacted nuclei has a hooked shape, like mouse spermatozoa [14]. In other words, protaminization of somatic cells produced diploid nuclei, with a gross morphology very similar to spermatids (Figure 15.1). The developmental potential to the blastocyst stage of oocytes receiving protaminized nuclei was twice that of control cells, meaning that protaminization also enhanced nuclear totipotency.

Therefore, it is plausible that "pre-treatment" of the somatic cells prior to nuclear transfer with the purpose of making artificial gametes could be used to enhance nuclear totipotency through heterologous expression of protamine 1.

Besides in vitro nuclear reprogramming treatments, the choice of the "haplodizing" recipient oocyte remains a challenge. The published data discussed above have demonstrated that both MII and GV stage oocytes are unsuitable for correct chromosome segregation. The additional complicating factor is that the nuclear reprogramming capacity – of fundamental importance as anticipated above – is very limited and unpredictable in MII oocytes, and totally absent in GV oocytes. The reprogramming activity is, in fact, concentrated in the GV, therefore, enucleated, or intact GV oocytes are devoid of nuclear reprogramming capacity [15]. We may thus assume that the reprogramming factors are released from the GV concomitantly with its breakdown and resumption of meiosis. Therefore, a suitable recipient oocyte might be a "selectively enucleated" GV oocyte.

Selective Enucleation

The selective enucleation (SE) approach was developed by Modliński [16], who used it for production of mouse haploid embryos. Using a very narrow pipette (tip ~1 μm), Modliński removed the nuclear envelope of one zygotic pronucleus (PN). The nucleolar precursor bodies (NPBs), probably together with other soluble PN components, were expelled into the zygote cytoplasm. The NPBs rapidly disappeared in the cytoplasm. No new PN formation has been reported. Follow-up studies have demonstrated that chromatin is firmly attached to the nuclear envelope and thus it is removed along with it. In 2006, the same study group reported a significant improvement of the nuclear transfer outcomes when eight-cell stage embryo

DNA/hPrm1-RFP

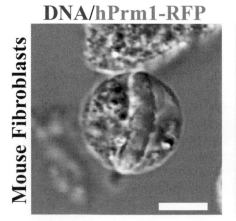

DNA/mPrm1-GFP

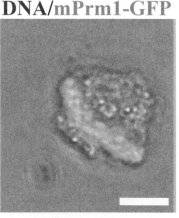

Mouse Fibroblasts

Figure 15.1 Nuclear remodeling of somatic cell nuclei expressing mouse and human Protamine 1 (Prm1). (A black and white version of this figure will appear in some formats. For the color version, please refer to the plate section.)

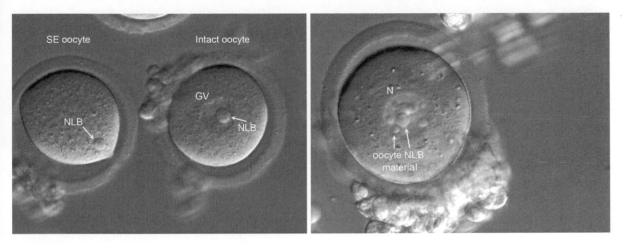

Figure 15.2 Meiotic resumption of SE GV oocyte receiving a somatic cell nucleus, following release from dbcAMP.

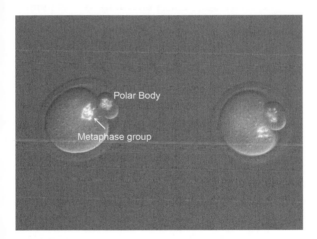

Figure 15.3 Left oocyte: selective enucleated oocyte versus control GV one. Right: nuclear remodeling of somatic cell nucleus following its transfer into SE GV (18 hours), meiotically blocked with dbcAMP.

nuclei were transferred into zygotes from which both pronuclei were removed by SE. No detailed characteristics of transferred blastomere nuclei in a new environment were reported; however, if completely enucleated (whole PNs removed) zygotes were used for NT, no blastocysts were obtained. On the other hand, when SE zygote cytoplasts were used, about 50% of reconstructed embryos reached the blastocyst stage and 7.8% of offspring was obtained. The authors postulated that PNs contain certain reprogramming factors that improve the process of reprogramming of the transferred nuclei [17]. These experiments were further expanded by the same group [18] showing that even 16-cell blastomere nuclei can support full-term development. At the same time, very limited development has been reported when fetal fibroblasts and embryonic stem cell nuclei were used.

Therefore, the published data suggest that SE GV oocytes might be valuable alternative recipient cytoplasts for nuclear transfer experiments aiming at generation of artificial haploid gametes. Thus, we were prompted to study the effects of SE cytoplasm on transferred somatic cell nuclei (cumulus cells, G0/G1) in more detail. Both structural and epigenetic parameters were analyzed in transformed somatic nuclei. The experimental setup included transfer of somatic nuclei to intact, completely enucleated immature cytoplasts and SE cytoplasts. The manipulated oocytes were then cultured overnight (18–20 hours) in the presence of dbcAMP to prevent disassembly of the transferred nuclei. Unlike the other types of recipient cytoplasts, only the SE cytoplasts were able to markedly remodel the transferred somatic nuclei and, in the best cases, the somatic nuclei were grossly indistinguishable when compared to normal GVs (Figure 15.2). Nucleoli from GVs were readily incorporated into transformed nuclei and the nuclear envelopes exhibited normal parameters. This remodeling was also accompanied by efficient transcriptional silencing and histone H3.3 deposition into the somatic chromatin. None of these effects was observed in the other types of cytoplasts or when the factors were sequestered in the intact GV [19,20]. This shows that the soluble GV content is critical for reprogramming. At the same time, the somatic histones H3.1 and H3.2 were not completely released from the somatic chromatin.

When the meiotic block was removed, the reconstructed oocytes began to mature and after about 5–6 hours they extruded the first polar bodies in high proportion (about 85%) (Figure 15.3). Encouragingly, the metaphase plates contained chromosomes with single chromatids and this indicates that DNA replication in transformed nuclei was prevented (Fulka, unpublished).

Thus, from these experiments we may conclude that the soluble GV content is the critical GV subfraction able to elicit favorable epigenetic changes in the transformed somatic nuclei. At the same time, the same fraction is responsible for the marked remodeling of the pseudo PNs, shaping them as control, unmanipulated GVs.

Future Directions and Conclusions

The data currently available on in vitro protaminization indicate that this results in better nuclear reprogramming, compared to untreated somatic cell nuclei. In our view, this is of primary importance for generation of "totipotent" haploid gametes by nuclear transfer. Also promising are the nuclear remodeling and epigenetic modification occurring in somatic nuclei (GO/G1) transplanted into SE GV oocytes. The two approaches, jointly applied, offer unprecedented opportunities to haploidize somatic nuclei in SE GV oocytes.

Un-replicating, protaminized G0 somatic cells undergo a first round of nuclear reprogramming, biologically validated through the increased developmental frequencies of oocytes reconstructed with protaminized nuclei. A second – perhaps more radical – reprogramming phase should take place, on the basis of our findings, following their transfer and prolonged permanency (20 hours) in the cytoplasm of SE GV oocytes. The morphological remodeling acquired by the somatic nuclei at the end of the reprogramming phase is truly remarkable. The extensive genomic remodeling/reprogramming should, in our view, allow for better centromere clustering during meiotic prophase, facilitating homologous chromosome pairing. Furthermore, such correct attachments between sister chromosomes and microtubules through the kinetochores should result in faithful chromosome segregation. While such speculation requires further investigation, we found telling the segregation of chromosomes in the meiotic divisions observed following release from the meiotic block. The metaphase plates appeared to contain single chromatids, thus indicating that DNA replication in remodeled/reprogrammed nuclei was prevented (Fulka, unpublished).

Certainly, further experiments are required before definitive conclusions can be drawn from the data reported here. Crucial information is required on the composition of the chromosome sets extruded/retained after first meiosis: does chromosome segregation occur properly in SE GV oocytes receiving protaminized cells?

What is the extent of nuclear reprogramming following the two rounds of remodeling induced onto the somatic cell nuclei, the first with protaminization, the second by GV remodeling factors released in the cytoplasm?

Finally, is the epigenetic asset correctly preserved following such extensive nuclear reorganization?

These questions are of overwhelming importance before pronouncing the final word on the possibility of deriving "artificial gametes" by haploidization of somatic nuclei, and their applications to treat human infertility. The answers will be provided by further investigation in vitro, but uppermost, from production of normal offspring following reconstruction of MII oocytes with haploidized somatic nuclei. It is of relevance to underline that the normalcy of the offspring should be thoroughly monitored, including adult life and senescence. Such a follow-up is compulsory, in our view, to exclude subtle epigenetic alterations with overt phenotypes later in life, leading to metabolic or psychological diseases.

Acknowledgements

This project received funding from the European Union's Horizon 2020 Research and Innovation Programme under the Marie Skłodowska-Curie grant agreements No. 734434. MC, LP, PAS and PL were supported by the project "DEMETRA" (MIUR) Department of Excellence 2018 – 2022. JF Jr. is supported from GACR 17-08605S and HF from GACR 20-04465S.

References

[1] Gurdon, J.B. (1962) The developmental capacity of nuclei taken from intestinal epithelium cells of feeding tadpoles. *J Embryol Exp Morphol.* **10**, 622–40.

[2] McGrath, J., Solter. D. (1983) Nuclear transplantation in the mouse embryo by microsurgery and cell fusion. *Science.* **220**, 1300–2.

[3] Surani, M.A., Barton, S.C., Norris, M.L. (1984) Development of reconstituted mouse eggs suggests imprinting of the genome during gametogenesis. *Nature.* **308**, 548–50.

[4] Willadsen, S.M. (1986) Nuclear transplantation in sheep embryos. *Nature*. **320**, 63–5.

[5] Campbell, K.H., Loi, P., Otaegui, P.J., Wilmut, I. (1996) Cell cycle co-ordination in embryo cloning by nuclear transfer. *Rev Reprod*. **1**, 40–6

[6] Loi, P., Ledda, S., Fulka, J. Jr., Cappai, P., Moor, R.M. (1998) Development of parthenogenetic and cloned ovine embryos: effect of activation protocols. *Biol Reprod*. **58**, 1177–87.

[7] Campbell, K.H.S., McWhir, J., Ritchie, W.A., Wilmut, I. (1996) Sheep cloned by nuclear transfer from a cultured cell line. *Nature*. **380**, 64–6.

[8] Wilmut, I., Schnieke, A.E., McWhir, J., Kind, A.J., Campbell, K.H.S. (1997) Viable offspring derived from fetal and adult mammalian cells. *Nature*. **385**, 810–13.

[9] Palermo, G.D., Takeuchi, T., Rosenwaks, Z. (2002) Oocyte-induced haploidization. *Reprod Biomed Online*. 4, 237–42.

[10] Fulka, J. Jr., Martinez, F., Tepla, O., Mrazek, M., Tesarik, J. (2002) Somatic and embryonic cell nucleus transfer into intact and enucleated immature mouse oocytes. *Hum Reprod*. **17**, 2160–4.

[11] Galat, V., Ozen, S., Rechitsky, S., Kuliev, A., Verlinsky, Y. (2005) Cytogenetic analysis of human somatic cell haploidization. *Reprod Biomed Online*. **10**, 199–204.

[12] Tateno, H., Akutsu, H., Kamiguchi, Y., Latham, K.E., Yanagimachi, R. (2003) Inability of mature oocytes to create functional haploid genomes from somatic cell nuclei. *Fertil Steril*. **79**, 216–18.

[13] Iuso, D., Czernik, M., Toschi, P., Fidanza, A., Zacchini, F., Feil, R., Curtet, S., Buchou, T., Shiota, H., Khochbin, S., Ptak, G.E., Loi, P. (2015) Exogenous expression of human protamine 1 (hPrm1) remodels fibroblast nuclei into spermatid-like structures. *Cell Rep*. **13**, 1765–71.

[14] Czernik, M., Iuso, D., Toschi, P., Khochbin, S., Loi, P. (2016) Remodeling somatic nuclei via exogenous expression of protamine 1 to create spermatid-like structures for somatic nuclear transfer. *Nat Protoc*. **11**, 2170–88.

[15] Gao, S., Gasparrini, B., McGarry, M., Ferrier, T., Fletcher, J., Harkness, L., De Sousa, P., Wilmut, I. (2002) Germinal vesicle material is essential for nucleus remodeling after nuclear transfer. *Biol Reprod*. **67**, 928–34.

[16] Modliński, J.A. (1975) Haploid mouse embryos obtained by microsurgical removal of one pronucleus. *J Embryol Exp Morphol*. **33**, 897–905.

[17] Greda, P., Karasiewicz, J., Modlinski, J.A. (2006) Mouse zygotes as recipients in embryo cloning. *Reproduction*. **132**, 741–8.

[18] Mohammed, A.A., Karasiewicz, J., Modliński, J.A. (2008) Developmental potential of selectively enucleated immature mouse oocytes upon nuclear transfer. *Mol Reprod Dev*. **75**, 1269–80.

[19] Fulka, H., Ogura, A., Loi, P., Fulka, Jr.J. (2019) Dissecting the role of the germinal vesicle nuclear envelope and soluble content in the process of somatic cell remodelling and reprogramming. *J Reprod Dev*. **65**, 433–44.

[20] Fulka, H., Novakova, Z., Mosko, T., Fulka, J. Jr. (2009) The inability of fully grown germinal vesicle stage oocyte cytoplasm to transcriptionally silence transferred transcribing nuclei. *Histochem Cell Biol*. **132**, 457–68.

Chapter 16

The Prospects of Infertility Treatment Using "Artificial" Eggs

Katsuhiko Hayashi

Overview

New methods for the production of eggs in culture from pluripotent stem cells will usher in a new era in reproductive biology and regenerative medicine. Such "artificial" eggs are expected to be a useful tool for reproduction and elucidation of the basic mechanisms underlying oogenesis, and as a potential cure for infertility. In an animal model, artificial eggs capable of full-term development were produced from embryonic stem cells (ESCs) and induced pluripotent stem cells (iPSCs). The latter source is more applicable, as iPSCs can be derived from adult somatic cells and the resulting artificial eggs are autologous. Technologies to produce artificial eggs, called in vitro gametogenesis (Figure 16.1), are being gradually but steadily applied to other animals, including humans. However, apart from ethical issues, there are still technological issues that should be cleared before in vitro gametogenesis can be applied to human beings. This chapter summarizes the current status of artificial eggs and possible future applications.

Developmental Trajectory of Egg Production In Vivo: A Roadmap for Artificial Eggs

Eggs are produced in vivo through a unique series of differentiation processes in the germ line. The differentiation commences in primordial germ cells (PGCs) by their specification from the pluripotent cell population soon after implantation [1]. PGCs initially locate at the posterior end of the embryo but eventually migrate towards the gonad though the hindgut. During migration, PGCs proliferate and undergo epigenetic reprogramming in which their DNA methylation is erased and their histone modifications reorganized at a genome-wide level [2]. This is an important step in the propagation of a founder population to produce a robust number of gametes. After

reaching the gonads, the PGCs interact with surrounding somatic cells and differentiate in a sex-dependent manner. In the female gonad, PGCs enter meiosis (thereby becoming primary oocytes) and then form an ovarian follicle structure with neighboring (pre)granulosa cells at the perinatal stage. After puberty begins, some of the follicles periodically undergo follicular development, which is characterized by proliferation of granulosa cells and maturation of theca cells [3]. During follicular development, the oocytes acquire de novo epigenetic modifications in the genome, which is essential for subsequent embryonic development after fertilization. When the follicle is fully developed, the oocyte(s) resume meiosis to reach the meiotic metaphase II (MII) stage and are ovulated with cumulus cells into the fallopian tube(s), where fertilization with sperm takes place.

The Current Status of Artificial Eggs

Reconstitution of PGC Specification in Mice and Humans

As each step of the germ cell differentiation process is important for conferring totipotency to the egg, artificial eggs must be made to advance through these processes as precisely as possible. For this reason, much effort has been made to reconstitute the differentiation process using pluripotent stem cells. Reconstitution of PGC specification is an initial and important step toward artificial eggs, as the quality of the PGCs, including the completeness of their epigenetic reprogramming, would reflect the developmental competence of the eggs. Briefly, in mouse embryogenesis, PGCs arise from the pluripotent epiblast in response to bone morphogenetic protein (BMP) 4 secreted from the adjacent extraembryonic ectoderm at around embryonic day (E) 6.5 [4]. During specification, a set of transcription factors, such as

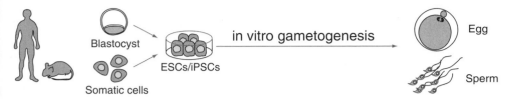

Figure 16.1 Scheme of in vitro gametogenesis. ESCs and/or iPSCs are the source of in vitro gametogenesis. By recapitulating each differentiation process of germ cell development, ESCs/iPSCs differentiate into egg and sperm. In mice, artificial eggs can be made by in vitro gametogenesis.

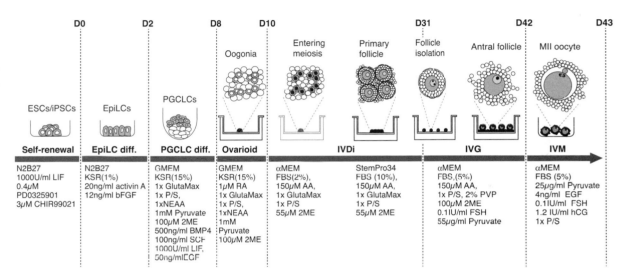

Figure 16.2 How to produce artificial eggs in mice. Shown are the condition of each culture term and days after differentiation from ESCs/iPSCs. IVDi, in vitro differentiation; IVG, in vitro growth; IVM, in vitro maturation. (A black and white version of this figure will appear in some formats. For the color version, please refer to the plate section.)

Blimp1/Prdm1, Prdm14 and Tfap2 c, orchestrate a PGC-specific gene expression program accompanied with epigenetic reprograming. A key feature of PGC specification is a unique responsiveness to BMP4, termed PGC competence, that is conferred temporarily to the pluripotent epiblast The PGC competence can be conferred to mouse ESCs/iPSCs by culturing with bFGF and activin A (Figure16.2) [5]. The PGC-competent ESCs/iPSCs, called epiblast-like cells (EpiLCs), can differentiate into PGC-like cells (PGCLCs) in response to BMP4. PGCLCs have gene expression and epigenetic reprogramming profiles that are highly similar to those of bona fide PGCs. Importantly, PGCLCs are capable of differentiating functional sperm and oocytes in the transplanted testes and ovaries, respectively [5,6]. PGCLC-derived sperm and oocytes have potency to develop to offspring that grow up without developmental retardation or premature death, and then become fertile

adults. These studies demonstrate that the culture system successfully reconstitutes the PGC specification process in mice. This technology was immediately applied to humans: derivation of PGCLCs from human ESCs/iPSCs was done at four years after the mouse model [7,8]. As in the mouse model, PGC-competence was conferred to human ESCs/iPSCs by culturing with a set of agonists, such as bFGF and activin A (or TGFβ) [7], or activin A and CHIR99021 [8] (see below in detail). Irrespective of which method is used, the PGC-competent ESCs/iPSCs are capable of differentiating into PGCLCs in response to BMP4, and the resulting PGCLCs exhibit gene expression and epigenetic reprogramming profiles highly similar to those of human PGCs in vivo.

Reconstitution of Oogenesis in Mice

Reconstitution of oogenesis after PGC specification is challenging, as the sex-dependent differentiation

155

process essentially requires surrounding somatic cells in the gonads. To reconstitute an environment sufficient for oogenesis, construction of an organoid system for ovaries, named the "ovarioid", is one possible option. In general, organoids are formed by mingling cells composed of the organ and develop in culture similarly to the way the organ develops in vivo. Accordingly, the ovarioid system to produce oocytes from mouse ESC/iPSC-derived PGCLCs can be achieved by mingling with gonadal somatic cells in E12.5 embryos [9]. In the ovarioid, the PGCLCs immediately start to express MVH, a late PGC marker gene, and then enter meiosis. The subsequent culture system is designed according to studies on organ cultures that succeeded in the production of functional eggs from residual precursors in neonatal ovaries [10] and fetal ovaries [11]. In the organ culture systems, secondary follicles were isolated from cultured ovaries and then the isolated follicles were further cultured until fully grown germinal vesicle (GV) oocytes. These GV oocytes resumed meiosis to become MII oocytes in culture for maturation and, importantly, developed to offspring after fertilization. Combining these findings, eggs can be made in the ovarioid by passing through three culture periods—in vitro differentiation (IVDi), in vitro growth (IVG) and in vitro maturation (IVM)—in which oogenesis proceeds to primary oocytes in the secondary follicle, fully grown GV oocytes and MII oocytes, respectively (Figure 16.2). Importantly, artificial eggs derived from the culture system were capable of fertilization and full-term development. Moreover, the pups from artificial eggs were apparently normal, as both female and male pups grew up and become fertile adult mice (Figure 16.3). However, it is evident that artificial eggs are not equivalent to eggs produced in vivo. For example, the gene expression profiles of artificial eggs and bona fide eggs were different: in the MII stage, the transcripts of 363 and 61 genes in artificial eggs were higher and lower, respectively, than those of bona fide eggs. The frequency of mispairing between homologous chromosomes in meiotic prophase I was higher (53.8%) in the primary oocytes in the culture system than in the primary oocytes in vivo (5.3%) [9]. Moreover, the frequency of aneuploidy was higher (22.2%) in MII oocytes in the culture system than in vivo (2.4%). Possibly as a result of these defects, the successful rate of producing offspring from artificial eggs was 20-times less than that from bona fide eggs. Interestingly, a detailed analysis of the differentially expressed genes suggested that artificial eggs precociously resume meiosis even though they are still immature. Therefore, further refinement of the culture condition is required, especially to improve maturation of the artificial eggs. Nevertheless, in mice, the entire process of female germ cell development can be reconstituted in culture, which yields a number of artificial eggs with potency for the full-term development.

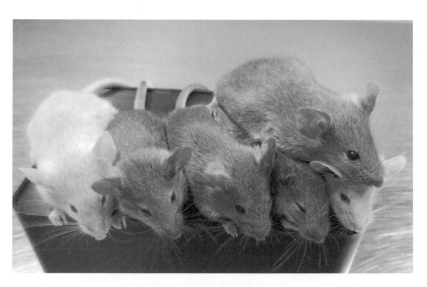

Figure 16.3 Mouse offspring from the tail. Shown are mice from artificial eggs derived from iPSCs that were established from adult tail-tip fibroblast. (A black and white version of this figure will appear in some formats. For the color version, please refer to the plate section.)

A Brief Manual for Making Artificial Eggs in Mice

This section provides a brief explanation of the production of artificial eggs in mice. For the complete protocol, readers are referred to Hayashi *et al*. [12]. As partially described above, ESCs/iPSCs are differentiated into PGCLCs as the initial step in producing artificial eggs. The process of PGCLC differentiation is composed of two steps: the first is to differentiate ESCs/iPSCs into epiblast-like cells (EpiLCs), which have a competence for PGCLC differentiation in response to BMP4, and the second is to differentiate the EpiLCs into PGCLCs. The key growth factors involved in each step are bFGF and activin A for EpiLC differentiation, and BMP4, LIF, SCF and EGF for PGCLC differentiation. For details of the PGC differentiation, please see the published protocols [13,14]. After PGCLC differentiation, PGCLCs must be reaggregated with somatic cells from fetal ovaries: usually 5,000 PGCLCs are reaggregated with 50,000 gonadal somatic cells to provide an ovarioid. Ovarioids are cultured under a series of IVDi, IVG and IVM conditions (Figure 16.2). There is a critical step between IVDi and IVG, which is the isolation of individual follicles followed by treatment with collagenase. Individual follicle structures should be carefully isolated from the ovarioid; otherwise the follicles would stop growing. The treatment with collagenase strips mural granulosa cells in the follicles, which allows the culture medium to reach the cumulus oocyte complex. Practically, at least in mice, the treatment is quite important to yield a high number of mature oocytes. After IVG culture, the cumulus-oocyte complexes can be picked up easily by a glass pipette and used for IVM culture. Then, the resulting MII oocytes can be treated, such as for in vitro fertilization, in the same manner as MII oocytes derived in vivo, although MII oocytes made in culture tend to be sensitive to osmotic stress and mechanical stresses such as ICSI.

Current Attempts to Apply Artificial Eggs to Humans

Would it be possible to apply the technology of producing artificial eggs to humans? Indeed, this would seem to be the case, as there are several reports of PGCLCs being derived from human ESCs (hESCs) either spontaneously or in response to BMP4 [15,16]. More recently, more organized methods for PGCLC differentiation from ESCs and human iPSCs (hiPSCs) were published [7,8,17]. Irie *et al*. cultured hESCs/hiPSCs under a 4i condition [7], and then conferred PGC competence to hESCs/iPSCs by culturing with TGFβ (or activin A) and bFGF. The PGC-competent hESCs/iPSCs differentiated into hPGCLCs in response to BMP4, SCF, LIF and EGF, which is the same set of cytokines seen for mouse PGCLC differentiation. Sasaki *et al*. cultured hiPSCs under a feeder-free condition with bFGF and then conferred PGC-competence by culturing with activin A and a GSK3β inhibitor. The PGC-competent hiPSCs were called incipient mesodermal cells (iMeLCs) and could differentiate into hPGCLCs in response to BMP4 [8]. Sugawa *et al*. also reported hPGCLC differentiation from hESCs/iPSCs via temporal induction of mesodermal-like cells with activin A, bFGF and a low concentration (5 ng/ml) of BMP4 [17]. Irrespective of which method is used, the resulting PGCLCs have gene expression profiles and epigenetic genome modifications that are similar to those of human PGCs in vivo. Although the function of hPGCLCs has not been critically validated, for example by transplantation into testes or ovaries, for both technical and ethical reasons, it is likely that PGCLCs have the potential to differentiate into further developmental stages of the germ cell lineage.

Based on the mouse system, the production of artificial eggs as functional gametes is achieved by a proper interaction between PGCLCs and gonadal somatic cells. It seems that somatic cells from fetal ovaries have a greater potential to support oogenesis than those from adult ovaries, as the follicle structures are formed around the neonatal stage. Unlike in mice, preparation of fetal ovaries from human embryos is not feasible. Even if human embryos can be obtained from, for example, aborted embryos, the sex and developmental stage of the embryos would be quite variable. Furthermore, based on the experiments in mice, it is impossible to completely remove residual oocytes that mingled in the gonad, such that the resulting ovarioid is chimeric with multiple sources of oocytes. Compensation of human gonadal somatic cells by cells from other species is an unlikely option, because oogenesis from hPGCLCs was shown to be arrested at oogonia in a reconstituted environment using mouse gonadal somatic cells. Therefore, it is essential to overcome this obstacle to prepare a number of somatic cells with the potential to fully support oocyte formation from hPGCLCs.

Even in the case that human ovarioids can be produced using PGCLCs and appropriate somatic cells, generation of artificial eggs would be still challenging, as there is no robust culture system that reproduces oocyte formation from PGCs. However, partial reconstitution in culture of oogenesis has been done using a piece of ovarian tissue. Remarkably, McLaughlin *et al.* reported that mature oocytes could be obtained in culture from human unilaminar (primordial or primary) follicles in the ovary [18]. Similar to the series of culture periods in mice, the culture system in humans was composed of four steps, each of which yielded secondary/multi-laminar follicles of 100–150 μm in diameter, antral follicles with cavities, cumulus oocyte complexes and MII oocytes. Although this is significant progress, the culture system is still far from being applicable to testing of the developmental potency because of the low efficiency and abnormal morphology of the MII oocytes—for example, their polar bodies are larger than those of MII oocytes in vivo, presumably because of an aberrant position of the spindle. These findings indicate that further refinement of the culture condition is needed, especially for oocyte maturation. Several studies have contributed data on the optimal culture conditions for secondary follicles in primates, including humans [19–22]. Based on these studies, 3D culture systems would be advantageous for the production of mature oocytes. In particular, alginate hydrogel would be suitable as a scaffold material in a 3D culture system to produce mature oocytes [23]. In this culture system, the concentration of alginate hydrogel is optimized according to follicular development. These ongoing efforts are expected to provide clues to establish a culture system to produce artificial eggs from hESCs/hiPSCs.

Prospects of Infertility Treatment Using Artificial Eggs

As described above, artificial eggs are produced in mice and may one day be produced in humans. What is the scientific and medical significance of such artificial eggs and the related technologies? One important consideration is that these eggs could provide a model system to improve our understanding of oogenesis. As the entire process of oogenesis can be reconstituted in culture, this can be a useful tool for investigations of the genetic and epigenetic involvement in germ cell differentiation. This would be particularly effective in humans, as many of the processes of oogenesis proceed in the embryo, which is hardly accessible. It is also favorable that artificial eggs originate from ESCs/iPSCs, which are extremely susceptible to genetic manipulation. This could enable us not only to determine gene function during oogenesis but also to identify causative genes of infertility. The latter could be achieved by deriving iPSCs from infertility patients, followed by induction of PGCLCs and oocytes from the iPSCs. In this context, it is also possible to compensate gene(s) causing the infertility to precisely determine a causal relationship between the gene function and the symptom.

Another significant application of artificial eggs, which is more important from a practical viewpoint, would be to use the eggs to produce offspring. The importance of this aspect of the technology would be more prominent if it could be applied to infertility patients. Based on the accumulating knowledge described above, and several technical obstacles notwithstanding, it is likely that an egg-like structure can be obtained from hESCs/hiPSCs within 10 years. However, there are several concerns to be dealt with before considering the application of artificial eggs. These concerns are concentrated on a simple question: how different are artificial eggs from bona fide eggs? As described above, the mouse model suggested that artificial eggs are inferior to eggs in vivo in many respects, including fidelity of meiotic pairing of homologous chromosomes, gene expression and developmental potency [9]. These findings provide a clear answer to the question of fidelity to bona fide eggs: namely, many of the artificial eggs are not equivalent to eggs in vivo. To improve these inferior differentiation process and developmental potency, it is essential to refine the culture conditions. Comparisons of the gene expression, epigenetic modifications and metabolism between oogenesis in vivo and oogenesis in culture will provide clues toward the refinement of the culture conditions. Such comparisons will also contribute to the identification of factor(s) regulating the robust production of eggs in vivo. On the other hand, it is also evident that some artificial eggs are potent to become offspring, which gives rise to a further and potentially more complex question: Are the offspring from artificial eggs sound? This should be carefully considered, as although it has been reported that the animal model successfully produced fertile mice from artificial eggs, the animals were not rigorously evaluated in terms of gene expression, epigenetic modification, metabolism, longevity and diseases. Even a short-term culture may affect epigenetic and metabolic states during development, especially in the placenta. Then, whether such alterations take place in offspring derived from artificial eggs should be evaluated to consider the applicability of the technology. To have a future evidence-based discussion of the utility of human artificial eggs, artificial eggs and their related technology must be examined in many species, including non-human primates.

References

[1] Saitou, M., and Yamaji, M. (2010). Germ cell specification in mice: signaling, transcription regulation, and epigenetic consequences. Reproduction 139, 931–942.

[2] Sasaki, H., and Matsui, Y. (2008). Epigenetic events in mammalian germ-cell development: reprogramming and beyond. Nat Rev Genet 9, 129–140.

[3] Pedersen, T., and Peters, H. (1968). Proposal for a classification of oocytes and follicles in the mouse ovary. J Reprod Fertil 17, 555–557.

[4] Ohinata, Y., Ohta, H., Shigeta, M., Yamanaka, K., Wakayama, T., and Saitou, M. (2009). A signaling principle for the specification of the germ cell lineage in mice. Cell 137, 571–584.

[5] Hayashi, K., Ohta, H., Kurimoto, K., Aramaki, S., and Saitou, M. (2011). Reconstitution of the mouse germ cell specification pathway in culture by pluripotent stem cells. Cell 146, 519–532.

[6] Hayashi, K., Ogushi, S., Kurimoto, K., Shimamoto, S., Ohta, H., and Saitou, M. (2012). Offspring from oocytes derived from in vitro primordial germ cell-like cells in mice. Science 338, 971–975.

[7] Irie, N., Weinberger, L., Tang, W.W., Kobayashi, T., Viukov, S., Manor, Y.S., Dietmann, S., Hanna, J.H., and Surani, M.A. (2015). SOX17 is a critical specifier of human primordial germ cell fate. Cell 160, 253–268.

[8] Sasaki, K., Yokobayashi, S., Nakamura, T., Okamoto, I., Yabuta, Y., Kurimoto, K., Ohta, H., Moritoki, Y., Iwatani, C., Tsuchiya, H., et al. (2015). Robust In Vitro Induction of Human Germ Cell Fate from Pluripotent Stem Cells. Cell Stem Cell 17, 178–194.

[9] Hikabe, O., Hamazaki, N., Nagamatsu, G., Obata, Y., Hirao, Y., Hamada, N., Shimamoto, S., Imamura, T., Nakashima, K., Saitou, M., et al. (2016).

[10] Eppig, J.J., and O'Brien, M.J. (1996). Development in vitro of mouse oocytes from primordial follicles. Biol Reprod 54, 197–207.

[11] Morohaku, K., Tanimoto, R., Sasaki, K., Kawahara-Miki, R., Kono, T., Hayashi, K., Hirao, Y., and Obata, Y. (2016). Complete in vitro generation of fertile oocytes from mouse primordial germ cells. Proc Nat Acad Sci USA 113, 9021–9026.

[12] Hayashi, K., Hikabe, O., Obata, Y., and Hirao, Y. (2017). Reconstitution of mouse oogenesis in a dish from pluripotent stem cells. Nat Protoc 12, 1733–1744.

[13] Hayashi, K., and Saitou, M. (2013a). Generation of eggs from mouse embryonic stem cells and induced pluripotent stem cells. Nat Protoc 8, 1513–1524.

[14] Hayashi, K., and Saitou, M. (2013b). Stepwise differentiation from naive state pluripotent stem cells to functional primordial germ cells through an epiblast-like state. Methods Mol Biol 1074, 175–183.

[15] Clark, A.T., Rodriguez, R.T., Bodnar, M.S., Abeyta, M.J., Cedars, M.I., Turek, P.J., Firpo, M.T., and Reijo Pera, R.A. (2004). Human STELLAR, NANOG, and GDF3 genes are expressed in pluripotent cells and map to chromosome 12p13, a hotspot for teratocarcinoma. Stem Cells 22, 169–179.

[16] Kee, K., Gonsalves, J.M., Clark, A.T., and Pera, R.A. (2006). Bone morphogenetic proteins induce germ cell differentiation from human embryonic stem cells. Stem Cells Dev 15, 831–837.

[17] Sugawa, F., Arauzo-Bravo, M.J., Yoon, J., Kim, K.P., Aramaki, S., Wu, G., Stehling, M., Psathaki, O.E., Hubner, K., and Scholer, H.R. (2015). Human primordial germ cell commitment in vitro associates with a unique PRDM14 expression profile. EMBO J 34, 1009–1024.

[18] McLaughlin, M., Albertini, D.F., Wallace, W.H.B., Anderson, R.A., and Telfer, E.E. (2018). Metaphase II oocytes from human unilaminar follicles grown in a multi-step culture system. Mol Hum Reprod 24, 135–142.

[19] Skory, R.M., Xu, Y., Shea, L.D., and Woodruff, T.K. (2015). Engineering the ovarian cycle using in vitro follicle culture. Hum Reprod 30, 1386–1395.

[20] Telfer, E.E., and Zelinski, M.B. (2013). Ovarian follicle culture: advances and challenges for human and nonhuman primates. Fertil Steril 99, 1523–1533.

[21] Yin, H., Kristensen, S.G., Jiang, H., Rasmussen, A., and Andersen, C.Y. (2016). Survival and growth of

isolated pre-antral follicles from human ovarian medulla tissue during long-term 3D culture. *Hum Reprod* **31**, 1531–1539.

[22] Yu, R.R., Cheng, A.T., Lagenaur, L.A., Huang, W., Weiss, D.E., Treece, J., Sanders-Beer, B.E., Hamer, D.H., Lee, P.P., Xu, Q., *et al.* (2009). A Chinese rhesus macaque (Macaca mulatta) model

for vaginal Lactobacillus colonization and live microbicide development. *J Med Primatol* **38**, 125–136.

[23] Xiao, S., Zhang, J., Romero, M.M., Smith, K.N., Shea, L.D., and Woodruff, T.K. (2015). In vitro follicle growth supports human oocyte meiotic maturation. *Sci Rep* **5**, 17323.

Index